PROGRESS IN BIOMECHANICS

NATO ADVANCED STUDY INSTITUTES SERIES

Proceedings of the Advanced Study Institute Programme, which aims at the dissemination of advanced knowledge and the formation of contacts among scientists from different countries.

The series is published by an international board of publishers in conjunction with NATO Scientific Affairs Division

A Life Sciences	Plenum Publishing Corporation
B Physics	London and New York
C Mathematical and Physical Sciences	D. Reidel Publishing Company Dordrecht and Boston
D Behavioural and Social Sciences	Sijthoff & Noordhoff International Publishers B.V.
E Applied Science	Alphen aan den Rijn, The Netherlands and Winchester, Mass., USA

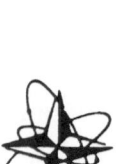

Series E: Applied Science – No. 32

PROGRESS IN BIOMECHANICS

edited by

Dr. NURI AKKAŞ

Associate professor,
Department of Civil Engineering
Middle East Technical University
Ankara, Turkey

SIJTHOFF & NOORDHOFF   1979
Alphen aan den Rijn – The Netherlands

Proceedings of the NATO Advanced Study Institute on
Progress in Biomechanics
Ankara, Turkey
July 10-21, 1978

ISBN-13: 978-94-009-9564-2   e-ISBN-13: 978-94-009-9562-8
DOI: 10.1007/978-94-009-9562-8

TABLE OF CONTENTS

VI

PREFACE

The purpose of this particular NATO Advanced Study Institute is to contribute to the dissemination of advanced knowledge and the formation of contacts between scientists from different countries. The Institute is meant to have a substantial teaching component while also providing a forum for discussion at the highest level.

The NATO Advanced Study Institute on Progress in Biomechanics was held July 10-21, 1978 in Ankara, Turkey and the Proceedings are presented in this volume. Sixty-four engineers, mechanicians, medical and biological scientists from fourteen countries attended.

Prof. R.M. Kenedi of the University of Strathclyde, Glasgow, Scotland and Prof. W. Goldsmith of the University of California, Berkeley, USA were the other members of the Organizing Committee. As Director of the Institute, I wish to thank them for their assistance without which the Institute would not have taken place. Time will show whether the Institute has served its purpose; namely, exciting interdisciplinary communications and developing a lasting and productive link from which significant academic and technological advances might emerge.

N. Akkaş

METHODOLOGY OF MULTIDISCIPLINARY COLLABORATION

Brigitte Eckstein

Technische Hochschule Aachen,
Aachen, Federal Republic of Germany

ABSTRACT. Increasingly, the multidisciplinary working team gains importance in research and development. However, up till now hardly any University or Polytechnic provides its leavers with the basic communicative and cooperative skills necessary for the functioning of working groups, leave alone interdisciplinary ones. Accordingly, multidisciplinary groups frequently get up with but poor results, or they become stuck altogether. due generally to person- and group-centered rather than task-centered problems. The basic attitude of mutual rivalry, constituent for a competitive society like ours, is incompatible with the cooperativity necessary for a team. Thus working groups habe to be facilitated to provide for their functioning.

Various means for facilitating multidisciplinary groups and to overcome the arising problems, are discussed in this paper. The problems arising in a multidisciplinary group difter from those common in any heterogeneous group essentially in intensity – they are much the same, but more thorough and more difficult to handle.

1. THE GENERAL BASIS - THE BEHAVIOUR OD THE PERSON IN MORE OR LESS STRUCTURED GROUPS

A multidisciplinary working team by definition is a "group" and is subject to all problems and all facilitations familiar with small groups. The methodology of multidisciplinary collaboration thus essentially is the methodology of small group facilitation.

2

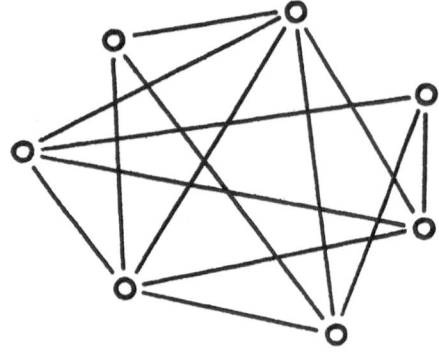

Fig. 1. The multilateral, essentially symmetric pattern of communication of a well functioning working group.

1.1 "Groups", structured and otherwise

A "group" can be defined as a social entity with a pronounced
feeling of "we" among the members, separating them from non-
members. The minimum number of members defining a group may be
taken either three or five. - According to this definition, a
class of say twenty students attending a lecture may represent
a group. However, there is an important difference between such
an audience and a discussion or working group of the same size.
In contrast to the "one-way" and highly asymmetrical pattern of
communication of an audience, the communication in a typical
small group is multi-lateral and - ideally - essentially symmetric. The "small group" actually is defined by this very communication pattern (Fig. 1). - The group temporarily may subdivide
into subgrounds (Fig. 2), easily leading to disintegration of
the original group. Within hierarchical institutions, symmetric
communication sometimes but with difficulties is established:
while not necessarily blocking the formation of a symmetric and
balanced group, a uni-directional flow of orders and information
surely does not foster it.

    In a newly starting working group (the more so in a settled
one), the aim generally is given, as well as the special tasks
connected with the single members, the ranges of their responsibility, the hierarchy, and perhaps even the detailed agenda. The
whole "setting" is highly "structured": the range of decisions
to be taken by the group is fairly limited. Most decisions are
pre-structured by rational reasons, hardly giving cause for the
members' mutual fight for status and power.

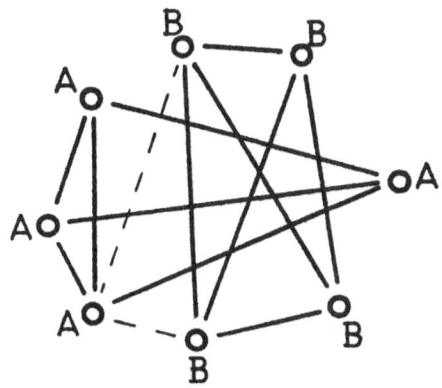

Fig. 2. Communication pattern of a group disintegrated in two but loosely linked subgroups A and B.

In contrast, the "unstructured" group situation is characterized by its lack of pre-defined goals, norms, roles, values,
hierarchy, and agenda. Every step of action first is due to a
multitude of decisions, occasion and cause for arguments, and
fights for status, power and allies. The group has first to
establish its social structure, defining roles and status attributed to each member, before being free to concentrate on a subject task. Many groups with insufficiently defined social structure fail in this critical first stage, and never reach a productive phase. Trouble in working groups generally stems from intragroup competition rather than from problems related to the subject task.

Structured and unstructured groups are but idealized limiting cases. No real group actually is totally "structured" or
totally "unstructured". The ranges of ambiguity and free decision markedly vary among groups (and, for that, for a given group
during its existence), and are an essential parameter regulating
the ongoings in the group.

1.2 The "leader-less" group

A group lacking a leader experiences a vast amount of uncertainty and ambiguity. Situations of undefined social structure generally are experienced as irritating or even threatening. "Leader-
less" groups and groups with a formal leader refusing "to exert
leadership" first undergo a most boring and frustrating phase of

fight for status, power, and leadership among the members. The
frustation and anxieties aroused may cause members to withdraw
mentally or even actually to drop out of the group. The group
may disintegrate totally, either by subsequent drop-out of members or with a clash. No subject task can be tackled, leave alone
accomplished, without the group having settled at least provisi-
onally its hierarchy and the way of decision-making.

Group norms and values (including person, rights, and
duties of the actual leader) eventually established, the group
enters a phase of of extreme conformism, lest the so painfully adjusted consequent may be risked. Individual traits and aims are not
admitted. Thus the group still is but limited in its potential.
By and by, the accomplished equilibrium is experienced as reliable, the members feel free to exert their own personality, and
the roles - e.g. the "actual" (momentary) leader, the "experts",
and the "outsider" (who represents the group's denied hopes,
fears, and goals) - shift among the members according to the
momentary situation. The proceedings are task- rather than per-
son- (status-) oriented, and the group can eventually deal efficiently with the subject task.

In this phase the subject output is generally quite satisfying. The members identify with the group and devote the whole
of their capacity to the common goal, not being diverted by
mutual competition. It is however a painstaking way of getting
a team to work, and the chance of failure before reaching that
phase is high. The comparatively long unproductive starting
phase, anyway frustating, may be intolerable when quick results
are needed. - Stringent need of immediate results sometimes helps
to overcome the initial phase, but outward pressure as well can
impede the group. Thus other ways of facilitating the team are
desirable.

1.3 The group and its formal leader

The troublesome starting phase of a leaderless group is essentially due to the ambiguity caused by a "leadership vacuum" in an
essentially competitive society. A formal leader may help a
group sooner to become productive. Within the limits given by
general conditions, task, ressources, and facilities, and by the
group members' personalities, capacities, and ambitions, he defines the group's aims, norms, and values, his own role and
function, and the roles of the members, mediates between subgroups, and safeguards minorities against being overruled.
Especially he settles the rules and patterns of communication,
including the flow of information, and the patterns of decision-
making.

Evidently, results are gained quickest by his deciding single-handed, perhaps not even consulting the group's experts. This "autocratic" style of leadership however does not pay in the long run. The members, dissatisfied by working under orders, don't identify with the decisions and become disengaged, investing but a fraction of their capacity in the group's aims, which they experience as the leader's aims rather than their own. Thus but part of the actual potential can be used. It generally pays well to strive for a group consent, thus getting the members to identify with the group and the aims.

The "counterpart" of directive, autocratic leadership style is the "laissez-faire" style. The leader, unwilling, uncapable, or too lazy or timid to "exert leadership", leaves decisions to the group without assisting decision-making. The group - lacking an "actual" leader - experiences the whole painful process of fights as any leaderless group, and may end up in anarchy and general frustations. - In case of doubt, autocratic leadership still is less harmful to a group than a laissez-faire "leader".

The most effective way of group-leading is the "social integrative" style. The leader offers as little structure and guidance as possible, but as much as necessary for the group not to become irritated. He helps the group to come to decisions, but he is not afraid to decide single-handed, if necessary. By knowing quick and effective ways of compromising, he helps to find a group consent without unduly stressing the members' patience. They feel content and hopeful, and are willing to invest their capacity for the benefit of the common goal. - This style however demands special knowledge and skills on the part of the leader, especially the command of techniques for deciding, compromising, and conflict-solving, achieved by a special training, which by now is offered hardly anywhere by post-secondary educational institutions.

1.4 On emotions, attitudes, and behaviour exhibited in a group

In our basically competitive culture, the fellow-human primarily is experienced as a possible rival, a threat for one's own strive for superiority and power, or as an easy prey. This deeply rooted attitude, is incompatible with mutual acceptance, esteem, and trust, which are fundamental for any cooperativity. Competition impedes cooperativity, and the internally competitive group achieves but mediocre results (if any). Intergroup competition may improve the work output moderately and temporarily. Intergroup competition however does not foster the autonomy and maturity of the group members, and hence in the long run fails to improve the group's efficiency.

A favourable group "climate" of mutual acceptance and esteem inhibits intragroup competition and mistrust, and forwards group's and members' maturity and autonomy. Establishing such a cooperative group climate is anything but trivial, and in contrast with our culture's basic values of individual superiority and mutual rivalry. Again, we have to learn and control our competitive attitudes, or we will not be able to master tomorrow's challenges of living in an increasingly overcrowded world without letal outbursts of violence and aggressiveness.

Competition - fight for superiority and power - in a working group generally goes camourflaged as a discussion about "subject matter". When the emotional engagement of the antagonists exceeds that justified by a mere difference in opinion, the actual topic is personal superiority rather than a subject problem. Scientific meetings offer ample opportunity to observe fights for personal prevalence, masked as a scientific argument, and using the discussion as a vehicle for hidden aims. Language then becomes a means to impress rather than to communicate, a weapon to threaten and to intimidate possible rivals and opponents.

When power and superiority are central values, weakness has to be concealed. Thus uncertainty, fears, affection, emotions in general are experienced as personal failure. Again, nobody can be permanently strong and infallible. The strive to live up to an unobtainable ideal becomes a source of anxieties. The drive for superiority and the fear of inferiority form a viscious circle, and lead up to mutual hostility based on fear. Thus in a disfavourable group climate, sudden outbursts of hostility and aggressiveness can occur and become rather frightening.

The group leader by his behaviour non-verbally defines norms of mutual connections and interactions. If he shows acceptance, openess, and cooperativity, the members will strive for the same attitudes. If he indulges in sarcasm, aggressiveness, and defense, he favours a hostile group climate. - Productivity and creativity, however, demand members feeling at their ease and free to make errors, impossible in a group of hostile and defensive climate. Hence striving for a permissive group climate is anything but sentimentalism, it is a vital condition for a group's productivity.

2. SPECIAL PROBLEMS OF MULTIDISCIPLINARY GROUPS

The multidisciplinary group is a special case of the "cross-cultural" group, as members of different disciplines in a certain sense represent different "subcultures", sometimes even definitely antagonistic ones. The normal problems of heterogen-

eous groups thus are intensified in the multidisciplinary
group, and may even lead to its disintegration. - The main
problems are those of interdisciplinary biases and prejudices,
of differing language, differing perception, differing norms and
values, and differing frames of reference. These differences
question and threaten the person's orientation and integration
in a puzzlingly multifold and ambiguous world. They are hence
irritating and hard to bear even in the case of mutual tolerance
and acceptance. In case of mutual mistrust and reserve, the experienced differences are taken as "proof" of the other person's
inferiority or even wickedness, thus increasing the mutual hostility and distorted perception. This viscious circle can be
overcome e.g. by certain group-dynamical exercises (see App.).

2.1 Biases and prejudices

Orientatation and action in a very complex and ambiguous world
demands for the person to take many things "for granted", thus
reducing ambiguity to a workable amount. Every culture thus
develops a set of assumptions, an arbitrarily chosen frame of
reference, to understand and to manage world and life. It is
transferred and firmly established by the socialization of the
person. To question, leave alone to change it, implies pain connected with an (at least temporary) loss of orientation, and
hence is strongly tabooed. Recently Kuhn [1] demonstrated the
effect of "systems of reference" - "paradigms" - in the development of science. Questioning or opposing a paradigm, as well as
any other basic assumption of a culture, leads to the status of
outsider, heretic, or scapegoat, and demands considerable mental
strength. The diverse sets of paradigms of different disciplines
cause barriers in interdisciplinary communication and cooperation.

Tolerating and understanding another culture's/subculture's
basic assumptions, implies the denial of the absolute validity
of the own culture's ones. Strong preoccupations concerning
members of other cultures are a safeguard against too much interest in the other culture's paradigms, and essentially counteract
anxieties connected with an anticipated need to change. The
stronger the claim for absolute validity of the own paradigms,
the more intense is the prejudice against outgroup members: the
prohibited ingroup hostility is projected on the outgroup, in-
tensifying the distortion of the mutual perception, which eventually becomes self-stabilizing and self-amplifying. The interdisciplinary prejudices in a group can be demonstrated by a
questionnaire (App. VII) and overcome by "segregation exercises"
(App. V).

2.2 Problems of different language

Effective group work depends on effective communication among
the members. Verbal communication is liable to misunderstandings.
The meaning of many words is ambiguous, the more so, when used
by members of different subcultures. Even within a discipline, a
lot of "scientific argument" is due to unprecise language
rather than to a real dissent. - It is a most common but erroneous assumption, that the meaning of words is clearly defined
and independent of the individual speaker. Especially in a multidisciplinary group, semantic misunderstandings can go unnoticed
for a long time, the members assuming a difference in opinion
rather than in language. While they - but poorly listening to
each other - try to convert each other, the dispute makes less
and less sense. Eventually everybody may be convinced of the
other oarty's stupidity, obstinacy, or lack of good will.

These barriers can be overcome by a purposeful alienation
of language, demonstrating its trickiness. The members thus become sensitized for the ubiquity of misunderstandings or at
least unprecise understanding, and learn to pay increased attention to be precision of their own statements. - The communication
can be improved by special exercise (see App. I). - Actually,
the belief in unambiguous communication is vital for a person
feeling at his ease. Thus most people thoroughly resist to realize the whole amount of ambiguity of language and its implications.

2.3 Differing perception

Beyond differently denoting given items, different persons even
perceive reality differently. Generally, "perception" is strongly
intermixed with inferences and interpretations [2, 3]. It takes
hard training to learn strictly and consciously to differentiate
the genuine perception from the resulting processed impression.
Even the "unprocessed perception" (unprocessed as far as ever
possible), differs individually, and it differs systematically
among members of different cultures/subcultures (different prof-
fessions).

In the processing of perception the overwhelming complexity
of the arriving impressions is reduced to workable, simplified
images. The whole of the permanent influx of information and
signals can't be handled by the brain but by reducing it to its
"important" and "necessary" points, transferring just a small,
arbitrarily chosen selection to consciousness. This very selection is individual, influenced by biographical data, especially
by the person's socialization, i.e. by cultural agreement.
Members of the same culture/subculture tend to perceive in an

characteristic way, still allowing however for vast individual
differences.

Actually a person deals with his perception or even image
of reality rather than with "reality" itself. Again, the reli-
ability of perception, the very existence of a common, percept-
ible, absolute "reality" is a basic demand for the human's
mental stability. Thus the cognition of "private reality" and
its implications, by most persons strongly is resisted. In case
on "non-identic reality" (differing perception of reality),
mutually stupidity, obstinacy, or ill will are assumed rather
than differing perception.

Special exercises as suggested by Abercrombie (see App. II)
help the members of multidisciplinary groups to become sensitized for possible differences in their perception.

2.4 Differing frames of references

In the mind the arriving perceptions become processed, classified, and filed according to the personal frame of reference.
Such a frame is a complex system, formed by the total of previous
"experiences" (which by themselves have been manipulated, arbitrarily selected, and processed by the person), cognitions, ex-
pectations, hopes, and fears. The personal frame of reference is
prestructured by cultural influence, including the person's profession (professional subculture), which controls his interests
and large parts of his experience. - In a multidisciplinary
group, the members differ broadly in their frames of reference,
both individually and according to their different disciplines.
Thus even in the fictitious case of identical perception, the
inferences and conclusions drawn from the perception would not
coincide.

The frame of reference controls the person's way of infer-
ing and reasoning, and by "implicit assumptions" regulates both
logical and ethical reasoning. - To attain effective innergroup
collaboration, it is essential to make evident the differing
implicit assumptions. Realizing one's implicit assumptions, however, might imply the necessity to correct or even to change
them altogether. Such a change of an essential part of the
personality, by most people is experienced as highly threatening and frightening. The confrontation with own and others' implicit assumptions is thus connected with deeply-rooted anxieties
and hence work on the very verge of psychotherapy.

Realizing the arbitrariness of any frame of reference, the
former "that is how things are" transforms into "that is how I
experience things", including a shift towards mutual tolerance,

and improved communication and cooperation in the group. By questions like "how do we know / why do we believe / can we check this idea?", implicit assumptions generally can be made explicit. Additionally, exercises of the Abercrombie-type help to make people aware of their frame of reference and its implications.

3. A THEORETICAL FRAME FOR DESCRIBING GROUP PROCEEDINGS

The proceedings in a group are determined by the group's task, (including all the working conditions), by the members' personalities (including their needs, fears, and their personal frames of reference), and by the mutual interactions among the members. Task, personalities, and "group process" (interactions) may be considered as "components" constituting the ongoings in a group. Ruth Cohn, a Gestalt psychologist and psychtherapist, hence suggested a representation of group proceedings in a system of triangular coordinates, the so-called "Cohn's triangle" 4 .

3.1 Cohn's triangle

The corners of Cohn's triangle (Fig. 3) respectively symbolize the task ("theme"), the personalities of every single member including his momentary needs, desires, and fears ("I"), and the mutual relations, connections, and interactions among the members ("we"). - In any given moment, the topic of a group is a well defined combination of subject task, personal concern, and mutual interaction. It can be represented by a point in the triangle. The smaller this point's distance from one of the corners, the larger is the share of the connected "component" in the momentary proceedings. In the idealized case of a group totally restricted to the subject task, the representing point coincides with the corner "theme". In therapy and encounter groups, the representing point keeps near the "I"/"we"-edge of the triangle.

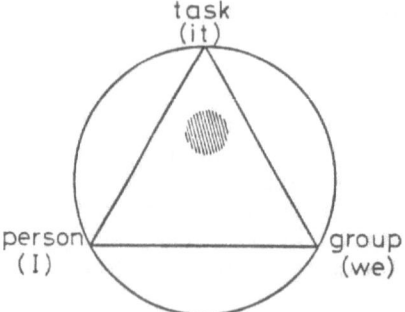

Fig. 3. Cohn's triangle, embedded in the "sphere" (the whole of outer conditions). Shaded the optimum working area for a team.

The center of the triangle represents equilibrum among subject task, personal concern, and group process. The region beneath the triangle's center ought to be left to trained facilitators and group therapists, as personal emotions and group process easily get out of control of an amateur group leader.

Besides evidencing the group's momentary concern, the representing point as well can give a mean value with reference to a whole working session or the total of the group's existence. Generally, the "averaged" representing point during a group's life shifts from a position nearer to the "I"/"we"-basis during the initial stages towards the corner "theme", according to the members' fading interest in personal status and group hierarchy.

Groups work within certain social, institutional, and material conditions. The total of these "outer conditions" in Cohn's representation is symbolized by an embedding circle (the "sphere"). The circle comprises both the ressources available and the limiting restrictions, which control the range of activities and decisions accessible to the group. Any group is wise before starting to work, to become aware of its conditioning "sphere", of the total of facilities and limitations.

A group's task in itself may be person- or group-oriented, e.g. in a managers' trainings course, or in working groups in humanities. Cohn's triangle then becomes asymmetric, the corner "task" approaching the "I"/"we"-basis.

3.2 The optimum working area

Even with a strictly ego- and group-distant subject task, the optimum working conditions don't coincide with the corner "theme". The person has got a body and a mind as well as an intellect, and thinking and reasoning are influenced by and intermixed with emotional factors and needs. Mutual sympathy and idiosyncrasy controls communication and the collaboration attainable, and by being denied they don't lose any of their effect. Ignored emotions and needs increase the tendency to rivalry and hostility, and thus decrease the groups's efficiency. Far from being wasted, time and effort invested to overcome emotional barriers, help to increase the group's work output. Indulging too far into emotions, however, distracts a groups from its subject task. A balance between task and feelings prevents trouble rooted in denied needs, as well as the "loss" of the task. The optimum working area for an interdisciplinary team, as indicated in Fig. 3, represents a mean value, and temporarily has to be left to overcome person- or process-centered hinderances, or to deal exclusively with the task.

Optimum working conditions are attained by manoeuvring the group proceedings within Cohn's triangle according to the momentary needs. The group leader can do so by emphasising the point neglected by the group. He either states a drift from the subject task, or he expresses his own feelings, or he states denied innergroup troubles, thus amplifying the group process. By asking the group to find some decision, the leader generally shifts the group towards the basis of the triangle: decision-making actualizes the question of personal influence and hence the struggle for power, thus also activating fears, temptations, and anxieties. By a question like "what is our present concern?/ are we still dealing with our task?" the group is brought back again from an overemphasised group process (Fig. 4).

4. THE RULES OF COMMUNICATION

Main function of the formal group leader - besides providing the necessary structure - is the assistance in conflict solution and decision-making, till the group attains efficient self-regulation. Implicitly or explicitly, the leader states the rules for the handling of disagreement and conflict, and for deciding among alternatives. The rules of communication from an essential part of the strategy of deciding and conflict solving.

4.1 The rules of communication

In the very beginning of the first group session, the leader - mostly implicitly - defines the rules for innergroup communication. The most common and least effective way of discussion is by a call-list, strictly following the sequence of interventions. The call-list inevitably deforms the "discussion" into a

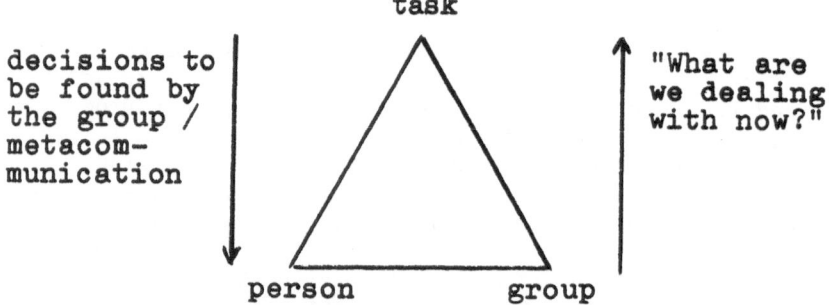

Fig. 4. Shifting the group proceedings towards or from the basis of Cohn's triangle.

series of monologues hardly related to each other. An effective
discussion in contrast needs rules which foster communication
rather than monologues. Ruth Cohn [4] offered a set of rules
which proved very effective in facilitating small group discussion. Considering that only the person himself can decide at
what moment he can make a meaningful and productive contribution,
Cohn explicitly leaves the decision about when to speak to the
member himself, relying upon his responsibility and discipline.

The whole set of rules essentially is implied in the very
first one: "Be your own Chairman!" - decide yourself when to
speak and what to say, considering and balancing your own needs
and those of the group. Speak for yourself and leave the other
person to speak for himself. Avoid the ambiguous and non-committal "we" or "one" in speech, but speak by the first person
singularis. Expose yourself as a person with clearly stated desires and idiosyncrasies, rather than hiding in anonymity and
ambiguity. - It takes some effort to shift from the non-committal
"one should ..." or "ought we not to ..." to the frank statement
"I would like to ...", but the improved communication is an ample
reward for this trouble. For similar reasons, questions ought to
be completed by a statement, which shows the person's concern
and interest in the question, and enables the partner better to
understand context and meaning and to answer the question to
the point.

The second rule, "priority for disturbances", essentially
is implied in the first one. A member who is distracted and momentarily unable to concentrate on the discussion, is to utter
this fact, lest he looses his connexion with the group proceedings and is lost as a contributor to the task. It pays well to
state the distraction, rather than sitting absent-mindedly while
the discussion goes on. Most distractions can quickly be settled,
or they are settled cathartically just by being stated. A distraction due to an unsolved conflict has to be dealt with in
greater extent, otherwise it might easily become self-amplifying.
It generally is better to invest the time needed to overcome
the underlying problem, rather than trying to ignore it.

During the first group sessions, the communication generally
is fairly asymmetric. Loquaciousness on the part of some members,
withdrawal on the part of others amplify. By focussing on the
asymmetric discussion, and by encourageing the more reserved or
timid members, the group leader helps towards a more symmetric
communication. He indicates the non-verbal signals showing a
person's desire to speak, and he points out when a member is interrupted or is not allowed to get a word in. With very obstinate
non-stop speakers (who mostly additionally complain on the
taciturn others), the leader may have to use special exercises,
or to keep them busy by extra tasks as running the record or

observing the group process. Fairly soon, the group learns
efficiently to handle the rules and thus to control itself
and to communicate freely.

4.2 Fostering decision-making

The "democratic" way of decision-making by votes, dividing the
members into "winners" and "loosers", proves inappropriate for
working teams. An outvoted participant can not identify with the
decision and devote the whole of his capacity to it. The members
of the majority realise that by the next voting they may be the
ones outvoted. The either/or-philosophy of a choice between
antagonistic alternatives, is very common but erroneous. For
small groups nearly always a workable compromise is attainable,
to which all members can consent. Finding it, rather than being
unduely time-consuming, is a quick procedure, if handled compe-
tently - the quicker, the better the group climate. Again, to
know that no member's needs will be outruled by a majority,
fosters a group climate of mutual tolerance. Disagreements no
longer are a cause of fight, as a compromise rather than a "win-
ner/looser-approach" is sought.

An appropriate first step in "no-looser decision making" is
the so-called "snapshot", quickly giving a survey of opinions.
The problem clearly defined and a short break given for consideration, each member in succession states his opinion by one
single sentence. Strictly sticking to the sequence and to the
limitation of one sentence per person, it is impossible to give
reasons or to argue, and the snapshot can not deform into an
argument. Within a few minutes, the thus obtained survey on the
ranges of opinions indicates the outlines of possible compromise.
After some more discussion and re-definition of the problem, a
new round of snapshot mostly produces consent.

Disagreeing minorities are often found willing to cooperate, provided their dissent be stated on record; or workable
conditions for their cooperation can be found. Ardent dissent on
a problem's basic philosophy often coincides with consent concerning the necessary course of action (especially in multidisciplinary groups), hence all problems better are approached from
their practical aspect. However, general consent is by no means
necessary for successful group work. Groups stand a vast amount
of dissent, as long as it is frankly stated.

A useful way of handling dissent is a temporary split of
the group. Various subgroups deal with different subtasks, or
pursue different approaches. The working results of the formerly
antagonistic subgroups often coincide, or the initial contrasts
otherwise just fade in the course of work, giving way to consent.

-Before parting, the various subgroups' (single members')
tasks, the expected results (e.g. verbal or written reports), the
time of reporting back, and time and topic of the next plenary
session clearly have to be stated. Lest the group disintegrates,
close contact has to be kept by regular exchange of the subgroup's
intermediate results in plenary sessions.

In larger (e.g. multidisciplinary) groups comprising more
uniform subteams, decision-making is facilitated by the "fish-
bowl"-technique, a type of "slow open panel", avoiding the split
into an eager panel and an increasingly disinterested audience.
Every subgroup (defined by discipline, rank or opinion) sends
some representatives into the bowl (panel). Any member from the
plenary, who wants to join in the discussion or feels misrepre-
sented by his representatives, can relieve a representative of
his own subgroup. Or the bowl contains some extra chairs to be
taken temporarily by a member from the plenary while making a
contribution, to be vacated again afterwards. Thus anybody is
free to present his opinion and hence can identify with the solution found, and the usual difficulties of plenary sessions are
still avoided.

Decisions are but rarely irrevocable - a fact important to
realize and explicitly to state. Compromises can be consented
on as "on trial", to be corrected if they fail to work. This
knowledge helps to make deciding a less tough problem.

In difficult cases of decision-seeking in small groups,
the following approach proves useful. The group splits into subgroups of four or five members. Every member notes down one
sentence essential to him with respect to the problem in question.
The slip is handed to the neighbour, who adds a commenting
sentence, and hands the slip on for a next comment to be added.
Eventually every statement is commented on by three other members. The subgroups then take notice of the thus provided content, which for a while is open to discussion. The slips then
are exposed on a notice board and discussed in a plenary session.
-By limiting both statements and comments to one single
sentence, the members are restricted to the essentials, and
have to become aware of what is essential to them. The "time-
consuming" process actually is time-saving by outruling insigni-
ficances and cutting down to the essentials.

4.3 Handling conflicts

Group leaders and members often are frightened by the idea of
an open group conflict. A frankly stated conflict however rarely
blocks a group. Only the denied conflict restricts the group's
potential, as any action might bring it to evidence and hence

implicitly is avoided. - Conflicts concerning dislike or prejudice among single members, by a trained facilitator can be handled
by an "alter-ego"-technique. Volunteering members role-play the
conflict on behalf of the actual opponents, who are bound to
listen silently and to postpone comments and corrections till
later. The substitute sotto voce adds to his speech what he
thinks the suppressed thoughts of the substituee, evidencing
the supposed blames, reproaches, and fears. The subconscious
sources of the conflict thus become evident and may be overcome
in a subsequent discussion, and the conflict generally is
settled. - Unexperienced group leaders however are strongly
warned against the technique, which demands knowledge and skills
of a highly competent trained facilitator. In tough cases of
mutual dislike the unexperienced leader rather ought to look for
professional help.

In less serious cases, he may ask the opponents themselves
to run their argument, however with exchanged roles. They thus
have to identify with the conflict partner, trying to understand
his position. Underlying misunderstandings become evident, and
the mutual resentments generally cathartically are resolved.

A conflict concerning the whole group rather than single
members is tackled in a sequence of steps:
1. Defining and stating the topic of conflict as clearly as
   possible.
2. Defining who has "got" the problem, who are the involved
   parties, and what interests are affected.
3. Collecting possible solutions by brainstorming (see App. VI),
   not classifying or evaluating any suggestion.
4. Evaluating the suggested solutions as more or less practic-
   able.
5. Seeking consent for the "best" solution.
6. Deciding the steps of action to be taken (who is when to do
   what?).
7. Checking the success of the solution after suitable testing.
Points 1 through 4 and 3 through 7 form loops which might have
to be passed twice.

The conflict sometimes proves to be different from what it
looked like initially, or a discomfort diffusely is felt, but
first can not be attributed to a stated conflict. The members
are then asked to complete sentences of the type "under all conditions, I want to .../ under no condition I will .../ we ought
now to .../ I am afraid we might .../ I would like now best
to ..." (the sentences to be adapted to the situation). - Exposing the slips with the completed sentences on the notice board
and discussing the results usually helps to realize the underlying problem. - Sometimes the reasons for the group's troubles
and difficulties can be evidenced by questionnaires (see App.

VIII). If and when a consented statement on the points of conflict is attained, finding a workable solution essentially is a
formality. It generally is facilitated by a statement on when
the consented solution is to be checked on its success and - if
need be - altered.

In tackling a conflict, it sometimes is useful to list up
the points of general consent and agreement in the group, to
give the members some reassurance by the feeling of prevalent
agreement. However, the group leader wisely does not try to mol-
lify the agitated minds or to pettify the trouble. It is better
frankly to state "you feel seriously disappointed / you are quite
angry now / this is a tough problem" - the members, feeling
understood rather than shook off, more readily will help the
empathic leader to overcome the problem.

5. GETTING A WORKING GROUP STARTED BY THE HELP OF SPECIALISTS

Getting a group to work has some features related to psychotherapy, a task most safely pursued by a trained facilitator, who
know to handle the members' fears and temptations concerning
the group and each other - mostly connected with fear of and resistance to change. As soon as the rules and norms are set, further difficulties are to be expected but temporarily - the most
critical phase of the group is the start.

5.1 Training by a preceding encounter group

Most of the problems connected with multidisciplinary teamwork
in one way or another are tackled in encounter groups. Their
topics are the personal and mutual feelings, emotions and fanta-
sies of the members in the actual group situation ("here and
now"). Attending an encounter group hence might be a suitable
training for multidisciplinary teamwork. However, such a prescribed gambit in most cases would raise disapproval and resistances on the part of most members. Up till then not having experienced the problems to be overcome, people generally are re-
luctant to undergo what they think to be "some dubious psycho-
training not immediately connected with the group's task". Besides, the practical profit is questionable anyway, as the transfer of experiences from the encounter group to every-day's professional work is neither trivial nor immediate. The encounter
experience might provide the participants with valuable information on their attitudes and behaviour in a group, but not
necessarily with the capacity of its application in the actual
situation.

Again, the formal leader rather than the whole group might

undergo an encounter training, thus rendering unnecessary a
trained facilitator. Joining an encounter group however hardly
provides the leader with all necessary knowledge, skills, and
experience. A facilitator's training is anything but incidental
or haphazard, and it takes more than the attendance to a chance
encounter group for learning to facilitate a group, and not to
panic in any possible emergency (e.g. instable members' emotional outbursts or even breakdown). Besides, role and status of the
facilitator ought not to be muddled with that of the formal
leader. Even if the latter happens to be a trained facilitator,
he is wise to restrict to "formal leadership", as one of the
facilitator's most important tasks is to help the members to
come along with the group leader.

5.2 A facilitator accompanying the group

The best approach is accompanying the starting group by a trained
facilitator, who comments on the group problems as they arise,
and offers remedy in case of need. His main strategy is "metacommunication" (communication on communication), focussing on the
communication in the group as it tackles its subject task. The
facilitator solves present problems rather than to deal with
anticipated problems and conflicts "in advance", and hence the
members are willing to follow his suggestions. Resistances thus
are avoided, and the suggested rules for communication accepted.

Videotaping the sessions allows for immediate confrontation
with the members' attitudes and behaviour as exposed on the
screen, a valuable base for metacommunication. No session however must be videotaped but with the group's consent, which
usually is given readily, when asked for in a casual way. Possible objections generally are eliminated in advance by mentioning that the tape is needed for facilitating the group process,
and will not be accessible to any non-participant. The tape
helps to demonstrate the individual differences in perception
and interpretation of the group process, which then can be dealt
with. - Generally, the members forget about the camera (as about
an audio-tape) after the first minutes of the session.

When a videorecorder is not available, feedback as a basis
for metacommunication can be provided by questionnaires. Variants
of the type shown in App. VIII B help to make evident the present state of group and members. Estimating the number of other
members' positive votes for each item, the participants are made
aware of the other members and their condition. They become sen-
sibilized for non-verbal signals, and for considering each
other's state and needs. Besides training empathy, the questionnaire helps to evidence neglected group problems (e.g. asymmetric communication) and unuttered dissatisfaction.

The central items of this type questionnaire are:
-- Do you agree with the present group proceedings (course of
the discussion)?
-- Can you contribute as you wanted to?
-- Do you feel at ease with respect to the other members?
Items to be added ad libitum (not surpassing a total of five
questions) are:
-- Are the proceedings dominated (manipulated) by some few
members?
-- Did the group essentially (successfully) deal with the sub-
ject task?
-- Was fair regard given to opposing opinions?
By varying the items, the questionnaire can be adapted to a large
choice of group problems, which thus become evident and hence
can be overcome.

Feedback can also be provided at the end of each working
session by a scaled questionnaire, rating on items as group climate, work efficiency, dedication to the task, leader's and members' behaviour, involvement, and similar topics according to
the actual needs. Mean values and standard deviations are computed and exhibited as a "group chart". Subsequently, some ten
to twenty minutes are devoted to a discussion of the results,
especially if these are less favourable. Even in the more mature phases of a group, it pays well to keep the last minutes of
each session to metacommunication, to stay aware of the mutual
reactions and interactions. During the initial group phases,
metacommunication and feedback might cause irritation, demanding for the facilitator's professional skill, lest it becomes
self-amplifying.

Especially, the facilitator intervenes in the case of
thoroughly asymmetric communication, of withdrawal, evasion,
antagonistic subgroups or members, or open hostility. He fosters
the sensibility for misunderstandings based on different perception, language, or frame of reference. He encourages the members
to be aware of their feelings, even those of miscomfort and
irritation (own as well as other participants'), and frankly to
state them, as well as their needs, wishes, and preferences. He
demonstrates the importance of a good group climate for the subject outcome. Especially he fosters mutual feedback ("that is
how I perceive and experience you"), indicating the difference
of feedback and inferences/interpretations ("you just can't
stand any authority!"). - In favourable cases, the group can
acquire the necessary cooperative and communicative skills even
without a facilitator, in infavourable cases however (instable,
excessively dominant, or rigid members) only a trained facilitator can prevent serious trouble.

While the members learn efficiently to communicate and to

cooperate, the permanent presence of the facilitator becomes unnecessary. By and by withdrawing, he ought to stay "available
on demand" for some more time, a "safety-valve" decreasing
anxieties and taking the edge out of possible conflicts. The
group thus gets along safely. Feeling abandoned, in contrast, a
group by self-fulfilling apprehension easily ends up with acute
need for additional professional assistance. - Regular rating
on the group climate and progress, and discussing the results,
helps the group to become independent on the facilitator. With
growing experience, the routine rating may be reduced to the end
of every working day, even of every week, but it ought not to
be abandoned altogether. Again, any member feeling need for a
rating by his own discomfort, always ought to be allowed to ask
for it.

6. FACILITATING A GROUP WITHOUT A FACILITATOR

Trained group facilitators generally are highly paid specialists
and not always available. They mostly offer the best advantage
in fostering multidisciplinary collaboration. When they are not
available, combinations of information on and methodical instruct-
ion for observing the group process offer at least some compensation for the lacking facilitator.

6.1 Written instruction, questionnaires, and exercises

Unfamiliar and unintelligible situations raise fear and even
anxieties. Experiencing a situation as inexplicable and threatening, increases the participants' readiness for irrational and
aggressive reactions. Intellectual understanding of a new situation may change feelings of threat into interest and curiosity.
Thus information on what is happening or might happen, decreases
the members' uncertainty, and hence decreases the chance of
trouble and conflict.

    In the very beginning, the members of a working team mostly
are not interested in "wasting" time on information and problems
not evidently connected with their subject task. The leader can
unobtrusively introduce non cognitive topics by asking for
suggestions on group decision making, or by suggesting Cohn's
rules. Either way he can ask the members about their experiences
with various ways of group communication, and how they liked
different types of groups with a more authoritarian or a more
tolerant climate, and what the work outcome was. He thus re-
activates their experiences on the connection between group
climate and work output. He then may offer Cohn's rules, and
relate them to Cohn's triangle. Adding a list of "dos"(App.
IX), he gives some more information on groups and group process

as an explanation. Denoting all of them as "experts' suggestions", protects him from most of the possible criticism. "To
test the advantages/disadvantages of the suggested rules", he
introduces questionnaires (emphasising that they just take some
minutes' time and help a lot for facilitating communication),
which again give opportunity unobtrusively to focus the attention on group proceedings. By and by he thus prepares the participants to accept additional written information on groups
- carefully selected, processed, and adapted to the present
group's and members' actual needs.

If group or single members be efficiency-ridden, metacommunication and information on group process strictly have to
be restricted to short periods. Only acute trouble (e.g.
blocked efficiency, failing decision-making, hostility among
members - which then are fairly sure to occur) increases the
members' willingness to deal with "non-subject-task" topics.
To overcome present difficulties, the leader may offer a brainstorming (see App. VI) on the possible causes, or by a questionnaire give a basis for metacommunication (using e.g. one of
the forms shown in App. VIII). If and when the importance of non-
subject ("mental") problems for the smooth functioning of the
group once is realised by the members, exercises on observation,
communication, and cooperation can be offered. "Informal meetings", taking advantage of the relaxation by a shared meal or
drink, are most appropriate for first discussions of group process and mutual interactions (avoiding to talk about absent
members - according to the general rule "talk with him, not
about him"). A suitable setting - seats fairly close together -
facilitates the communication and fosters a favourable group
climate.

Rating the group climate and work efficiency as a routine,
again is advisable as a quick and efficient way to confront the
members with the group's progress and their own integration/lack-
ing integration in the group. Sometimes the rating is to be evaluated according to single subgroups (e.g. various disciplines
or various ranks) rather than to the total of the group, when
the ratings of an unhappy and a content subgroup combine to an
acceptable mean value.

With the members' increasing awareness of and interest in
the group process, the leader by and by can intensify metacommunication, and offer additional information on groups. Referring directly to present group's or - worse - members' trouble
easily raises defences. The leader wisely avoids too direct a
reference to the ongoings in the group, but discusses the problem
better in a more general way: "What might cause a group/ a member
to act in this way?". The members anyway subconsciously realise
the connection with their own group problems. - The leader -

having a double function as a formal leader and a facilitator -
regresses with his suggestions to "experts' advice", "we just
as well may try it"; a way to deflect criticism from himself to
some absent "psychologists".

Assuming a favourable combination of participants, and
sufficient social skills of the leader, the group thus may get
along splendidly and never need psychological assistance. Power
ridden, authoritarian, excessively ambitious, or irritable members however may be a heavy burden for a group, and irritating
pecularities or irritability of members by a mental clinch can
totally block the group's work efficiency. When a leader does
not get along with such a "difficult" group, professional help
by a trained facilitator is vital. Generally, the chances for
good working results are the better, the less ambitious (promo-
tion-oriented) and the more interested in the subject outcome
the members are. In selecting the members of a team, it generally pays well to take the more cooperative one rather than the
famous expert, whose belief in his own outstanding importance
is a permanent challenge to less self-oriented co-workers:
Successful teamwork is an emotional as well as an intellectual
problem and demands social as well as intellectual skills of
the team members.

6.2 A multi-media approach

"Trigger films" (stimulating films of but two or three minutes'
duration) on key situations and interactions in a group, combined with instructions on observation, written information,
and subsequent discussion, are a convenient way of facilitating
a group's start without the aid of a trained facilitator. The
group's first official meeting could be devoted to such an "introduction into group work". Scaled questionnaires on various
aspects demonstrated by the films could be filled in by the
members, and compared with the substantiated written comments
of the producers. They form a base for the future routine rating
of the group's own proceedings, using the same questionnaires.
The participants thus are provided with the basic knowledge on
what might happen in a group, its possible causes, and the ways
of overcoming trouble. In contrast to most written information
on the same topic, a film demonstrating typical group situations generally is readily accepted, and very useful to trigger
the discussion on group proceedings and to raise interest in
more information.

There is but one disadvantage with this otherwise most promising approach in group facilitating: up till now, multi-media
material - trigger films, instructions, questionnaires, exercises, comments - has not been produced. It ought to be a chall-

enge for a multidisciplinary team of psychologists, facilitators, sociologists, educational technologists, and producers of
instructional films. They even might use for demonstration cuts
of their videotaped working sessions, to show the problems they
themselves experienced in starting and running the team. - In
some more years, this like material will be available for facilitating group work without a trained facilitator.

Altogether, a multidisciplinary working team is subject to
difficulties stemming from mutual competition and rivalry,
amplified by interdisciplinary differences in perception, reasoning, and language. A formal group leader familiar with basic
knowledge and techniques, and of considerable mental stability,
using written information, questionnaires, and special exercises, generally can deal successfully with the problems arising especially during the first stages of a working group, if
a trained facilitator is not available. With "difficult" groups
or members however, professional help may become necessary and
ought to be provided.

APPENDIX

I. Improving communication

The exercises of "active listening" and of "controlled dialogue"
are run in groups of three members, and best repeated with a
different grouping, e.g. first all partners of the same, then
all of different disciplines. - Audiotaping and playing back the
tapes intensifies the effect.

Active listening [5]. A member taking the role of "speaker"
reports to the "listener" on a topic of personal concern to the
speaker, while a third party acts as "observer". At suitable intervals, the listener states what he understood to be said; the
speaker either confirms or corrects him. - After seven to ten
minutes, the roles rotate among the members, till everybody
acted once as listener, speaker, and observer. - Subsequently
ten minutes' discussion in the small groups, then discussion in
the whole group.

Controlled dialogue. Again the third party acts as observer, while the other two run a dialogue, including active listening: Before making his own contribution, each party has to
summarize (not to repeat word by word!) what has been said by
the partner, who has to confirm the correctness. If the momentary listener fails correctly to summarize, he gets a second try,
if he still fails, the speaker has to repeat his contribution.
If he himself fails, observer or audiotape are consulted. Rotation of roles, small group discussion, and discussion in the

whole group as above.

The parties here have to split their attention between listening/summarizing and answering. - The probability of misunderstandings grossly increases with topics connected with preoccupations of one or both partners.

The first two Abercrombie-exercises also help to improve communication.

II. Abercrombie exercises [3]

The exercises result in a confrontation with the ambiguity of perception, reasoning, and language. - Some "stimulus" (e.g. a list of words, a text, a graph, a picture, a trigger film) is offered to the members, who for some ten minutes silently note down their perception and the inferences, trying to different-iate between "perception" and "inference". An unstructured dis-cussion (not guided by the leader) follows and exhibits the differences in the various individuals' perception, inferences, use of words, and sets of implicit assumptions, norms and values.

List of words. The members are asked to define the meaning of given key-words as "normal / average / random - - equivalent / coinciding / comparable / similar - - probable / possible / undoubted / proved".

Texts. The members are given a text of about a page, and either asked what the author meant by words as the above, or by the whole text. The text may or may not be collected before the noting down.

Graphs. The members are given a graph, e.g. Fig. 5. They are to note down all information on the relation $y = f(x)$ they take from the graph. This graph is appropriate for all data-collecting and data-processing disciplines.

The "impossible object". The members are to note down the feelings and emotions associated with Fig. 6, which generally raises quite a lot of irritation and defences. The discussion exhibits the members' tendency to prevent the perception of ir-ritating reality (to minimize the "cognitive dissonance"), a fact of central importance in dealing with preoccupations.

With very rigid, unbalanced, or aggressive participants, Abercrombie exercises - especially the "impossible object" - may cause difficult group situations.

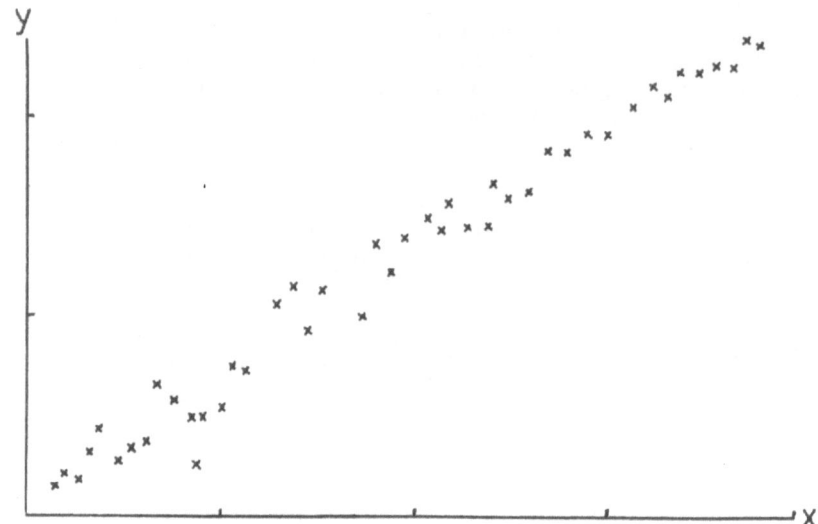

Fig. 5. A graph for Abercrombie exercises.

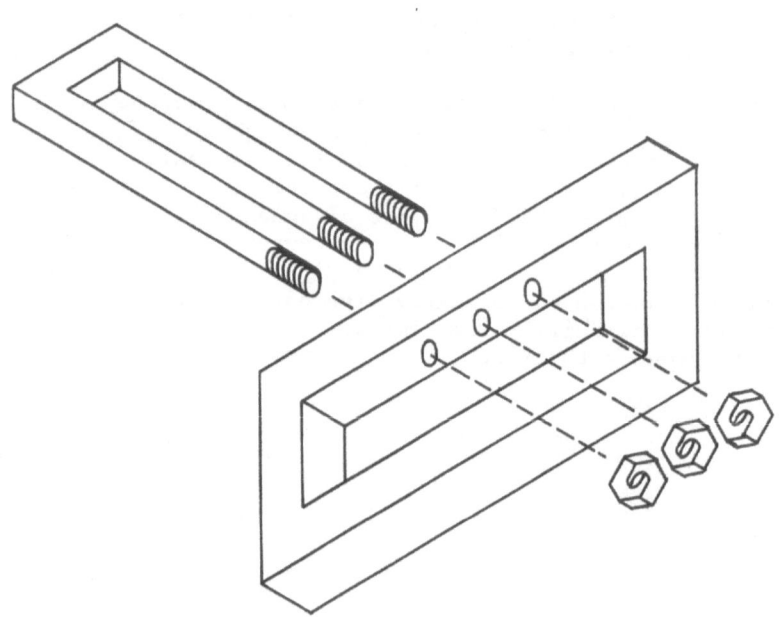

Fig. 6. "Impossible objects".

III. Improving cooperation

Material: as many jigsaw (puzzle) games (about 50 pieces per
game) as members. - The group is subdivided into competing teams
of three or four members, each team seated around a table. The
pieces of the - different - puzzles are distributed arbitrarily
among the members of the team. Winner is the team which first
has finished all the puzzles. No speaking, no direct interfering,
no taking pieces off a partner or offering to him, no correcting
a partner. Pieces not needed by a party are deposited in the
center of the table; all pieces laying there to be taken by any
team member ad libitum. - Subsequently some minutes' discussion
in the teams, then discussion in the whole group.

IV. Compromising and conflict-solving

A training in compromising and conflict-solving either is gained
by role-playing a conflict not acute to the actual group, or by
settling a conflict of but minor importance for the group. The
role-play might concern the distribution of assumedly scarce
facilities (laboratory technicians, clerical service, computer
time, experimental outfit) among the members, to whom well-de-
fined roles - different from their actual profession and rank -
are attributed. Subsequently, the participants rate the handling
of the conflict according to the questionnaire VIII C. The role-
play is videotaped (if ever possible), and the tape played back
in the subsequent discussion, which concerns the process of conflict-solving, the quality of the solution, and the satisfaction
of the members as shown by the questionnaire, and the application
to possible conflicts in the group.

Petty conflicts for the training of conflict solving are
provided by the "group Rorschach test". The group gets some eight
Rorschach tables and has to find an interpretation consented to
by all members for every table, in altogether 15 minutes' time.
Rating, videotaping, and discussion as above. - Maximum group
size seven; for eight and more members subdivide into smaller
groups working in parallel and in mutual competition.

If Rorschach tables or similar material are not available,
the members first fill out questionnaire VIII C on the last
session, or rate on some controversial topic (newspaper article,
political issues) offering some five different aspects, or on
five different controversal topics. The forms then are collected
and the members asked to consent on estimated mean values for
all the items. Videotaping, rating the conflict-solving, and discussion as above.

V. "Segregation" (overcoming sub-grouping)

The formation of sub-groups (due e.g. to interdisciplinary pre-
occupation) can be overcome by a segregation exercise. - For an
hour, the members are distributed and arbitrarily re-distributed
every ten minutes into subgroups, discussing the same topic of
interest to the group (e.g. "what is the central problem of our
group?" / "how might we overcome the group's present difficulties?"). - Patterns for splitting the group hardly can be too
bizarre, e.g. smokers vs. non-smokers / male vs. female / col-
oured vs. whites / engineers vs. medics / members older vs.
members younger than 30 / northerners vs. southerners. - The
last split according to the formerly unintegrated or antagonistic subgroups. - Subsequent discussion of the experience with the
whole group.

VI. Brainstorming

1. All participants for some minutes note down all the associations / suggestions they get to the given keyword / problem.
2. All suggestions / associations are collected on the blackboard without judging or classifying, not criticising or refusing any, as bizarre or absurd as they might seem.
3. Add suggestions / associations stimulated by what has been
offered till then.
4. Structure and classify, discuss inferences and feasability.

VII. Making evident interdisciplinary preoccupations [6]

Variants of the following exercise are suitable to make evident
preoccupations between two different (groups of) occupations /
disciplines (here - engineers vs. medics).

    Each member quickly is to tick the items of the following
form. Then the number of ticks given to each item by the members
of each subgroup are counted and shown on the blackboard. Subsequent a discussion according to Abercrombie.

You are outlining character and behaviour of a "typical" engineer and a "typical" (medical) doctor for a television play as
lifelike and convincing as possible. From the list below, tick
in the left (right) column the items more probable to characterize the engineer (the doctor). - Tick the items quickly without long considering!

More probable to charact-   more probable to characterize the engineer   erize the doctor

is empathic
is a heavy smoker
works long hours
is amiable
is well paid / well off
leads a happy family
    life
is dependable
is good-looking
has a lively sense of
    humour
is slightly feminine
is competent
is imaginative
is ambitious
gambles
is happier dealing with
    things than with
    persons
is pedantic
is authoritarian
would like to cheat
    with his income-tax
likes open-air life
is sociable
is somewhat dull
likes luxury
enjoys close logical
    argument
is generous
is interested in arts
likes to work in a team
is avaricious
is highly intelligent
is a "leading citizen"
helps his wife with
    household chores

VIII. Questionnaires

The items of these three model questionnaires are to be varied
and adapted according to the actual group's needs and situation.

A. Eliciting the cause of sluggish discussion / work

Please tick the reasons (a maximum of five reasons) you think
important for the sluggish progress of the discussion (the work)
in this group!

	number of ticks
1. Topic not clearly defined	...
2. No concern for the topic	...
3. Insufficient knowledge of topic	...
4. No concern for the group	...
5. Discussion too theoretical	...
6. Discussion too general	...
7. Level of discussion too low	...
8. Repeatedly in vain tried to speak	...
9. Some members too eloquent	...
10. Discussion runs in circles	...
11. Theme is exploited	...
12. Some members monopolise the group by running a fight	...
13. Hostile climate - people become attacked or ridiculed	...
14. Members interested in their personal status rather than in the task	...
15. Tiredness / headache / other causes not connected with group or task	...
16. _____	...
17. _____	...

Number of participants: .....

(The blank lines are preserved for items suggested by the group.)

B. Eliciting ignored group problems

yes-votes
yes? est. actual

1. i Do you agree with the group's proceedings
in this session (during the last minutes)? ...
   ii How many yes-votes do you expect to result?   ...   ...

2. i Could you participate as you wanted to?   ...
   ii How many yes-votes do you expect to result?   ...   ...

3. i Did single members dominate (manipulate)
the proceedings?   ...
   ii How many yes-votes do you expect to result?   ...   ...

4. i Do you feel at ease with respect to the
other members?   ...
   ii How many yes-votes do you expect to result?   ...   ...

5. i Was fair regard given to opposing opinions?...
   ii How many yes-votes do you expect to result?   ...   ...

Session ...   Number of participants ...

C. Rating the group proceedings

Ratings: +2 "very good", +1 "satisfying", + 0 "passable"
         -1 "poor", -2 "very disappointing"

Please rate the following items for the past session:

	your value	group's mean
1. Group climate	...	...
2. Group's work efficiency	...	...
3. Members' dedication to the task	...	...
4. Communication among the members	...	...
5. Allowance for divergent opinions	...	...
6. Your own contribution to the pro- ceedings	...	...
7. Leader's assistance to the group	...	...

IX. A list of "dos"

1. Be aware of your feelings and emotions, express them, but don't act according to them.
2. Be aware of the role you are playing, of your aims, and of the presentation of yourself you are giving in the group. Are you acting as you actually want to?
3. In discussing a suggestion, first list its advantages. If you start by noting the disadvantages, any proposition will be dismissed as unfeasible.
4. Note down the suggestions / propositions, using preservable posters (brown paper) rather than the blackboard, that soon is wiped clean again.
5. Give positive feedback (encouragement, confirmation) whenever possible.
6. Try "active listening" to prevent misunderstandings.
7. Avoid to interprete, patronize, dominate, convert, judge, fight, manipulate, or ridicule a member.
8. Beware of perfectionism - you are not obliged (nor capable) always to win, or to find the very best solution.
9. Take your time and don't loose patience - groups mostly have a slow start, but then go on steadily.

REFERENCES

1. Th.S. Kuhn, The Structure of Scientific Revolutions. The University of Chicago Press, Chicago, 2nd ed., 1970.
2. R.L. Gregory, The intelligent eye, Weidenfeld and Nicolson, London, 1970.
3. M.L.J. Abercrombie, The Anatomy of Judgement, Penguin Books Ltd., Harmondsworth, 1974.
4. R.C. Cohn, Journ. Group Psychoanalysis and Process Vol. 2 (1969/70) No. 2.
5. Th. Gordon, Parent Effectiveness Training, Peter H. Weiden Inc., New York, 1970.
6. L. Hudson, Frames of Mind, Penguin Books Ltd., Harmondsworth, 1970.

REHABILITATION MEDICINE AND REHABILITATION ENGINEERING :
ITS CORRELATION, PARTICULARLY IN BIOMECHANICS

Victor M. Santana Carlos

Medical Director
Rehabilitation Medicine Centre
Alcoitao - Estoril, Portugal

1. INTRODUCTION

In attempting to say something about rehabilitation engineering,
particularly when we wish to consider its correlation with
rehabilitation medicine, we think it becomes indispensable to
refer some basic elements of the latter, that is to say, we should
remember what rehabilitation medicine is, the technicians that its
adequate use requires, and its humanitarian and socio-economic
value. This will certainly justify its progressive improvement in
a number of countries, particularly for the last decades, whenever
completed, as it should be, by vocational rehabilitation and the
integration of the disabled in the community.
    Then, it is our purpose to mention rehabilitation engineering,
with particular incidence on biomechanics, drawing attention to
the fact that it is a doctor and not an engineer who is approaching
this important subject, leaving for this reason everything considered
more relevant and specific to the engineer competence. In short,
our purpose is just to give general ideas on rehabilitation medicine
and rehabilitation engineering, rather than to go thoroughly into
a specific matter.

2. MEDICAL AND VOCATIONAL REHABILITATION

Till the beginning of the 20th century, the role of the doctor was
almost exclusively that of saving lives. This responsability
generally ended when the acute case, either medical or surgical,
had been solved. Changing gradually and enlarging its scope in a
more human and social sense, medicine has thus been acquiring new

perspectives, so that "the doctor's responsibility does not end
when the acute illness is ended or surgery completed; it ends only
when the individual is restrained to live and work with what is
left". Therefore, independently from the unquestionable benefits
of preventive medicine and of curative medicine and surgery, medical
services started also to develop in what some authors called the
third phase of medical care: rehabilitation medicine. There are,
of course, elements of medical rehabilitation in "preventive medicine"
and "curative medicine and surgery", just as elements of the latter
are always present in rehabilitation medicine. This basic concept
of doctor's responsibility can properly function whenever rehabilitation is truly considered an integral part of the medical services.

   In rehabilitation medicine the treatment is total, that is to
say, it should satisfy not only the needs of purely physical
character of the patient, but have also in consideration his
psychological, educational, social, professional, economic problems,
and any others which may, to a greater or lesser extent, be
originated by disability.

   Having in consideration what has been said before, rehabilitation can be defined as the restoration of the handicapped person
to the utmost in his physical,mental, educational, social,professi-
onal and economic aspects. This concept lets us foresee that the
rehabilitation process must be the attribute of a team of conveniently
specialised technicians who act in the closest possible collaboration,
the patient himself participating and the doctor assuming the main
responsability. This is the only way of considering, as one should,
all the problems caused by handicap and not a sole one: that of
purely physical disability.

   The number of members who compose a rehabilitation team can
vary, either according to the needs of the hospital service where
they must act, or the type of patients to be considered. In many
of these services or departments, the doctor, the nurse, the
therapist and the social worker are enough. In others, such as
medical rehabilitation centres, mainly when teaching and research
activities must be carried out there, the above mentioned team
should be more complete and constituted as far as possible by
carefully selected and more experienced technicians.

   In the application of techniques and rehabilitation methods,
the doctor will have the greatest responsibility. He will examine
and follow the patient, will evaluate the degree of his disability,
will prognosticate and decide when the patient should be discharged
and be able to return home or to work. As the head of the team,
the doctor shall coordinate the efforts of all its members and
direct it in such a way that the purpose of rehabilitation, with
regard to the particular case of each patient, be more efficiently
attained.

   One must ask, however, which doctor should assume such
responsibility? In principle, we defend the idea that every doctor
should be interested in rehabilitation medicine, since it starts
in the place of the accident or in the patient's bed. At least as

regards anything related with preventing the appearing of complications or contributing to a possible aggravation of the disability, every doctor should have a basic knowledge of rehabilitation medicine when he graduates and leaves the Medical School. The practical application of the knowledge acquired may be an excellent contribution to reduce to the minimum the inevitable complications resulting sometimes from the ignorance of simple current techniques in rehabilitation. Such complications not only cause the patient to stay an incomparably larger number of days in internment, and consequently increase the financial charges, but also frequently contribute to a much larger functional devaluation of the patient.

If it is true that every doctor should have some basic knowledge of rehabilitation medicine, it is not less true that this medical speciality demands as a large knowledge, which has to be increased day by day due to the introduction of new techniques and new methods of rehabilitation. Therefore, in order that the doctor may be able to observe, prescribe and orientate the rehabilitation of the disabled in all its aspects, whatever the cause of this disability, and also to co-ordinate the efforts of a team of specialist paramedical staff, we have to admit the necessity of their careful preparation, of their specialization generally during a period of not less than three years, in adequate institutions of recognized scientific value. As a rule, the speciality is called physical medicine and rehabilitation, or simply rehabilitation medicine, or even physiatry, and the specialist doctor, physiatrist.

Other important members of the working team are the nurse, the physiotherapist, the occupational therapist and the speech therapist. Rehabilitation nursing is a specialization of a trained nurse with the general certificate which can usually be obtained after a three-year course. In Portugal, the post-graduate course of rehabilitation nursing lasts for an academic year, and that of therapist three years.

The rehabilitation nurse is responsible for the treatment prescribed by the doctor, and for the application of specialized nursing techniques, teaching the disabled patient to keep a correct position in bed, so as to avoid possible deformities, to turn, to sit, to get up, to walk, and taking care of the patient's personal hygiene, etc. The physiotherapist evaluates the functional possibilities of the patient, and under medical prescription uses physiotherapy, such as heat, light, electricity, water and also therapeutic exercises, teaching the patient to move, to go up or down the stairs, ramps, with or without braces, crutches or wheelchairs. The occupational therapist directs a specialized programme of functional activities with the purpose to improve or compensate a functional deficiency, and to awaken in the patient his interest in activities which may contribute in the future, to guide him in the learning of a new profession, if necessary.

The speech therapist, besides informing herself of the degree of importance and of the disfunction areas of the patient, both as regards speech and hearing, trying to find the unscathed means of communication, is responsible for the especialized treatment of the alterations found.

The rehabilitation nurse, the physiotherapist and the occupational therapist, besides their specific work, will also deal with the patient's training in activities of daily living (A.D.L.), trying to take him to perform them in a way as near the normal one as possible. For example, the disabled should be trained to get up from bed, wash, dress, eat, write, etc.

There are, however, other members of the working team whose role in the patient's rehabilitation is also important. Experience tells us that, as soon as the patient realizes, after the desease or the accident, the importance of disability, he will promply concentrate the best of his attention on the disability and the problems connected with it. The patient's thoughts will concentrate on himself, and as a rule they will tend to orientate themselves towards disability, treatment, environment, altered relations with his family, employer, friends, society and consequently his problematic future. To lose important parts of the body, or mere body functions is, naturally enough, very depressing, but it is not less so the humiliating dependence in which the patient will find himself because he needs the others' help, even to perform the most elementary daily activities.

Such situations of depression or, what may also happen, agitation and revolt, are frequent, and they should be expected and understood by the different members of the rehabilitation team. They have a great influence on the capacity of active participation, or decided motivation of the patient in the team work, and this is of the utmost importance so that the best results may be obtained. The patient is thus wisely considered member No.1 of the rehabilitation team. As a matter of fact, whatever his race, skin colour, religion, politics, social life standard etc., we should always be concerned with the dignity of the human person and consider him as an irreducible whole, and not only as a simple paralized or amputated member. If these principles must be taken into consideration by the above mentioned members of the team, others are still frequently called to a greater activity by the patient, so that the total aims of rehabilitation may be more securely attained. These are the social worker, the psychologist, the vocational counselor, and the placement officer.

Particularly in rehabilitation centres where, together with ambulatory patients, there is an in-patient service, the respective work-team includes also other technicians, such as the prosthetist and the orthotist. The existence of departments or workshops where prosthesis, braces, special shoes, corsets and other technical aids can be made and repaired is indispensable in a good rehabilitation centre. Special education and recreation, including sports, should also be a must in such centres.

The co-ordinated work of the team members we referred to is a valuable contribution to the solution of the main problems of

the disabled, who after evaluation has shown the necessary
rehabilitation potential. Nevertheless, medical rehabilitation
alone will be of little value if it is not immediatly followed
by a careful vocational evaluation, and then by appropriate
vocational training for a new profession, if it is no longer
possible for him to carry on the one he had before disability
occurred. As a matter of fact, although conveniently trained, and
helped by all technical aids, the different values of rehabilitation, including its cost, will be entirely useless if, once
medical rehabilitation has terminated, we do nothing but leave
the patient at the door of the rehabilitation centre. Should we
so behave, in most cases, if the individual without crutches,
prostheses or wheelchair, begged or consummed public assistance
funds, he wil do it now at a higher cost, with those devices,
without having the problem satisfactorily solved. Such an active
and as extensive as possible participation of the disabled in the
life of the community is not only just but indispensable as well.
As the United Nations Universal Declaration of Human Rights
proclaims, "all human beings are borne free and equal in dignity
and rights." "The handicapped person is an individual with full
human rights which he shares in common with the ablebodied".

"Regardless of the employment situation and the economic
fluctuations", says Jochheim, "rehabilitation services must be
available to enable all disabled persons to enjoy their rights
and develop their full potentialities ... Sooner or later the
development of social security will exceed the production capacity
of the younger generation, which is decreasing in number, if the
disabled - despite their disability and age - do not participate...
Rehabilitation is not only a humanitarian duty towards the disabled,
it is at the same time the only possibility of making bearable
the rapidly increasing costs for healt services and social security".

From the foregoing, Industrial Rehabilitation Units, Vocational Training Centres and Sheltered Workshops are indispensable
organizations for evaluation of abilities, training for a profession at an accelerated pace, and for sheltered employment when
competitive work is not yet possible for psychological and social
reasons or others such as a great slowness in the performance of
a given task. The possibility for more severe cases of home-
making employment should also be considered. This is the way of
attaining a total rehabilitation which allows the disabled to
obtain a job later, to fulfill his duties without frustration
and to occupy in the society the place he is entitled to.

As to the job, and according to experience, we stress that
ont only is it possible but it has also been found that the jobs
can successfully be held. Followed-up studies of disabled persons
rehabilitated through the State-Federal Vocational Rehabilitation
Programme, in the United States, made after rehabilitation, show
that 80% to 85% of rehabilitants :
   a. Continued to work;
   b. Are in the same or better job;
   c. Increase their earnings just as other workers do.

A two-year study comparing 11,000 handicapped workers with 18,000 unimpaired workers shows that the handicapped workers are:
   a. Adaptable. - They adjust quickly and satisfactorily to the conditions of the job;
   b. Productive.- They are equal and sometimes superior to other workers in their job performance;
   c. Careful. - They make job safety records equal or superior to their fellow workers;
   d. Regular. - They tend to have job attendance records as good as other workers on the same jobs;
   e. Reliable. - They are not job-hoppers;
   f. Capable. - They can do any kind of work where their impairments are not handicaps.

Obviously, for the cases of extreme disability, even after the use of up-to-date rehabilitation medicine, such disabled will need to be admitted in residencial social centres or homes for the irrecoverable where the cost per bed will be much lower. To keep their living, which is generally difficult to manage in their own homes, and try to grant them a rather reduced minimum of simple personal activities are, among others, two of the objectives of these social organizations.

It should be remembered that during the whole rehabilitation process the role of the community must never be forgotten. The community must, indeed, be involved in this continuing process even in the extent of considerable adaptation in both working and living environment and particularly where the residuals of disease and disability are accompanied by poverty and economic problems.

Useless to say that the role of the engineer in the course of the whole process of medical and vocational rehabilitation and also after the latter, in the job, in the performance of a given task, and also in adequate integration of the disabled in society, is of the greatest importance for the valuable contribution he can give, particularly in the cases of severe disability. Besides the great variety of devices or technical aids to be adapted to rather different situations, and to be improved, one must count upon the frequent changes to perform in the home where the disabled is going to live, and with the numerous problems the architectural barriers impose on the disabled in the social environment where he shall have to move and live.

We should like, however, before referring more in detail in this paper to rehabilitation engineering, to justify the reasons why the rehabilitation of disabled has been and continues to be necessary and compensating, when adequately carried out.

3. HUMANITARIAN AND SOCIO-ECONOMIC VALUE OF REHABILITATION

The rehabilitation of disabled has unquestionably a humanitarian, social and economic value. In trying to preserve or restore the dignity of the disabled person, the sense of his independence,his

confidence and active participation in community life, rehabilitation contains an intensively human aspect, contributing to increase
the individual's value, and, with him, the society he belongs to.
However, the need for medical and vocational rehabilitation still
results from the existence of a high number of disabled, and the
nember is increasingly growing. A study made in Canada revealed
that among the population of twenty two million there are a million
and a half of permanently disabled people. In the United States a
survey based on 1970 Census data showed a total population of
121 million in the typically accepted employable age-range of 16
to 64 years old. Not included were those in institutions or those
in military service. Women made up 51 percent of the number. The
Census also showed there were 11,265,000 persons in the same age-
range with disabilities which existed for six months or longer.
Excluded were persons in institutions. Women made up only 47% of
the handicapped population. One in every 11 Americans - over nine
percent - were handicapped.

In a simpler and generalized way, Susan Hamermann states, in
an excellent report on "The Social and Economic Implications of
Investments in Rehabilitation", made at the request of the United
Nations, that "at least 10 percent of the population of any
country suffers from some form of mental or physical disability".

Hobson refers on his turn that recent estimates made by the
Social Security Administration (SSA) and the Swedish Institute for
Handicapped (National Research Council, 1976) indicate that between
10 and 12 percent of the population in the U.S. are handicapped.
Using the lower figure and estimating on the conservative side
means that there are approximately 20 million handicapped individuals
in the United States. The SSA figure also indicate that about 8
million are able to work either normally or in a limited capacity
and 7.5 million are unable to work at all. By education, says
Hobson, the remaining 4.5 million must be comprised of those from
the young and geriatric populations. The loss of productivity plus
the financial burden borne by federal and state programmes are
estimated to be in the billions of dollars. Of course, these
financial burdens are in addition to personal losses suffered by
physical handicapped individuals resulting from their inability
to participate in many aspects of life-losses that cannot be
measured in dollars, as Hobson rightly says.

In a chartbook on Work Disability in the United States,
published by the Social Security Administration, Department of
Health, Education and Welfare, one can find the latest available
information on the socioeconomic and medical status of the disabled
in that country. The usefulness and the social importance of the
data collected led us to report them very shortly in this paper.
More than 15 million of noninstitutionalized Americans aged 20-64
are limited in their ability to work because of chronic health
conditions and impairments. Total disability increases sharply
after age 55. The disabled are older than the nondisabled. The
median age of the nondisabled adult population was 38; the partially
disabled averaged 47 years, and the totally disabled, 53. The

totally disabled are least likely to be married. The higher the
degree of disability, the lower the level of education. Most
disabled persons are limited in their ability to move freely. Of
the totally disabled reporting limitation in mobility, more than
half were confined to the house; most of the rest needed help with
transportation but could otherwise get around outside without
assistance. The disabled have the greatest difficulty with
movements of the legs. Stooping, crouching, or kneeling posed
problems for them. Almost as many had trouble walking. About 2
million must depend on others for help in movement and personal
care. These 2 million people stand for less than 2 percent of the
working-age population. Yet their individual and collective losses
may be considerable because they must include personal and economic
losses to spouses and children as well as to the totally disabled
themselves. Musculoskeletal and cardiovascular problems produce
more than half of all disability, from a list of 39 disorders.
The totally disabled were almost three times more likely than the
partially disabled to report mental disorders as the major disabling condition. The totally disabled are 2 to 4 times as likely
to be hospitalized. A third of the totally disabled spend $500 or
more annually for healt care, and this was more than two times
the proportion of nondisabled having similar costs. The totally
disabled spend 3 times more per person, most of it for hospital
care. The disabled have less insurance coverage resulting in higher
out-of-pocket costs. Large proportion of the disabled are unemployed
or out of the labour force. The totally disabled who remained in
the labour force were not able to work regularly although 12 percent
of the men were working full time when the data were collected.
Average income for the totally disabled is half that of the nondisabled. Totally disabled persons, especially the nonmarried, are
most likely to be poor. Disabled married persons depend most on
earnings; disabled nonmarried persons, on public assistance.
    We would like to stress now the importance of the reflexes
that the physically disabled population, not rehabilitated, may
have in the economy of a country. As a matter of fact, disability
has significant economic repercussions within any community. Its
effects, though more apparent for the persons directly affected,
also fall, and sometimes to a great extent, on the society in general.
Individually, disability "reduces the patient's capacity to absorb
education, to be productive in work and to function independently".
Therefore, disability also results in a loss of national income
which will no doubt have to be covered by the economically active
section of the population.
    It is known that the mortality rate has decreased, particularly
in more developed countries as regards public healt and economy.
The progress found within preventive medicine and healt care, and
also in therapeutics, both medical and surgical, caused an
appreciable increase in longevity, translated in an important and
progressively growing increase in the number of individuals who,
in a given section of the population reaches older ages. Such

progress had also repercussions on the group of individuals who
compose the opposite end of human life: childhood and adolescence.

The increase found in the above mentioned extreme groups,
that is to say, on one hand, that of sixteen-year-old persons,
on the other, the group of 64 or over this age, who are practically
considered as groups of non-productive ages, is not always
accompanied at the same pace by that of ages considered as productive or economically active, particularly in the countries where,
together with an increase in the longevity average, an increase
in birth-rate is also found.

The economically active group has to be responsible for the
non-productive. Therefore, the people who form the non-productive
groups will be in a dependent situation, the charges caused by this
dependence being supported by those of the active group in as
larger a scale as the number of people who compose it is lower.
If we have in consideration, on one hand, the progressive rise in
old people, the higher and higher specialization forcing young
people to a longer technical preparation (therefore to a dependence
situation) and, on the other, if we think of the considerable
percentage of people with physical disabilities existing in the
active segment of population, we are led to conclude that the
number of those who compose the economically active group will tend
to decrease and consequently the charges per person will tend to
increase.

Medical and vocational rehabilitation may contribute , to a
great extent, to reduce the unevenness between the two groups
considered, increasing the number of active persons, and thus to
raise the economic potential of the country. By using up to a
useful maximum the human energy left intact by the accident or the
disease, improving it and orientating it towards the fulfillment
of a profession, not only will it contribute to increase productivity
and the taxable income through contributions, but will also determine
a reduction of the growing draining of funds or subsidies, inevitably
required by the dependent, non-productive population. For the above
reasons we may consider the rehabilitation of a disabled as a fair,
compensatory investment of capital.

The expenses its adequate application involves are by far
financially repaid. As an example, we wish to sum up some statistical data presented by the State-Federal Vocational Rehabilitation
Programme, in the United States, concerning the fiscal year ended
on 30 June 1962. In that year, 102,396 persons were rehabilitated.
Of these, one in six received, before starting rehabilitation,
subsidies from public assistance, totalising 18 million dollars per
year. After rehabilitation, they became active members of the
community, their earnings being computed only in the first year
after rehabilitation, in 33.5 million dollars. Obviously, to this
benefit others should be added, such as the sum of 18 million
which ceased to be spent by public assistance, the income of taxes
from discounts in salaries, and an important number of working
hours, per person, to add to national productivity.

Considering particularly the decline in public assistance
as a result of an adequate rehabilitation of disabled, Conley
reports that data collected in the United States of America in
connexion with the analysis of free-and post-rehabilitation service
earnings of disabled clients indicated that between 1958 and 1967
the percentage of clients receiving public assistance at acceptance
for service ranged from 12 to 13%. At closure of rehabilitation
service, this was reduced on the average to between 5 and 6%. The
estimated annual reduction in public assistance payments, as a
result of the federally funded state vocational rehabilitation
programmes, was $9.6 million in 1961, and by 1967 this figure had
not risen to $16.4 million.

It should be remembered that disabilities can be congenital
and acquired, resulting in the latter case, from the disease or
the accident. They can also be physical or mental nature. It is
found that the great cause of disability is the chronic disease.
It is followed by accidents (work, traffic and war) and finally by
congenital conditions. The greatest amount of disability is found
among older persons. However, one must bear in mind that disability
is no respecter of age. Rheumatic fever, cerebral palsy, epilepsy
and still, sometimes, poliomyelitis, for the most part, cripple
the very young, not to speak of children born, for instance, with
partial or total lack of members or other anomalies. Among chronic
diseases, the most frequent cause of disability is cardio-vascular
disease, such as the cerebro vascular accident and myocardial
infarction. Peripheric vascular diseases, which are the origin of
situations leading to amputation, are also very frequent, followed
by mental retardation, those of neurologic origin, the arthritis,
various sensory disorders etc.

4. PREVENTION OF DISABILITY

From all that has been said up to now one can see the importance
and the severity of the problems imposed upon the society by
disability, and for the solution of which the public authorities,
private organizations and technicians are required to give the best
of their effort and collaboration. In order to reduce the problem
of disability and its effects, a lot of progress has been achieved.
Nevertheless, we are still far from attaining the level of results
that should be desired, mainly if we remember that over 400 million
people in the world are disabled and that it is estimated that not
less than 3 million persons would be added to that total each year
taking into account population increase, improved longevity,
industrialization, progressive increase in traffic and other
factors. Thence the need to intensify the research into the causes
of disabling conditions and into methods of preventive and remedial
care of such conditions; to obtain funds so that it may be possible
to take rehabilitation programmes to those who it is not possible
to help today; to intensify the training of rehabilitation technical
staff, including that of bioengineering, trying to give financial

support to the existing training institutions required to produce
the additional personnel needed; to create more facilities for
providing rehabilitation services of all types to the disabled;
extension of disease and accident prevention programmes, encouragement of community organization to widen public understanding and
to solve the problems of the disabled concerning their social
integration or reintegration, including extension of educational
efforts to increase employment acceptance of the handicapped.

It is therefore an important and necessary programme which,
in view of its wide scale, we cannot develop, but one aspect of
which we would like to stress, although briefly: prevention.
Disability prevention includes all action taken to reduce the
occurrence of impairment and its development into function
limitation and further fixation of the latter into disability.

An impairment is a permanent or transitory psychological,
physiological or anatomical abnormality or loss of such a degree
that it may create disability. Example: an amputated limb, hypertension, mental retardation etc. Impairment may cause functional
limitations which are the partial or total inability to perform,
normally, those activities indispensable for motor, sensory or
mental functions, such as walking, seeing, speaking, making contact
with surroundings etc. A functional limitation may be temporary,
permanent or reversible.

Disability, when progressively caused by functional limitation
and/or impairment, means a limitation in the functional ability
to perform activities which, according to age, sex and social
role, would be regarded as important components of life. Example:
activities of daily living, such as ambulation, dressing, feeding,
etc., social activities, including family activities, recreational
and professional activities.

Concentrating now on two examples, the above mentioned
expressions, (impairment, functional limitation and disability)
we could quote two cases, one of hypertension and another of
amputation. So, a 60 year-old person with hypertension for several
years, suffers a stroke (cerebro vascular accident) resulting in
right-side hemiparesis and aphasia. Impairments : hypertension
and some disturbance of brain function; function limitations :
inability to talk, decreased ability to walk and use right hand,
fatigue through low physical endurance; disability : inability
to work, partial inability to look after himself, inability to
communicate and interact with surroundings.

Another example would be the one of a 25 year-old man, who,
after a traffic accident had an amputation above the knee. The
impairment is the loss of leg; the functional limitation is
decreased ability to walk, and the disability will be decreased
abilities to work, to enjoy normal social activities (sports,
dancing) and to make social relationships.

Nevertheless, a point should be stressed. The expressions
impairment, functional limitations etc., may reflect a negative
side of a person. We all know that what is more important to the
functional valorization of the disabled is not what he lost in

consequence of the accident or the disease, but all that was left
intact. It is then the positive side which should count more in
rehabilitation. And still in this case it is convenient to bear
in mind that even for almost similar functional limitations the
degrees of handicap can be different . As a matter of fact, disability and handicap may not be exactly the same thing. Hamilton
quotes the example of two persons who had undergone amputation of
the left index finger approximately at the same level. From the
medical point of view, the disability is similar, or even the same.
Nevertheless, if one of the persons is a professional violinist
and the other a driver, we can easily see that the degrees of
handicap resulting from similar disabilities are entirely different.
Therefore, it is advisable that a full description of a patient
should thus include both his abilities and disabilities.

5. REHABILITATION ENGINEERING

From all that has been said before we could say that the value of
the medical and vocational rehabilitation of the disabled and his
adequate integration in the community is sufficiently great and
compensating to enable us to invest, without fear, in everything
that may contribute for a progressive development of techniques,
methods and work programmes. These must be, as far as possible,
adapted to the cultural and economic standards of living of the
country they are intended for.
    In such conditions, a balanced technological investment will
in all probability permit that not only a higher standard in
rehabilitation of disabled in general should be reached, but that
we make this rehabilitation possible in many of those more severely
attained cases. These would, otherwise, have to take shelter in
homes for unrecoverable, or, owing to inevitable complications,
lose their lives.
    "In accordance with Hobson, a conservative estimate is that
technology can be potentially beneficial to at least 50 percent
of the physically handicapped population. Through a judicious
application of technology it is quite possible to increase the
independence of individuals, thereby reducing cost of care and
increasing their involvement in productive job activities".
    This is why the engineer is called to a closer association
in the life sciences, and consequently to an active collaboration
with the doctor. He will thus be able to contribute a great deal
to the well-being of the disabled patient, improving his functional
possibilities and therefore the general requirements of his daily
life, thanks to the application of an advanced technology. This
makes the engineer's collaboration very important and quite
desirable.
    It is found, however, that the traditional role of the engineer,
who applied his skills almost exclusively to military needs, and
a little more to civil needs in the late 18th century and the early
19th century, has gradually developed, as otherwise happened with

other sciences, namely medical sciences. Therefore, new specific
areas develop, namely the one concerning mechanical engineering.

In the latter part of the 1950's the recognition Committee
of the Engineers Council for Professional Development proposed
the following definition: "Engineering is the profession in which
a knowledge of the mathematical and physical sciences gained by
study, experience and practice, is applied with judgement to
develop ways to utilize economically the materials and forces of
nature for progressive well-being of mankind". Therefore, and in
agreement with Renato Contini, "if knowledge is to be applied for
the progressive well-being of man-kind, knowledge is necessary as
to what constitutes this well-being. This implies knowledge of
what affects the physiological and psychological states of man".

Besides, in ancient history of humanity, the association of
engineering with medicine had already been demonstrated. In some
countries, namely Egypt and Peru, trepaning, or the surgical removal
of a small part of the skull to relieve pressure on the brain,
were found in excavations there.

The Romans associated engineering and medicine whenever they
tried to solve problems of draining of marshes and the availability
of potable water. They could thus be considered as pioneers of
public-health engineering. Leonard da Vinci (1452-1519), a great
artist, also quoted by Contini, was not only an engineering genius,
but an outstanding anotomist and physiologist who applied his
knowledge of physical law to explain physiological phenomena, even
to attempting to describe the circulation system. And Geovani
Boreli (1609-79), pupil of Galileo, applied the laws of mechanics
to the movements of animal and wrote the first treatise on biomechanics (Contini).

As a matter of fact, a great deal of example could be given
to show that scientists of the most varied branches of science,
including artists, great painters, sculptors etc., thanks to their
genius, were able to give their pioneer contribution, demonstrating
the important value of engineering when adequately applied to
medicine.

Near our century, wars have greatly contributed, owing to the
number of amputated they have caused, to the development of prosthetic
devices. The Franco-Prussian war, towards the end of the 19th
century, was an example. The collaboration of engineering with
medicine was already necessary in those days for the solution of
some of the most difficult problems of the amputated. However, in
the course of World War I and World War II, and during the periods
that immediately followed them, the collaboration of engineering
with medicine became gradually indispensable, the interdependence
of the engineer with the behavioural and life scientist being
entirely justified. But it was in the course of the period which
preceded Space Age and beyond, that a new branch of engineering,
commonly called bioengineering appeared, although it has also been
occasionally designated by the some scientists as biotechnology,
medical engineering and biomechanical engineering. With these
expressions they tried to mean an association of the engineering

scientists with the medical scientists.

Medicine, on its turn, is usually defined as the art and the science of preserving or restoring health or due physical condition as by means of vaccines, drugs, surgical operations and appliances, devices or technical aids. Medicine is responsible for prevention whenever possible; for the diagnosis of the disease, as much as possible at its onset; for cure, when prevention had not been possible; and finally for the functional restoration of occurred disabilities, with a view to an integration or reintegration of the patient in the community.

In any of the above mentioned stages, the bioengineer may give a very important contribution, such as designing or perfecting for the physician some particular device or technical aid. The bioengineer may also be consulted by the physician who suggests the need for equipment to perform some specific function. He can also work together with the doctor and other members of the rehabilitation staff such as the nurse, the therapist, the prosthetist or the orthotist, and, in team work, understand better the patho-physiology of a given clinical problem, so as to allow him to suggest more easily a more adequate and efficient rehabilitation device for the disabled patient. Contini quotes, as an example, a study made by him on pressures within the socket of the amputees. "A number of fitting techniques have been developed on the basis of different hypotheses as to what occurs at the stump-socket interface. This study was conceived to evaluate a variety of these techniques to investigate pressures, and changes in pressure within the step cycle during the day and diurnally. Consultation with the physician for the possible causes of the observed variations may eventually result in a better understanding of socket shape, and the effect of fitting and of alignment.

The bioengineer may also act as project director, and initiate the research, which, of course, does not imply the absence of the physician, particularly whenever this is necessary. Obviously, to collaborate effectively in team-work with the doctor and other paramedical staff, in the rehabilitation of disabled, the engineer must acquire the specialized knowledge he does not have when he leaves the engineering school. A multidisciplinary collaboration among technicians from two quite different scientific disciplines, engineering and medicine, cannot be achieved without great difficulty. Besides good human relations, which are always indispensable, the knowledge of behavioural and life sciences, I would say of bio-engineering, is a must, particularly when related to the rehabilitation of disabled, a medical area in which engineering has had the widest scope till now.

A Committee of the Engineers' Joint Council, in the United States, defined bioengineering as "the application of knowledge gained by a cross-fertilization of the engineering and biological sciences so that both will be more fully utilized for the benefit of man".

According to Robert Kenedi, Bioengineering Unit, Wolfson Centre, University of Strathclyde, in Glasgow, U.K., whose philosophy of

bioengineering education we follow, that definition includes four
major areas, namely: bionics, applied biology, biomedical engineering
and environmental health engineering. Biomedical engineering is
one of the most important areas, covering "the application of
engineering to medicine in basic studies of the human body and of
the man-machine relationship, in the provision of replacements
for damaged structures, and in the design and construction of
diagnostic and therapeutic instrumentation" (Kenedi).

Not less important, particularly to people too severely
disabled to make use of self-help devices, is the environmental
health engineering, that is "the use of engineering to create and
then to control environment optional to life". According to Donald
Selwyn, "this science, the redesign of environmental facilities
to permit their use by severely handicapped people, is termed:
Rehabilitation Engineering". Nevertheless, although we consider
such science as extremely important, we believe that it must be only
a part of all the aims that rehabilitation engineering may have.
Depending upon the degree of the remaining abilities - age, personal
preferences, motivation, etc. - usually and as far as the environmental area of his activity is concerned, the engineer may have to
solve the three basic problems: on-the-job physical performance,
low cost and relativaly independent living, and transportation. No
doubt the solution of these problems nearly always represents hard
work to the engineer, even when he is helped by his team members,
specially the doctor, the adviser and the client himself. But in
spite of the importance and necessity of this type of work, the
whole rehabilitation engineering cannot concentrate only on it.
We will refer to rehabilitation engineering in more detail later.

The first academic programme in bioengineering was started
in the U.S.A. in 1952. Given the non-existence of financial problems,
many other postgraduate courses followed. Since 1960, the National
Institute of Health has provided fifteen major universities with
training grants for post-graduates in biomedical engineering. In
the U.K. too, three important centres, among others, of biomedical
engineering established postgraduate programmes succesfully (The
Imperial College and the Universities of Strathclyde and Surrey).

It makes sense that most of schools still require as a
condition for admission into a postgraduate course in bioengineering
that the candidate is a fully trained engineer. The courses are thus
orientated to enhance engineering know-how and to provide the
necessary life science background. A good feature common to most
centres, both in the U.K. and in the U.S.A., is the requirement
for the student to undertake a bioengineering project of practical
significance.

Kenedi rightly stresses that "the principle of team effort
must be accepted as a basic "tenet" in the practice of biomedical
engineering. Thus, he says, the basic philosophy of a postgraduate
course must be orientated to producing a member of a team (in place
of an 'all-knowing' hybrid) highly competent as an engineer on the
necesssary sophisticated level and equipped with the appropriate

multidisciplinary background. This background is to be designed
to assist the biomedical engineer (a) to understand and appreciate
the problems in their medical as well as in their engineering
context, (b) to be able to communicate with the other members of
the multidisciplinary teams, and finally (c) to be prepared in a
broad educational sense to meet the moral, ethical and social
problems associated with medicine today, and originated to some
extent by the applications of the developments of technology".

We certainly also feel, in agreement with McLaurin, of Toronto,
Canada, that the postgraduate training must include an "exposure to
real patients and clinical problems on an internship basis" as an
indispensable part of the engineer's training.

The principles indicated are too important not to be wisely
considered by the engineer during and after his postgraduate course.
They must be not only retained but truly lived by the engineer, if
he wants to acquire, as it becomes indispensable, an appropriate
multidisciplinary background. The lack of this background may lead
not only to serious ethic situations, such as the ones thay may
occur when dealing with artificial joint replacements and/or
natural transplants, but also to those in the origin of frustrations
and of pure waste of time and money without any advantage to the
patient.

We think that the following example may confirm the importance
of Kenedi's basic philosophy of the postgraduate course. Traub and
Leclair, director and deputy director, respectively, Rehabilitation
Engineering Programme, R.S.A., U.S.A., report that in the middle of
1960's, efforts were made to use U.S. space and defense anvanced
technological developments. A joint programme with the National
Aeronautics and Space Administration (NASA) was developed, to obtain
unclassified technological advances in hopes of applying them and
resolving complex rehabilitation problems. "Several rehabilitation
centres joined the effort. NASA organized five biomedical applications technology (B.A.T.) teams which visited each centre to identify
problems that might be solved by the information stored in NASA
computers. Once located, the B.A.T. team submitted a written report
to the centre for evaluation and possible application. After 8
year's experience, however, the programme terminated and engineers
and clinicians failed to communicate effectively their problems
and solutions, thereby blocking the successful transfer of technology to rehabilitation practice".

This example seems to indicate that not always has a truly
integration of the engineer in team-work been found. He has rather
been operating as one of its members, in equally active collaboration
and responsibility, in relation to his team colleagues, all of them
having obviously in view the well-being and the maximum functional
improvement of the patient.

This tendency to a peripheral work, in the hospital or in the
rehabilitation centre, creates a solitary situation with clear
damage to the engineer, the doctor, and particularly to the patient.
The unquestionable humanitarian, social and economic value of rehabilitation we have already referred to, could thus be highly spoilt if

such situation would continue to be the rule.

In order to avoid such situations, which are harmful to the communitary objectives of rehabilitation, we should like to stress the great importance of an efficient teamwork.

J. Foort and his colleagues, in a recent article, states that "it is the inclusion of engineers that creates both expectation and dismay among team members who are not really prepared for the dichotomy between the medical and engineering role". And they point out as major differences, among others, the following ones: 1) Medical people see the patient as a problem; 2) Engineers see the patient as an example of a problem; 3) Medical people want an immediate, unique and complete solution to a particular-patient's-problem, while engineers want general solutions for populations.

No doubt that if such differences are always found in the practice, the team-work will be seriously harmed, since the vision of the problems and the ends to be reached may not be exactly the same. A coordinated team-work requires, first of all, that its members speak the same language. If the engineer has not some clinical input and the physician and the allied health professionals do not know at least a minimum of the basic principles of applied biomechanics, it will be difficult, or even impossible, to obtain helpful results to the disabled patient. Besides, we assume that, beyond professional competence, there is always a total disponibility and a mutual respect for the rights of the human being, among those who compose the work-team and the patient himself. If conditions are found, we believe to be possible that, with more probabilities and efficiency, the team may work together toward real solutions of the problems shown by the disabled patient.

Fortunately, a more realistic approach has been placing engineers, physicians and related scientists together in an aduqeate clinical arrangement to work directly on patient problems. In the United States, the Rehabilitation Service Administration (RSA) in fiscal year 1972, undertook a major programme commitment in rehabilitation engineering and related sciences for improving the vocational and self-care goals of the severely handicapped.

Under Traub and Leclair, the Rehabilitation Services Administration, whose programme is different from the one under the National Institutes of Health, the following areas of interest were outlined: 1) Artificial limbs - both internal and external prosthetic replacements; 2) orthopaedic braces - both internal and external orthopaedic assistive systems; 3) amputation and recons-tructive surgery; 4) mobility aids for orthopaedic disabled persons -wheelchairs, automative systems, etc.; 5) mobility and communica-tion aids for the blind and deaf; 6) architectural barrier removal for the severely disabled; and 7) fundamental studies directly goal -orientated to rehabilitation in the above areas.

Under the Biomedical Engineering Programme of the Institute of Health, the following areas of interest were considered: 1)Life -saving devices, that is, artificial hearts, renal dialysis, heart -lung machines, etc.; 2) facility engineering-automated hospital and patient monitoring equipment; 3) surgical and medical instrumentation, etc.; and 4) implantation materials for vessel and organ synthetic grafts, covering for electrode implants, etc.

Many areas of RSA research use products of the National Institutes of Health, such as materials for maxillo-facial prostheses, artificial kidney machines, and others. Besides, there is a close collaboration of the RSA with other scientific Foundations or Organizations, and particularly with the Veterans Administration.

The words "rehabilitation engineering" were new in 1970. In accordance with Leclair and Reswick, such words were coined by James Garrett, Chief of Research and Demonstration Programmes, and Joseph Traub, who is Director of Rehabilitation Engineering in RSA, and they are now of a world-wide acceptance.

With the signing of the Rehabilitation Act of 1973, Rehabilitation Engineering has become one of the primary priority of the agency. Project research programmes and the establishment and support of Rehabilitation Engineering Research Centers, to develop innovative methods of applying advanced medical technology, scientific achievement, and psychological and social knowledge to solve rehabilitation problems, including cooperative research with public or private agencies and organizations, are some of the important goals to be attained by the mentioned Rehabilitation Act.

At present, there are at least eight rehabilitation engineering centres in U.S.A.. In accordance with Leclair and Reswick, the objectives of the rehabilitation engineering centres are as follows:
1. To improve the quality of life of the physically handicapped through a total approach to rehabilitation, combining medicine, engineering, and related sciences;
2. To perform research and development in pioneering areas in which a Centre has developed unique capabilities;
3. To collaborate with laboratories and industy to carry out new devices and techniques through all phases of research, development, and clinical evaluation to active production and patient use;
4. To make available new devices and techniques to patients referred to the centre;
5. To educate clinicians and other professionals to use these new developments and the need to provide these services and techniques to patients throughout the nation;
6. To cooperate with other Centres in the clinical evaluation of their developments;
7. To provide an environment for education of physicians, engineers and other professional persons involved in related life,physical, and social sciences;
8. To cooperate, coordinate, transfer and exchange research findings and information with related centres and other institutions on a continuing basis.

Traub and Leclair point out that the research issues developed since 1972 in Research Strategies for each year have proposed a broad-scale attack upon many problems of the target populations of R.S.A.. The current research strategy (1975-1979) presents the following variables for study: Physical and vocational requirements of the disabled; available technologies and how they can be adapted to the needs of disabled; evaluation systems; sense delivery systems. The first two variables require high concentration of effort immediately to determine what the disabled needs, can accept, and can use. Evaluation systems are necessary to identify successful research and move it as soon as possible toward the service providers. New and improved service delivery systems must be designed that will provide the estimate in rehabilitation potential, while, at the same time, reducing costs of individual programmes in order that the total population in need of these services can have them available, and the technology be used, so that those benefitting from services become more employable.

It is worth knowing the figures representing the number of persons in the United States, located throughout the nation who constitute the target populations: the best estimates, based on several surveys, for the spinal cord disabled, place them between 500,000 and 1,000,000; amputees 375,000; paralyzed and/or deformed: 3,000,000; blind: 1,280,000; deaf: 1,705,000; and deaf-blind:40,000.

In order to consider the present activities carried out namely in the U.S.A., we will mention some of the existing ones and their respective action areas:

1) The Rancho Los Amigos Hospital, University of Southern California, has a programatic emphasis on functional simulation in patients with motor neuron diseases, and specially in stroke patients. It is well-known that in the centres of rehabilitation medicine with polyvalent character of admission, one of the disabled patients more frequently admitted for treatment is the hemiplegic as a result of a cerebro vascular accident (CVA). Quite a few hemiplegic patients cannot walk, mainly because they can't support their body weight due to weakness of the extensor muscles of the knee and the hip and of dorso-flexors of the foot. Ambulation therapy programmes are often postponed until the patient gains strength, because in these programmes both surgery and bracing were found to be unsufficient. Electrical stimulation of the quadriceps, gluteus medius and gluteus maximus during the stance phase of gait of some marginally ambulatory patients by means of a 3-channel stimulator has allowed ambulation at a level not possible without stimulation. Besides serving as a functional device, it hastens the provision of normal therapy and provides a training effect in itself by strengthening muscles and facilitating the patient's own response through sensory feedback. Patients who respond only during Functional Electrical Stimulation (F.E.S.) but not afterwards are screened for possible permanent implantation of a neuroelectric stimulation that was developed jointly by the Rancho R.E.C. and Medtronic Corp. The implant is more easily managed by the patient and is more reliable for long term use. Leclair and Reswick also report that approximately 150 patients have been treated using the 3-channel FES device in the last years. Three patients have been implanted with devices to gain hip stability, while four have been implanted for knee stability. The Rancho R.E.C. also developed a floated bed (MUD bed) which permits patients to lie on

their pressure sores without being turned at night while the wounds
continue to heel.

2) <u>The Moss Rehabilitation Hospital</u> has carried out studies
with the objective of determining weight line in humans. It has
developed a Limb Load Monitor to assist patients with ambulatory
deficiencies by training or retraining them on the amount of loading
or weight to apply to achieve a correct and proper weight-bearing
level.

To determine the weight line, signals from strain-gauges
attached to a platform on which a person stands are processed to form
a vertical line on a cathode ray tube. The vertical line, which
represents the location of the weight-line in a given plane, is
super-imposed on the image of the person viewed through the lens
of a camera. A photograph can be taken for a permanent record, or
the arrangement can be used for visual observation under clinical
conditions, such as alignment of an artificial leg or lower-limb
orthosis. It was thus possible to develop in the Moss Rehabilitation
Hospital R.E.C. a polypropylene ankle-foot orthosis, that has
revolutionized the treatment of drop-foot and other foot-ankle
impairments.

3) <u>The Texas Institute For Rehabilitation and Research</u> has
made its studies of rehabilitation engineering fall mainly upon
the pressure evaluation pad, which is a means of clinically
evaluating and observing the effectiveness of pressure relief
devices, or cushions, traditionally prescribed for patients with
spinal cord injuries.

Decubitus ulcers, bed sores or pressure sores are a frequent
and costly complication for the spinal cord injured patient and,
therefore, their prevention is of extreme importance for all
physicians interested in his rehabilitation. Through the use of
pneumatically controlled transducers or contacts, bony and soft
tissue pressure distribution is observed and recorded. By varying
the air pressure in the evaluation pad and photographically recording
which lights on the display box are illuminated in a sequence of
pressures, we can construct a pressure contour map which ultimately
enables us to individualize the cushion to the specific patient
needs.

4) <u>The Harvard - M.I.T. Rehabilitation Centre</u> seeks to rehabili-
tate handicapped people by applying highly sophisticated engineering
technology and theory. As part of the endeavour, the gait analysis
laboratory at Children's Hospital Medical Centre has developed a
system for acquisition, processing and analyzing the three major
measurable parameters of gait: all limb segment motion, muscle group
activity, and foot-floor reaction forces. Using a PDP 11-10 minicom-
puter and incorporating technological advances and in-house development equipment, the system directly measures, or indirectly
calculates, the biomechanical parameters of gait in real-time. The
forces, velocity, and displacement of the dynamic centre of body
means in relation to each limb segment and the energy transfer between
them is determined. With such objective measures, a better understanding of the neural control and complex dynamics of gait in the

handicapped patient can be achieved and lead to the development
of simple treatment programmes and uncomplicated assistive devices.

Presently, the laboratory is conducting a series of clinical
research projects in children with cerebral palsy, myelo-meningocele,
and scoliosis to determine the pathophysiology and efficacy of
various treatment programmes. A completed project on the patho-
dynamics of back-kneeing in children with cerebral palsy provided
an understanding of its creation and the validity of the effectiveness of a simple, lightweight plastic fixed-angle below-knee orthosis
in its correction.

Though requiring highly engineering technology and much
engineering-medical work, the ultimate goal of the research phase
at the Harvard Centre is to provide techniques and devices which
can be implemented simply and easily in any medical community.

5) Northwestern University - The Rehabilitation Engineering
Programme at this University concerns mainly the replacement of
damaged or diseased points with artificial components. Considerable
scientific and engineering effort is being expended to improve the
materials, designs, and the techniques or implantation of this kind
of prostheses, so that the surgical replacement of hips, knees and
other joints may improve the already obtained successes. Therefore,
the effort made in this field is divided into four main areas.
These are a study of current successes and failures of implants with
emphasis on the knee prosthesis; the design and development of
devices and techniques to solve identified problems; the identification of material problems and their possible solutions; and a basic
study of how joints function, with special emphasis on the supporting
structures that contribute to stability or instability.

6) Bioengineering Unit at the University of Strathclyde - As
regards the internal joint replacements, as otherwise research
work in other fields of engineering in connexion with medicine, we
cannot help referring to Bioengineering Unit at the University of
Strathclyde, in Glasgow, U.K. The application of engineering techniques to the study of medical problems, started in the University
of Strathclyde (then Royal College of Science and Technology) in
1957 when members of the staff of the Department of Medical Engineering and doctors from a local hospital became interested in the
creation and control of profound hypothermia in man. A little later
an experimental study of the mechanics of the skin was initiated and
the success of these and similar activities led to the creation
in 1963 of a Bioengineering Unit in the University. Research
activity in the unit follows the early established pattern of
applying engineering techniques, particularly those of mechanics,
to a wide variety of clinical and surgical problems. A further
important development in the Unit has been the introduction of
post-graduate courses for graduates in engineering and the physical
sciences which are intended to provide advanced training in the
application of these sciences to medical and surgical problems. In
1972, the National Centre for training and Education in Prosthetics
was established as part of the Bioengineering Unit. The research
activities of the Unit are conducted in 5 major groups:rehabilitation

engineering, tissue biomechanics, artificial organs, clinical
engineering and data analysis techniques. The development of
signal processing techniques on the Unit's PDP 12 computer is also
under way. The analogue input facilities of this machine have
enabled the design of systems for processing data from new devices
measuring cardiac function, from tissue testing equipment, from
test on lower limb function in normals and amputees and from
television cameras viewing the locomotion of normal and disabled
test subjects. This research involves close links with clinical
measurement, tissue and biomechanics divisions.

7) <u>University of California Los Angeles (UCLA) and Astronautic
  Company</u> - Traub and Leclair quote the example of the rather
important contribution of research for a greater independence of
epileptics. This type of patient no doubt looks forward to the
day when he can cross a busy street, operate an engine of a vehicle
and, particularly, when he can obtain and retain a suitable job.
A research project with the University of California, Los Angeles
School of Medicine, and Mc Donnell-Douglas Astronautics Company
was recently in the final stages of validating an epileptic seizure
warning system which would have a significant impact for the
epileptic's becoming more independent. The warning system consists
of a small electronic device slightly larger than a hearing and
which buzzes when an impending seizure is about to occur.

8) The <u>San Francisco Rehabilitation Centre</u> is particularly
concerned with sensory substitution and the development of sensory
aids for the blind and deaf. Projects include a tactile vision
substitution system, which delivers an image from a small television
camera to the skin of a blind person, enabling him to perceive
information that is normally accessible through vision. With training
the blind person uses visual means to analyze the information. This,
says Leclair, includes perspective, parallax, looming, zooming,
depth cues, and subjective spatial localization. A compare system
delivers spoker information from a microphone to a deaf person
through an array of electrical stimulators in contact with the
skin of the abdomen. The S. Francisco Rehabilitation Engineering
Centre has also taken an active part in the development of sensory
vocational aids.

These are some of the examples of the enormous, helpful and
humanitarian activity developed in the field of rehabilitation
engineering in U.S.A. and in U.K.. However, in various other
countries great attention has been given to the problems concerning
the rehabilitation of disabled, in which the collaboration of the
engineer with the doctor is of paramount importance. Supported by
the U.S. Rehabilitation Services Administration, other centres
work with the same objectives: in Poznan, Poland; in Ljubljana and
Belgrade, Jugoslavia; and in Cairo, Egypt. In Canada, France, West
Germany and Sweden, among other countries, a great activity has been
equally developed. We think that the great Rehabilitation Medical
Centres particularly interested in admitting both in-and-out-patients,
should be, as far as possible, and in accordance with the economic
possibilities of the country considerated, provided with a department

of rehabilitation engineering. Our point of view has tried for
long to materialize in Portugal, in our first 252 bed-rehabilitation
medicine centre (Alcoitao-Estoril), where there are excellent
possibilities for its installation, and medical and paramedical
staff eager to develop their activity in the field of research,
particularly in the scope óf biomechanics. It has not yet been
possible to reach this goal. Our action has, therefore, been
confined to useful, although unsufficient contacts with the
"Instituto Gulbenkian de Ciência" (Gulbenkian Institute of Science),
whose director, Mr. Correia da Silva, engineer, graduate in Biophysics by the Imperial College of Science and Technology, University
of London, and a member of the Group of Biomechanics, of the above
mentioned Institute, has given us the best collaboration. Although
it is difficult to foresee the annual increase in expenditure with
the functioning of a department of rehabilitation engineering, even
if it is a modest one and particularly devoted to biomechanics,
it is worth reporting the result of a study carried out by the
Veterans Administration (U.S.A.), concerning amputees only, and
quoted by Mc Laurin: "The expenditures of a little over $1,000,000
per year in research and development have not only resulted in
better service to the amputee, but also in overall saving of
$28,000,000 over a period of 25 years". And no doubt it was a great
contribution to the vocational potential and to the quality of life
of the disabled amputee.

However, the above mentioned examples concerning the already
developed activity and the technical achievements attained, suffice
to show us that the scope of rehabilitation engineering became
broader than the traditional focus of prosthetics-orthotics, although
the latter is, and should always continue to be considered of extreme
importance. This traditional incidence of the role of the engineer
in the solution of the problems of the amputee was entirely justifiable. In fact, and in accordance with McLaurin, "about one-tenth
of the physical disabled persons (U.S.A.) are amputees. Because
of an extensive private artificial-limb service, and because of
enlightened research and development projects that have been
sponsored by Veterans Administration and the Department of Health,
Education, and Welfare for the past 25 years, nearly all amputees
are assured not only of a good functional prosthesis but also of
a good overall programme in surgery and training as well"."Unfortunately", says McLaurin, "the same kind of service is not usually
available to the remaining 90% of disabled persons. Since World
War II, a continued and coordinated programme of research,
development, evaluation and training has been funded by VA and HEN
and other government agencies on behalf of the veteran and civilian
amputee". Till 1971, at least, some of the efforts carried out
have been directed toward bracing, but not to anywhere near the
extent that is indicated by the scope of the problem".

However, in the U.S.A., with the Rehabilitation Act of 1973,
the scope of the engineer in collaboration with the physician
became, as we have said, wider, concerning all aspects of rehabilitation technology and of the handicapped individual's life.

Experience has been showing that with this profound knowledge
of mechanics, chemistry, electronics and the materials normally
used in rehabilitation, the engineer's contribution has been of
the utmost value. This may occur either in improving or in inventing
new types of technical and sensory aids, or even in finding solutions likely to make it easier to overcome architectural barriers
or difficulties preventing the disabled from utilizing the current
means of transport.

Although engineering and the physical sciences have already
in our time a wide scope of useful application in rehabilitation
medicine, experience also shows that their valuable contribution
to the restoration of improvement of a function when the function
has been totally or partially lost, is more frequently considered
solely in some of its aspects, such as mechanics, materials and
electronics.

Although the application of the technology of electronics is
very important and has developed gradually and swiftly as regards
both diagnosis and treatment, we would prefer to refer only some
points concerning biomechanics, not because it is in the progmatic
line of this Institute, but also because, according to Foort "the
biomechanics clinic is the prime arena for rehabilitation engineering".

In order to keep as much as possible within the subject of this
lecture - Rehabilitation Medicine and Rehabilitation Engineering -
we shall limit ourselves to little more than quoting a few definitions and examples of some of the basic principles of biomechanics
which may be of interest to rehabilitation medicine.

6. SOME BASIC CONCEPTS ON BIOMECHANICS

Mechanics is that branch of the physical sciences which deals
with energies and forces, and their effect on bodies in terms of
movement and equilibrium.

Biomechanics is the science that deals with the effect of
energies and both internal and external forces on the living human
body whether in movement or at rest. Biomechanics covers a broad
spectrum, from theoretical study to practical application. The
fundamentals of theoretical mechanics, like anatomy, physiology and
kinesiology of the locomotor system, are used to relate the forces
in muscles, bones and joints to externally applied load which may
result either from pull of gravity, water resistance, elasticity of
materials, friction, stationary structures or even manual resistance
on the body parts.

Gravity, the most common load on the body, provides a line
of force in a constant direction. Both the weight and position of the
exercise resistance and of the body part are important when determining the effect of gravity. Pulley systems are used to change
the line of pull of the body. These may be set up to offer resistance
or to aid in support of movement, and may act in any direction. The
force of gravity may be reduced or neutralized by immersing the body
or body part in a tank of water. In this case, the gravitational

force is balanced by the force of buoyancy, since the body is buoyed
up by a force equal to the weight of the volume of water it dis-
places. However , water also offers resistance, directly opposing
a body part as that body part moves through it. The knowledge of
these physical properties is used in physiotherapy to facilitate
and make more efficient the training in the swimming-pool of disabled patients, who have paretic muscles. Another method often used
in physiotherapy, which also reduces the effect of gravity, uses
suspension in slings. It was originated by Guthrie-Smith in 1943.

A variety of elastic materials (such as springs, rubber bands,
etc.) are often used to provide resistance for muscle exercise. The
line of resistance force lies along the length of the elastic
material. Many other exercises devices make use of frictional
resistance as load for the muscle contraction. Some devices provide
a line of force which is perpendicular to the bony lever throughout
the range of motion. Stationary structures may provide resistance
for isometric contractions, whereas manual resistance can offer
isometric resistance or can give a wide range of resisting loads.

Applied biomechanics is concerned with the more practical
problems of improving movements and posture in rehabilitation
medicine and in activities of daily living. This happens frequently
with the sequela of cerebro vascular accidents (CVA), conditions
of a neurological origin, like cerebral palsy, multiple sclerosis,
muscular distrophy, etc., with arthritis, or again, situations
arising from inadequate use of prosthesis after amputation of a limb,
or of orthosis in the case of paralysis or muscular paresis.

Occupational biomechanics has been added to the understanding
of the complex mechanisms of interaction between the worker and the
industrial environment. The latter, as opposed to work environment,
is purposefully designed to maximize economic efficiency of human
performance. Particularly those who are responsible for the maintenance of occupational safety and healt have to overcome many
biomechanical, physiological and behavioural hazard vectors likely
to be overlooked in the design of the industrial environment.

The entire subject of mechanics covers two basic areas: statics
and dynamics. Dynamics in turn may be subdivided into kinematics
and kinetics.

Statics deals with bodies at rest or in equilibrium as a
result of forces acting upon them. A person standing upright and
relatively motionless, is an example of a static condition, in
which forces caused by gravitational pull of the earth are borne
by musculoskeletal system and transferred downward onto the floor.
All the downward forces are just exactly countered by the upward
forces and the body is said to be in equilibrium.

Dynamics deals with moving bodies and the force that acts to
produce the motion. A person walking illustrates both dynamics and
kinematics.

Kinematics deals with the relationships that exist between
displacements, velocities and accelerations in translation or rotational motion. It does not concern itself with the forces involved,
but only with the description of the movements themselves.

  Kinetics deals with moving bodies and the forces that act to produce the motion.

  The motion of a body is the result of work having been done on it by an expenditure of energy. Two very important component parts to be considered are mass and force.

  Mass is a quantitative measure of inertia, or the quantity of matter which a body contains. Inertia is a property of matter which causes an object to resist change in velocity, that is, if the body is at rest, it tends to stay at rest, and if moving, it tends to resist being speeded up or slowing down. Matter is anything that occupies space and has weight.

  In biomechanics we often deal with the quantity of matter, or mass, to which the force of gravity is applied. This mass may be an object, such as a wheelchair, or it may be the entire body or a segment of the body. The appliance of the principles of mechanics to human movement demands the constant use of the centre of mass of the object. The centre of mass is that point at the exact centre of the object's mass. It is also known as centre of gravity. Every part of an object has weight and as such will be attracted downwards by earth, and every part can be represented by a vector force. All these forces will be parallel to each other. The total weight of the object will be the resultant of all the forces. The point of application of the resultant will be the centre of gravity of that object. The centre of gravity is, consequently, the point in the body through which resultant force of gravity acts.

  When the mass of an object is symmetrically distributed, the centre of gravity is at the geometric centre of the object. But if the distribution of the mass is asymmetrical, as it is the case of the limbs of the human body, the centre of gravity will be nearer the large and heavier end. The centre of gravity of the entire human body when the limbs are straight as one usually stands in the anatomical position lies within the pelvis in front of the upper part of the sacrum. This point may vary in position from person to person according to body build, age and sex, as well as also vary within any given person when the arrangement of the segments shifts, as in walking, running, or sitting. And, of course, since this point represents the centre of the total mass, it will shift when weight is added to or substracted from some part of the body as with the addition of a cast or brace or following amputation of an extremity. It is, therefore, important to remember that a rigid object behaves as if its entire mass were acting, or being acted upon, at its centre of gravity.

  The line of gravity, an imaginary vertical line passing, in the human body, through the second sacral vertebra down to a point between the feet, when standing in the anatomical position, will fall in an area called base of support, in order to maintain the equilibrium. The base of support is very important to the stability of an object and it is obvious that the longer the base, the easier it will be to maintain the centre of gravity over it. The smaller the base the more difficult. In a man whose weight is entirely supported by his feet the base of support includes not only his two

feet but the space in between. Therefore, when the feet are
separated, the base is widened and stability improves. However, if
the feet are farther apart than the width of the pelvis the legs
will be in a slanting position. If this is accompanied by unsufficient friction between the feet and the supporting surface , then
this does not make for greater stability. This is what happens
when a patient stands on a slippy floor, wearing leather-soled
shoes.

A patient on crutches will further increase his base of support
and thus increase his stability. This can be done in different ways,
but, when improving lateral stability, if the crutches are lifted
off the ground the patient's stability will decrease as his centre
of gravity has been raised by the addition of the weight of the two
crutches. The use of a cane will also increase stability.

In patients with spinal cord lesions and those with muscle
weakness of the trunk and lower limbs, balancing the centre of
gravity over the feet becomes a critical problem. A paraplegic must
be able to balance the movements of the head and shoulders which
he can control through his muscles and his pelvis which he cannot
control. He must be able to control his head by moving it backwards
or forwards to help place the pelvis in the right position so as
to maintain the centre of gravity within his base of support, and
place the lower limb but correctly as for walking, climbing stairs,
etc. It is the physiotherapist duty to help the patient to work out
the most stable position at rest and in movement.

It is found that the speed of movement is closely associated
to the requirements of balance, since it is far easier to balance
on a quickly moving way than when moving slowly. This is why
patients with a precarious sense of balance hurry along in order
to decrease the requirements of a lateral stability.

Matter occupies space and has weight. Space and weight are two
other basic concepts, to be considered in biomechanics.

Space - The forces that we deal with may act along a single
line in a single plane or in any direction in space. In order to
locate our forces along a line, in a plane, or in space, it is
necessary to provide some reference system. In the two dimensional
system we do this by dividing the plane into four quadrants by
means of two perpendicular lines or axes, generally labeled X in
the horizontal direction (abcissa) and Y in the vertical direction
(ordinate). The point of intersection of the two axes is known as
the origin of the system. Measurements along the X axes to the
right of the Y axes are positive. Those of the left of the Y axes
are negative. Measurements along the Y axes above the X axes are
positive, below are negative. Any point on the plane can now be
defined by being assigned X and Y values. These numbers which
determine the point location, are called the coordinates of the
point. In order to locate points in three dimensions a third axis
must be introduced. This passes through the origin and is perpendicular to the X-Y plane in which the two original axes are found.
The third axis is usually labeled Z. All points in front of the
original X-Y plane are positive, while those behind the X-Y plane

are negative. Thus we have the means of locating any point in space.

In setting up such a system of coordinates for the purpose of describing human motion, it is convenient to place the origin at the centre of gravity of the body, which is approximately anterior to the second sacral vertebrae. Three cardinal planes may then be visualized in rotation to the X, Y and Z coordinates: frontal, dividing the body into front and back positions (X-Y plane); sagital, dividing the body into right and left halves (Y-Z plane); and transverse (or horizontal), dividing the body into upper and lower positions (X-Z plane).

Weight is the pull of gravity exerted by matter.It is the force with which matter is attracted towards the earth. To find the weight of an object is to measure the attraction of the earth for that object. The weight of an object depends upon two things : 1) the mass or quantity of matter it contains, and 2) the amount of gravitational attraction the earth has for it. The relationship between weight and mass is derived from equation and is expressed as W=Mg, where W=weight of the object, M=mass of the object, and g=acceleration effect of gravity.

The famous Sir Isaac Newton's laws of motion (law of inertia, law of acceleration and law of reaction),are basic laws involved in the area of statics, kinematics and kinetics. To illustrate Newton's laws, Wirta and Taylor, consider a wheelchair with a patient in it. To move the patient to some new location, a person would have to exert force to get the wheelchair into motion, in accordance with Newton's first law. The magnitude of the force is proportional to the mass of the wheelchair plus the patient (plus the force needed to overcome friction) and proportional to the acceleration imparted to the mass, in accordance with the Newton's second law. Since the inertia of the wheelchair and patient resist a change in velocity, there is an opposite reaction force developed against the action force supplied by the person pushing the wheelchair, in accordance with Newton's third law.

Force is one of the basic concepts in mechanics. It is the physical action of one body upon a second body which tends to change the position in space. It may be either a push (compression) or a pull (tension). Considering the concept of a force as a vector quantity, the force vectors must be specified by magnitude (indicated by length of a particular force arrow), sense of direction (indicated by the arrow head), the line of action (indicated by location of the shaft of the arrow), and the point of application (indicated by the point at which the force is applied). The force, whether it is a load or the force involving reaction stress can only be completely defined when all these characteristics are supplied. Any variations in any of these characteristics will produce a different result.

In addition to having four characteristics necessary to define it, force may act on bodies or systems in the following four different ways:

1. Linear, in which all the forces occur along the same action;
2. Parallel, with all the forces parallel and occuring in the

same plane but not acting along the same action line;
3. Concurrent, in which all the forces meet at a point;
4. General, with all the forces in a plane but not arranged
as in any of the other three.

In solving biomechanical problems we must take into account
all the forces that are acting upon the object. The problem may
consist of analyzing a single force system or a combination of
force systems. We can do it by two procedures. First, the composition of forces method is used when we have two or more forces
acting in the same plane (coplanar) and on the same point (concurrent), and we wish to show the resultant. Second, occasionally
we must replace a single force by two or more equivalent force
components. This process is called the resolution of forces. Both
approaches may be solved by graphic or algebric methods. The graphic
method uses precise measurements of magnitude and direction to
obtain the resultants of many vectors or the components of a vector.
The algebric method makes use of algebric equations and utilizes
trigonometric concepts.

In any case, to measure force one has to know both its
magnitude and direction. This is known as a Vector Quantity.
Quantities which have no particular direction but only magnitude,
such as volume, density, length, temperature or time are Scalar
Quantities. Similar example can be given as regards concepts of
motion. These involve considerations of speed, velocity and
acceleration, all consisting of a displacement in space with respect
to time. However, though speed and velocity are sometimes used
interchangeably, speed is a scalar quantitiy and velocity is a
vector quantity. Hence, speed is a measure of magnitude only,
whereas velocity includes both magnitude and direction. Acceleration is the rate of change of speed or velocity per unit of time.
As an object moves from one place to another, its velocity (rate
of displacement) may not be constant over the entire distance. The
magnitude of velocity may increase or decrease relative to its
straight line of displacement, or the direction of velocity may
change. As it is well known these phenomena are commonly known as
acceleration or deceleration. Because deceleration is essentially
negative acceleration, mathematically, only the term acceleration
needs to be dealt with.

To illustrate the resolution and composition of forces, Wirta
and Taylor consider the point in the gait cycle when heel strike
occurs. At that instant there is a force,F, transmitted down the
leg and onto the ground. Equal and opposite to the transmitted
force, F, is a ground reaction force, R. The force F may be thought
of as consisting of two component forces, namely, a vertical force,
V, and a horizontal force, H. This consideration of the single
force as a product of the two component forces is the process of
resolution of forces. Consider, on the other hand, that the same
subject is walking in a laboratory equipped with a force plate to
measure the vertical (V) and horizontal (H) forces; then the two
forces can be combined vectorially to determine F. This process
is known as composition of forces.

Forces may act between bodies which are not in contact with each other, as for instance the attractive force of gravity and the attraction and repulsion of electrically charged particles and magnetized materials. There are three primary kinds of forces: 1) compressive or pushing together forces; 2) tensile, or pulling apart forces, and 3) shearing, or forces which make one part of the body slide with respect to an adjacent part.

In mechanics the forces involved are both external and internal. The external forces outside the structure, called loads, are those such as the forces of gravity, air resistance, water resistance, inertia, muscle action, and ground reaction. The internal forces within a structure, reacting to these loads, are called stresses. Stress is therefore the internal resistance of a material which reacts to an externally applied load. Practically, stress is the ratio between the force and the area upon which it acts, i.e., force per unit area. Stress is often used synonimously with strength, but the term has little value unless the kind of strength, i.e., tensile, compressive, etc., is indicated. Stress is generally computed in terms of pounds force or kilograms force per unit area. Besides producing stress, when a force is applied to a body, it also produces strain, that is, a change in the linear dimensions of the body, causing in this a major or minor deformation (lengthening or shortening). Strain can be recorded as percentage, inches/inch, centimeters/centimeter, etc., since there are no standard units of measurement for it. Strain can be visible, as in stretching of a rubber band, but stress, which is only the ratio between force and area, is always invisible. When stress is plotted against strain, a stress-strain curve is obtained. The modulus of elasticity is a measure of the stiffness of a material, not its elasticity, as it could be assumed from the name. Elasticity is the property of a material that allows it to return to its original dimensions after the removal of a force or load.

The method of choice in determining the tensile or compressive strength of a material is to make a test specimen of a standardized size and shape and test it under a pure tensile or a pure compressive force. Under these conditions the cross-sectional area of the specimen is known, or can be easily computed, and only one force - tension or compression - is involved. If the specimen is tested like a simple beam (i.e., supported at the ends and loaded midway between the supports) and bending occurs, tensile, compressive and shearing forces are all involved. Tensile forces develop on the convex side of the bent specimen while compressive forces occur on the opposite (concave) side. There are also shearing forces which, like the tensile and compressive forces, are not uniformly distributed over the cross section of the specimen. The bending forces in the neck of the femur, as a result of the load applied to the head of the bone, have been determined by Zarek.

Pressure is an important aspect of force. It indicates how the force is distributed over an area. Being defined as force per unit area, pressure is calculated by dividing the force by the area over which it acts. This would give an "average" pressure. Pressure is seldom uniform, and its variation is often indicated

by a series of pressure vectors. Where both force and pressure
vectors are shown on the same diagram, the force vector indicates
the "resultant", that is the sum of the effects of the distributed
pressures in a particular region.

We would like to stress the importance of the pressure in
biomechanics, by mentioning the two following examples:

1) **Pressure in the fitting of prosthesis** – Pressure must,
indeed, be carefully taken into consideration in the fitting of
prosthesis for lower extremities amputees, especially those with
ischial weight-bearing devices or end-bearing stumps, because the
magnitude of pressure between the stump and socket is one of the
major determinants of comfort in a prosthesis.

To minimize discomfort, it is important to avoid excessive
pressure on the stumps. One way of reducing pressure is to have
the socket designed so that the contact force is distributed over
a large skin area. In practice it is not quite so simple because
the tissues of the stump are not uniform in firmness, and some
areas of the stump tolerate pressure quite well while other areas
are relatively sensitive to pressure. Even though, both of these
factors can be accommodated by adequate design of the contours
and shape of the socket.

In accordance with a physical general concept, the pressure
of a steel bar resting on top of a cube is equal to the weight
of the bar divided by the area of the cube's upper surface. However,
if the same bar is being supported, not only on the original cube,
but by two additional cubes identical to the original and at equal
distances from it, the pressure on the middle cube will be only
one-third as great as before, since the supporting area is three
times greater. This example illustrates the application of a basic
principle in prosthetic fitting, that is, to utilize as much area
of the stump as possible to distribute the force applied by the
socket to the stump.

In order to have pressure evenly distributed over the tissues
regardless of different degrees of their firmness, modifications
of socket contour with respect to the stump become necessary. If
three cubes had the same dimensions, but differed in their relative
firmness, the pressure would not be distributed evenly. If, for
example, the middle cube were made of steel and the other two were
made of soft rubber, the steel cube would support most of the load.
By cutting a slot, or relief, in the steel bar, a more even
distribution of pressure would be obtained, in spite of the
differences in relative firmness of the steel and rubber cubes.
However, in case the rubber cubes were much too soft, the relief
alone might not be enough to produce the desired distribution. To
illustrate, suppose the steel bar weighed 100 lbs. and the rubber
cubes were so soft that a force of 10 lbs. compressed them so that
the steel bar came to rest firmly on the steel cube in the middle.
Then the steel cube would have a force of 80 lbs. applied to its
surface, compared to the 10 lbs. applied to the surface of each
of the rubber cubes. To improve the weight distribution we would
have either to cut a deeper relief in the steel bar, which is not

64

advisable because it might weaken the bar, or to add two "build-ups" to the bar. Thus, if the relief were cut to the proper depth and "build-ups" of the proper thickness were applied, an even distribution of pressure would be obtained.

These biomechanical principles are important and frequently applied to a prostheses for the indispensable comfort of the patient. When the stump is not of uniform firmness, if the socket were shaped to match the stump accurately, the pressure on the stump would not be evenly distributed. A more even distribution of pressure could be obtained by purposely modifying the socket, making reliefs in the socket over the firm areas, which take relatively more of the load, and bulging the socket inward over the soft areas, that take relatively less of the load.

The same principles applied to differences in relative firmness can be used to compensate for different tolerance to pressure of the various areas of the stump. But, of course, the purpose is now different. Instead of producing an even distribution of pressure, the goal is to produce a selective loading of the tissues so that more of the weight will be supported by the pressure-tolerant areas and less weight will remain on the pressure-sensitive areas. Sockets for below-knee prosthesis, for example, should be designed to apply the biomechanical principles that have been referred to.

2) Pressure in traumatic transverse lesions of the spinal cord - A great number of disabled patients admitted to medical rehabilitation centres are paraplegics, most of them as a result of traumatic transverse lesions of the spinal cord. Paraplegics are quite prone to develop pressure sores. Most of them may be developed within the first few hours after the accident occurred. They may be due to intrinsic and extrinsic factors.

The most important intrinsic factor is the lowering of tissue resistance to pressure because of the loss of vasomotor control which leads to a lowering of the tone in the vascular bed of the paralyzed part of the body, especially the lower limbs. A pressure which under normal conditions will not produce blockage of the blood supply resulting in ischaemia, will do so under these circumstances. Another important intrinsic factor is the loss of sensation in the paralyzed parts. Normally, afferent impulses arising from an area exposed to pressure, causing blockage of blood circulation, elicit discomfort which in turn readily leads to a change of position. However, in transverse cord lesions, the normally existing sensations are abolished, and, if appropriate measures are not taken to change the patients position, ischaemia with all its harmful consequences on the tissues inevitably occurs. Other intrinsic factors occurred are: 1) the distance of the bony weight-bearing prominences from the skin and the thickness of padding tissues such as fat and muscles between bone and the skin; and 2) the spasticity of the paralyzed lower limbs, especially adductor spasms, which is responsible for the development of sores on the inner surface of knees and inner ankles as a result of producing shearing stress to the covering skin by continuous rubbing.

As far as the extrinsic factors are concerned, according to Guttmann, they are three: pressure , maceration from exposing the skin to moisture (urine), and cold, particularly in later stages of paraplegia. "Of these, pressure, says Guttmann, is of decisive importance, because causing blockage of the vacsular supply represents the immediate cause in the development of sores". The degree and extent of the harmful effect of local pressure in parap-legia causing ischaemia of skin and deeper tissues are determined by its intensity, duration and direction. As to the direction, one must distinguish between purely vertical pressure and shear-stress, of which the effect of shear-stress is much disastrous for its cuts of larger areas from their vascular supply. There can be little doubt that the forces resulting from shear-stress, acting parallel to the surface of skin and sliding the upper layers relative to the lower, play an essential role in determining the shape and size of a sore. With regard to the duration of pressure in producing death of tissues, Trumble (1930) found that pressure of more than 1.5 lb. per in^2. (about (80 mmHg) over a long period is likely to cause death of tissues.

From the foregoing, we can say that pressure is the main factor to consider in the prevention of pressure sores. This is why the patient must be turned day and night, every two or three hours in order to prevent the break-down of the skin over bony prominences such as the trochanters and/or sacrum during the bed-fast period. Besides, a perfect hygiene of the skin and the bedsheets, which must be kept dry and powdered, should be observed. To facili-tate the frequent turning of paraplegics, which otherwise requires a team of at least four people, the Egerton-Stoke Mandeville electrical turning bed was developed. The bed is divided longitudi-nally into three. When a button is pressed, two of these sections elevate to a maximum of 70^0. The remaining third can be slightly raised to maintain the patient in position. The four-button variety will also tilt head and foot down to 15^0. The Guttmann head traction unit can be fitted to the bed if necessary, and is so constructed that the weight is maintained as the bed turns. In the case this or other similar type of bed is not available, it is necessary to lift the patient with a team, maintaining a correct spinal alignment, every two or three hours, and position him with pillows and sandbags, particularly with double pillows, to relieve pressure over the most susceptible areas, that is where bony prominences are close to the skin. The skin must be inspected at every turn, and if there is any evidence of excessive pressure, no matter how minor (such as redness which does not fade on pressure, blistering, bruising, local swelling or induration, grazing), all pressure must be relieved over that area until it is healed. For example, if the sacrum is involved, turn side to side. It should be remembered that pressure is intensified when bed linens are wrinkled and when food crumbs and other foreign particles are present.

Once the patients are permitted to be ambulatory they must be indoctrinated with the importance of lifting themselves periodi-cally while in a wheelchair, getting out of their chairs every two or three hours for a rest of from 20 to 30 minutes, keeping their trousers dry and smooth, and carefully avoiding trauma while transferring to and from wheelchairs.

Needless to say that maintenance of the patient's general condition, including appropriate high-protein, high-caloric and high-vitamin diet, as well as frequent and consistent fluid intake, is very important and should be adequately combined with the relief and redistribute of pressure. However, a large percentage of paraplegics admitted for rehabilitation are already afflicted with pressure sores, among other complications. At our Rehabilitation Centre, at Alcoitão-Estoril-Portugal, the Special Unit, directed by Evaristo da Foncesa, by July, 1972, had reached the stage of having in one of its wards, 25 paraplegics (out of 40) who had a total of 67 pressure sores. This was a great problem to solve, not only because of the difficulties in their daily treatment and time consumption, but also because the increased days of hospitalization entail considerably greater financial cost.

Experience has shown that once pressure has developed, its treatment, both local and general, is usually rather slow and sometimes frustrating, even if aggrevating factors, such as anaemia, spasticity, hypoproteinemia, infection, etc., are not present. Plastic surgery, in turn, even if it may produce good results when carried out by skilled surgeons, is not always advisable, namely when the general condition of the patient is precarious or when the extension and localization of the pressure sore do not permit to anticipate a good result. It is also found that "in spite of all possible pre-operative care, infection and sutural dehiscence set in quite frequently".

Various different treatments have been recommended with greater or lesser success. Although bearing in mind that "once sores have developed, the principle of preventing pressure has to be enforced, and this represents the cardinal local treatment of sores", we should refer that E. da Foncesa has initiated in the Spinal Unit of our Rehabilitation Centre intensive research somewhat based on the hyperbaric oxygen system. We would like to have used the hyperbaric chamber, which has been used in the U.S.A. with success. However, its high cost prevented us from doing it. Thence the idea of trying to resort to a more economic process which would allow us to reach satisfactory results. This was achieved after a few years research carried out in the Rehabilitation Centre. Dr. Foncesa based his research on Paul Bert's experimental studies. These proved the existence of the phenomena of cellular respiration in an isolated tissular particle (consumption of oxygen and elimination of carbon dioxide) the knowledge that life is possible without hemoglobin provided the plasma contains enough dissolved oxygen, the acquaintance with the laws governing the solubility of gases in aqueous solutions and the study of cellular metabolic mechanisms, led us to suggest research into the hypothesis of speeding up the healing processess by the use of ambient air enriched with oxygen. This method, because it uses oxygen and air (OX_ from Oxygen, and AR - the Portuguese word for "air") is called

"OXAR". The first tests were carried out in 1972, then discontinued, and resumed in 1974. The first results obtained with the use of OXAR were presented in a Symposium of the Portoguese Society of Physical Medicine and Rehabilitation, held in June, 1976.

A ventilator expelling unheated air was used. This was fitted to a plastic tube, into which a second tube, of smaller diameter, for the supply of non-humidified oxygen, had been inserted. In the case of bedridden patients, regular position change and other routine nursing care involving hygiene, nutrition, etc., were maintained without introducing special standards. All pressure sores were measured and photographed once a week.

Once the OXAR treatment had been initiated, topical applications, such as antibiotics, enzymatic products, healing agents, etc., were systematically discontinued. Before administering the OXAR treatment, the pressure sore was gently washed with a solution of Cetavlon, an isotonic sodium chloride solution or hydrogen peroxide.

The parameters from which Dr. Fonseca started his investiga-tion have not changed and consist of the daily administration of air enriched with oxygen (6 days a week) for a period of 60 minutes at an oxygen flow rate of 10 liters per minute. After administering the OXAR treatment, a dry dressing of oxygenated gauze was applied and maintained for 24 hours until the next treatment. Gentle massage was applied daily to the tissues surrounding the ulcer. None of these pationts received blood transfusions.

Before we go any further, I would like to point out as a reference to Biomechanics of Pressure Sores, the importance of a book on the proceedings of a seminar on Tissue Viability and Clinical Applications, held at the University of Strathclyde, Glasgow, in 1975.

In the following, four cases concerned with the application of the OXAR are discussed in detail.

The first is the case of a 25 year-old male patient who, as a result of a traffic accident, became tetraplegic in consequence of traumatic shinal cord lesion at C_5 level, on 18th April, 1970. He was admitted to our Medical Rehabilitation Centre only on 8th January, 1974, after almost 4 years of treatment of urinary and other complications, such as pressure sores. On admission to our Centre, he had a complete examination, showing an ulcer in the sacral region, with a diameter of approximately 6 cms. touching another ulcer with a diameter of approximately 3 cms, and reaching the underlying bone in depth, both formed over many months. The pressure sores were treated with OXAR as from the 2nd of November 1974, to the 1st of January, 1975, therefore for two months. The result was: complete healing and a minimum of adhesions to the deep layers.

The second case is the one of a patient aged 30. Run over by a lorry, he became paraplegic as a result of a traumatic spinal cord lesion at D_{12} level, on the 20th of July, 1976. He was admitted to, and thoroughly examined in our Rehabilitation Centre on the 21st of September, 1976. He exhibited a deep ulcer, measuring approxima-tely 8 cms.x4 cms. with greenish exudate covering a large area of necrotic tissue. Treatment applied as from the 23rd of September to the 25th of November, 1976. Result: Complete healing in slightly over two months.

The third case refers to a 25 year-old male patient who suffered, as a result of a motor car accident, traumatic spinal cord lesion at D_{11} level, on the 25th of September, 1976, becoming paraplegic. He was admitted to, and examined at the Rehabilitation Centre, on the 27th October, 1976. Besides other pressure sores in sacral, calcaneal and heel regions, he showed another one on the outer surface of the right leg, approximately 6 cms. long and 3 cms. wide, adjoining a second pressure sore measuring approximately 4 cms. x3 cms., with peripherical macerated tissues. Treated with OXAR as from the 28th of October 1976, to the 1st of February,1977, therefore slightly over two months, all pressure sores were completely healed.

And finally, the fourth case is the one of a patient aged 34, who, right after falling off a staircase, became paraplegic in consequence of traumatic spinal cord lesion at D_{11} level, on the 1st of July, 1976. He was admitted to the Rehabilitation Centre on the 21st of September, 1976. He showed one pressure sore in the sacral region, with a diameter of approximately 10 cms. and two others with a diameter of approximately 3 cms. Treated with OXAR as from the 28th September, 1976, to the 4th of January, 1977. By the 18th October, 1976, the two smaller ulcers had healed. Deep ulcer on the right heel, measuring approximately 5 cms. x 3 cms., with a peripheral area of macerated tissue was also treated with OXAR as from the 28th September to 29 November, 1976, one the result was complete healing.

The results of the research already undertaken in this field, though still in its initial phase, allow us, however, to foresee that the OXAR technique is a very simple way of speeding up the healing processes in pressure sores, allowing the patient to initiate an earlier intensive rehabilitation programme. On the other hand, from the economic standpoint, by means of the OXAR treatment, great advantages can be obtained, such as: shorter periods of hospitalization, much cheaper treatments, no need for the use of local drug therapy, and the time spent by the nursing staff being considerably less than that required by other techniques usually used in the treatment of pressure sores.

Besides, comparatively to the use of hyperbaric oxygen systems, OXAR has the advantage of being a less costly technique, since the equipment required is much simpler; the patients do not run the risk of claustrophobia, and they are not subject to sudden decompression. Taking into account the mentioned advantages, OXAR may render greater benefits in any hospital, particularly in those away from large cities where more facilities are available, or even in developing countries.

7. CONCLUSIONS

Besides the basic concepts and practical applications indicated,
indispensable in biomechanics when related to medical and vocational
rehabilitation, other equally important principles could be quoted.
But, because the development of their practical applications would
take us far beyond the objectives of this lecture, we will mention
only, among others, those concerning the static equilibrium,
particularly the conditions of equilibrium (linear, concurrent,
parallel, lever and general force systems), friction, dynamics
(especially the work-energy approach), and the body segment parameters.

The engineer, with a thorough knowledge of these concepts
and of their practical applications, in a good collaboration with
the doctor, has contributed, and he can contribute even more in
the future, so that many of the problem of rehabilitation medicine
may find a more favourable solution in favour of the disabled
patient.

It is believed that the engineer, suitably trained in bioengineering, mainly within the field of rehabilitation of the
disabled patient, and therefore being of high-level professional/
technical competence, is a rather indispensable member of the
rehabilitation team. The determined cooperation of the doctor and
other allied health professionals and technicians, is surely equally
indispensable, and here too, can the engineer contribute to spread
physical principles or increase the knowledge of the doctors and
other members of the staff in all forms of applied physical sciences,
particularly as regards biomechanics.

The task to be carried out by both the doctor and the engineer
is not at all easy. In spite of the competence and determined good-
will that they may have, in order to find adequate solutions we
must accept that, after all the efforts carried out in the research
undertaken, some problems remain such as they were at the begining
of our work. As Contini rightly says, "research in this area is
not full of dramatic success". "As a matter of fact, most of this
research is dull, tedious and painstaking. It implies the accumula-
tion, reduction and interpretation of mountains of data. The human
organism is not as compliant, nor as willing to be experimental
with,for research purposes, as are the physical things to which the
engineer has become accustomed. These data will usually have a
greater variability, the number of subjects will be more limited;
and even more when the research is such as to assure or evaluate
some aspect of human effort, the psychological overlay may mask the
true meaning of the physical or psychological data. Engineering
research in this field requires dedication and should not be
undertaken in the search for glamour or instant reputation". We
must therefore be prepared, after long and hard efforts, to find
ourselves before deceiving situations.

In spite of that, many of the problems that have been considered without solution, could and should constitute a challenge
to the working capacity and the creative imagination of the

scientist. According to Leprince-Ringuet, the scientific pole of the human being is demanding. "In order that it works in full, it is necessary that man acquires a whole of qualities for a long and serious ascesis. These qualities are: honesty, team mind, balance between creative imagination and over-scrupulous patience between intellectual activity and manual work, and above all a two components way of mind, disponibility or reception mind, and criticism of readiness to question, to challenge anybody's and one's opinions".

From the foregoing, we think that rather than a presumptuous or an arrogant way of behaving, we will all benefit if we adopt a more modest attitude of mind. In fact, and as a simple example, we all know that in spite of the great progress and constant improvement achieved, for example, as regards prostheses of the upper extremity, there is none which can entirely replace the irreparable loss of a hand or of part of it.

Also, and following Contini, "we may in many instances prolong life, a life however, limited to the radius permitted by the length of tube or cable connecting the patient to his machine". Having these considerations in mind and remembering the great advances already obtained in the field of rehabilitation engineering, we certainly hope that the efforts to be made in the present and in the future by engineering and medical scientists, besides being a must, will also be a remarkable contribution for the well being of mankind in general and the disabled patient in particular.

ACKNOWLEDGEMENTS

I wish to express my best appreciation to Professor Robert M. Kenedi (Glasgow) for his assistance, and to Mr. Warren Springer (New York City) and Dr. Evaristo da Foncesa (Alcoitão-Estoril) for their helping in collecting some of the data for this paper.

REFERENCES

1. Anderson, M.H., Bechtol, C.O., Sollars, R.E.: Clinical Prosthetics for Physicians and Therapists, Charles C. Thomas Publisher, Springfield, 1959.
2. Breig, Alf.: Adverse Mechanical Tension in the Central Nervous System, John Wiley and Sons, London, 1978.
3. Burdette, M.E., Frolich, P. and Posner, I.: Work. Disability in the United States, Office of Research and Statistics, Social Security Administration, U.S. Dept. of Healt, Education and Welfare, 1977.
4. Chigier, E.: New Dimensions in Rehabilitation, Based on the XIII Congress of Rehabilitation. International, Gomeh Scientific Publications, Ben-Noon Press, Tel Aviv, 1978.
5. Comarr, A. Estin: The Practical Care of Spinal Cord Injuries, Journal of the Indian Medical Profession, 4: 1560-1585, Bombay, India, 1957.

6.   Contini, Renato: Engineering in Medicine, Bulletin of
     Prosthetic Research, Fall, 1967.
7.   Da Foncesa, Evaristo: Research into a Technique of Treatment
     for Pressure Sores, paper read on 6th May, 1977, at the
     Symposium of the Portuguese Society of Physical Medicine and
     Rehabilitation.
8.   Da Silva, K.M.C.: Biomechanics Research at the Gulbenkian
     Institute of Science, Oeiras, Portugal.
9.   Da Silva, K.M.C.: Neuromuscular Activity and Respiration
     Dinamics in the Cat, Ph. D. Thesis, Univ. of London, 1971.
10. Da Silva, K.M.C.: Biomecânica, engenharia biomédica e medicina,
     Expresso, 21.6.1975.
11. Drillis, R., Contini, R., and Bluestein, M.: Body Segment
     Parameters, Artificial Limbs, Spring 1964.
12. Dubleton, J., and Black, J.: An Introduction to Orthopaedic
     Materials, Charles C. Thomas, Publisher, Springfield, 1975.
13. Evans, F.G.: The Mechanical Properties of Bone, Artificial
     Limbs, Vol. 13, No.1, Spring, 1969.
14. First World Congress of the ISPO: Needs in Prosthetics and
     Orthotics Worldwide,Report of a Workshop held at Les Diablerets,
     Switzerland, 1975.
15. Fisher, B.H.: Treatment of Ulcers on the Legs with Hyperbaric
     Oxygen, The Journal of Dermatologic Surgery, Inc., Vol.I,
     No.3, October, 1975.
16. Foort, J. Hannah, R., and Cousins, S.: Rehabilitation Engineering
     as the crow flies, Prosthetic and Orthotics International,
     Vol.2, No.1, April, 1978.
17. Frankel, V.H., and Burstein, A.H.: Biomechanica Ortopedica,
     Editorial Jions, Barcelona, 1973.
18. Fung, Y.C., Perrone, N., Anliker, M.: Biomechanics. Its
     Foundations and Objectives, Prentice Hall, Inc., New Jersey,
     1972.
19. Guttmann, Prof. Sir Ludwig: Spinal Cord Injuries - Comprehensive
     Management and Research, Black-Well Scientific Publications,
     Oxford, 1973.
20. Guttmann, Prof. Sir Ludwig: On Health Deviation and Rehabilita-
     tion in Spinal Paraplegia and Tetraplegia, Community Health,
     Vol.8, No.4, May, 1977.
21. Hammerman, Susan: Social and Economic Implications of Investments
     in Rehabilitation, Department of Economic and Social Affairs,
     United Nations, New York, 1977.
22. Hobson, D.A.: Rehabilitation Engineering - a developing speciality,
     Prosthetics and Orthotics International, Vol.1, No.1, April,1977.
23. Hofstra, Peter, C.: The Clinical Engineer and the Spinal - Cord
     - Injured Person, Bulletin of Prosthetic Research - Fall, 1974.
24. Huckstep, R.L.: Simple Appliances for Developing Countries,
     Papers and Reports: P. 4, Rehabilitation International, New
     York.
25. John, V.B.: Introduction to Engineering Materials, The
     MacMillan Press, Ltd., London, 1977.

26. Kenedi, R.M.: Bioengineering Education and Training, Bio-Medical Engineering, March, 1967.
27. Kenedi, R.M.: Bioengineering Horizons, Bio-Medical Engineering, Vol.7, No.11, December 1972.
28. Kenedi, R.M.: Perspectives in Biomedical Engineering, Proceedings of a Symposium organized in association with the Biological Engineering Society and held in the University of Strathclyde, Glasgow, The MacMillan Press, Ltd., London, 1973.
29. Kenedi, R.M., Gibson, T. Evans, J.H. and Barbenel, J.C.: Tissue Mechanics, Phys. Med. Biol., Vol.20, No.5, 1975.
30. Kenedi, R.M., Cowden, J.M. and Scales, J.T.: Bed Sore Bio-mechanics, proceedings of a seminar on Tissue Viability and Clinical Application, The MacMillan Press, Ltd., London, 1976.
31. Komi, Paavo, V.: Biomechanics (V-A and V-B), University Park Press, Baltimore, 1976.
32. Kwatny, E., and Zuckerman, Ronnie: Devices and Systems for the Disabled, Krusen Centre for Research and Engineering at Moss Rehabilitation Hospital, Phyladelphia, April, 29th and 30th, 1975.
33. Leclair, R.E.: Rehabilitation Engineering : A Plan for Continued and Accelerated Progress, American Rehabilitation, Vol.3, No.2, Noc.-Dec., 1977.
34. Leclair, R.E., and Reswick, James, B.: Looking at Engineering Centres, American Rehabilitation, 1977.
35. Lehneis, H.R., Frisina, W. Marx, H.N., Sowell, T.T.: Bio-engineering Design and Development of Lower Extremity Orthotic Devices, Bulletin of Prosthetics Research, Fall, 1973.
36. MacDonald, F.A.: Mechanics for Movement, G. Bell and Sons, Ltd., London, 1973.
37. MacGregor, J.: University of Strathclyde Bioengineering Unit, British Journal of Hospital Medicine, May, 1972.
38. MacKenzie, W.C.: The Action of Muscles, Paul B. Hoeber, New York, 1921.
39. Martin, J. Purdon: Disorders of Locomotion due to Diseases of the Central Nervous System, Physiotherapy, Vol.50, No.6, June 10, 1964.
40. McLaurin, C.A.: On the Use of Engineers in Rehabilitation, Utdrag ur Inter-Clinic Information Bulletin, October, 1971.
41. Montan, Karl: R and D and World Cooperation: Situation ... but not Hopeless, Rehabilitation World, Vol.3, No.1, Spring (April), 1977.
42. O'Connel, A.L. and Gardner, E.B.: Understanding the Scientific Bases of Human Movement, The Williams and Wilkins Co., Baltimore, 1972.
43. Paul, J.P.: Forces Transmitted by Joints in the Human Body, Proc. Instn. Mech. Engrs., Glasgow, 1966-1967.
44. Paul, J.P.: Approaches to Design.-Force actions transmitted by Joints in the Human Body, Proc. R. Soc. Lond. B. 192, 163-172, Glasgow, 1976.

45. Paul, J.P.: Loading on Normal Hips and Knee Joints and on Joint Replacements, Engineering in Medicine, Vol.2, Springer-Verlag, Heidelberg, 1976.
46. Pearson, J.R.: Need for Research in Fundamental Biomechanic Studies, Artificial Limbs, Vol.11, No.2, Autumn, 1967.
47. Pratt, Rosalie: Nursing Care of Paraplegic Patients, MacMillan Journals, Ltd., London, 1971.
48. Radcliffe, Charles: The Biomechanics of the Canadian - Type Hip - Disarticulation Prosthesis, Artificial Limbs, Autumn, 1957.
49. Radcliffe, Charles W.: The Biomechanics of Belowknee Prosthesis in Normal, Level, Bipedal, Walking, Artificial Limbs, June,1962.
50. Rehabilitation Engineering Conference, WAFA WA AMAL, Proceedings of the Conference, Cairo, Egypt, June, 1975.
51. Reswick, J.B.: Some Thoughts Relative to the Rehabilitation Engineer, Rancho Los Amigos Hospital, California.
52. Roberts, T.D.M.: The Mechanics of the Upright Posture, Physiotherapy, October, 1969.
53. Rushmer, R.F.: Medical Engineering, Academic Press, New York, 1972.
54. Rusk, Howard, A.: Rehabilitation Medicine, The C.V. Mosby Company, Saint Louis, 1964.
55. Santana Carlos, V.M.: Aspectos Médicos e Profissionais da Reabilitação de Diminuidos Fisicos, Lisboa, 1963.
56. Selwyn, Donald: Rehabilitation Engineering for the Severely Handicapped, Rehabilitation, Number Sixty-four, January—March, 1968.
57. Shaw, A.: The bio-engineer - his role today, Engineering in Medicine, Vol.6, No.2, April, 1977.
58. Staros, Anthony: Plastics and Prosthesis, Papers and Reports, P.5, Rehabilitation International, New York.
59. Staros, Anthony and Peizer, Edward: The Clinical Engineer, Mechanical Engineering, 18 June, 1974.
60. Staros, Anthony: Education and Training Directions, Orthotics and Prosthetics, Vol.31, No.2, 1977.
61. Staros, Anthony and Sheredos, Saleem: The Rehabilitation Engineer, VA Prosthetic Center, New York.
62. Staros, Anthony and Rubin, Gustav: The Orthopedic Surgeon and Rehabilitation Engineering, VA Prosthetic Center, New York,1977.
63. Swanson, Sav: Engineering and Arthritis, Engineering in Medicine, The Institution of Mechanical Engineering, Vol.6, No.1, January,1977.
64. Tichauer, E.R.: Occupational Biomechanics, Rehabilitation Monograph No. 51, Institute of Rehabilitation Medicine, New York, 1975.
65. Townley, Charles, O.: The Anatomic Total Knee : An Up-dated Report, Medical Arts Building, Port Huron, Michigan 48060.
66. Traub, Joseph E., and Leclair, Richard, E.: The Rehabilitation Engineering Program, American Rehabilitation, 1976.
67. Who, Reports on Specific Technical Matters : Disability Prevention and Rehabilitation, A29/INF.DOC/1, 28 April, 1976.

74

68. Williams and Lissner: Biomechanics of Human Motion, W.B.
    Saunders Company, 2nd edition, Philadelphia, 1977.
69. Wirta, R.N. and Taylór, Jr., D.R.: Engineering Principles in
    Rehabilitation Medicine, Handbook of Physical Medicine and
    Rehabilitation, by Krusen, Kottke and Ellwood, Chapter 40, W.B.
    Saunders Company, Phyladelphia, 1971.
70. Wooldridge, C.P. and McLaurin, C.A.: Biofeedback - Background
    and Applications to Physical Rehabilitation, Bulletin of
    Prosthetic Research - Spring, 1976.

BIOMECHANICAL BEHAVIOR OF SOFT CONNECTIVE TISSUES*

A. Viidik

Department of Connective Tissue Biology, Institute of
Anatomy, University of Aarhus, Denmark

ABSTRACT. The main function of soft connective tissues is mechanical, to transmit or resist forces and to provide stability to the
organs without "skeletons of bone". The biomechanical properties
of these tissues are derived from those of their components. The
behavior is related to the morphological structure from the molecular to the macroscopic level. The lecture includes the following
sections: 1. Introduction. 2. Biomechanics of parallel-fibred connective tissue, 2.1. Tensile strength characteristics, 2.2. Stress-
-strain relationship, 2.3. Visco-elasticity and plasticity. 3. Interrelation between structure and function of collagen. 4. Remarks
on experimental techniques (measurement of original length and
cross-sectional area, specimen clamping, importance of specimen
storing and testing milieu, previous stress-strain history, testing machine set-up and errors). 5. Biomechanics of complex tissues, 5.1. Influence of geometrical configuration, 5.2. Influence
of non-collagenous tissue components. 6. Concluding remarks.

1. INTRODUCTION

The tissue in the mammalian body that is regarded to have the
greatest mechanical strength and the most pronounced stiffness is
bone, which is an "ossified connective tissue", for review see
Evans [1]. The skeleton of bone provides a major part of the general structural stability that the mammalian organism as a whole
has. Most of the organs in the body, however, lack frameworks of

---

*This work has been supported in part by the Danish Medical Re-
search Council, project no. 512-6637.

bone and their internal structural stability is instead provided
by "skeletons" of soft connective tissues. These tissues are also
important components in most types of links, which join the bones
of the skeletal system with each other (for review see Harkness [2,
3], Elliott [4], and Viidik [5,6]). There are considerable differences between the mechanical properties of the different types of
these "hard" and "soft" tissues, not only when the two groups of
tissues are compared with each other but also when comparisons are
made between tissues in one of the groups (for comparative review
see Yamada [7]). These differences are caused by variations in the
proportions and types as well as in the geometrical configurations
of the components that constitute the various tissues. It must
therefore be taken into account, when analysing the mechanical properties of a particular tissue, that the properties measured are
highly dependent on the characteristics of its morphological structure on all the levels from the macroscopic one "down" to the molecular (cf. Viidik [6]). The complexity of the analysis increases
further, when a functional unit consisting of different types of
tissues is studied.

The purpose of this chapter is to discuss the biomechanical
functions of soft connective tissues. The properties of bone, which
are dealt with in other chapters in this monograph, will only be
touched cursorily here for comparative purposes, when the soft connective tissues and their roles in larger functional units are discussed. The important physiological functions of dense and mostly
parallel-fibred soft connective tissues, such as muscle tendons
and joint ligaments, are primarily mechanical and related to forces arising either from internal or external sources. One of these
functions is to transmit forces from muscle to bone or from bone
to bone. Another one of them is to protect other components in
joints and consists of stabilization of joints and prevention of
overextension in them. The systems of collagen fibers are morpho-
logically dominant in most of these tissues. However, in a few of
them, e.g. ligamentum nuchae and ligamentum flavum, also elastic
fibers play a significant role. The function of the three-dimensional fiber framework in skin, which is dominated by collagen but
also contains some elastic fibers, is mainly protective. The non-
cellular part of the framework in blood vessels, which consists of
elastic and collagenous components, has also a protective function
but participates further significantly in the rheological response
of the vessel wall to the pulse wave. The system of fibrous rings
around the orifices of the heart ventricles provides the mechanical constriction necessary for the function of the valves. In soft
internal organs, such as the liver and the kidney, the stromata
and organ capsules of soft connective tissues constitute "skeletons".

Because of the structural variations in and complexity of
most of the organs containing soft connective tissues it is ne-

cessary, for the assessment of the biomechanical performance of the body or parts of it, to have a detailed knowledge of the characteristics of the components constituting the system(s) studied. Also a structure constituted "only" of connective tissue is complex enough to warrant an analysis of its various components separately. The starting point should be to evaluate characteristical properties of the different participating fibers per se and thereafter to proceed to an analysis of how they interact with each other and with the surrounding ground substance.

All connective tissues contain fibers of collagen, which is unique as a protein with regard to tensile strength and it has the main responsibility for the mechanical behavior of most soft connective tissues. Its molecular and primary structures, biochemical properties and aggregation into fibrils and fibers are resonably well known (for review see Ramachandran [8], Gould [9], Ramachandran & Reddi [10], Viidik & Vuust [11]). It is easily available for biomechanical analysis in a geometrically uncomplicated form as parallel-fibred muscle tendons and joint ligaments, which besides collagen contain only small amounts of ground substance and cellular elements (cf. Viidik [5]). The biomechanical characteristics of these tissues will therefore be discussed first.

2. BIOMECHANICS OF PARALLEL-FIBRED COLLAGENOUS TISSUE

Most interest was for a long time, when studying the biomechanics of tendons and ligament, focused on the ultimate tensile strength of these tissues. This parameter, synonymous with failure and breaking strengths as well as with maximum stress, is also of importance for the characterization of parallel-fibred collagenous tissue as a material. However, when forming a tendon or a ligament, this tissue never functions alone but always as a part of a functional unit and thus in interaction with other tissues. Stress values of the magnitude of the breaking strength for collagen are never reached in such units under physiological conditions (cf. Elliott & Crawford [12]). It is questionable whether such values are reached even in cases of sports traumata such as skiing accidents and "rupturing" calcaneal tendons when jumping. It is thus evident that a set of parameters must be measured in order to characterize this tissue:

(i) Tensile strength and the corresponding strain values.
(ii) Stress-strain relationship from the relaxed state to the point of failure.
(iii) Presence of time-dependent (viscous) and irreversible (plastic) components and how they interact with time-independent and reversible (elastic) components within the physiological range of tissue function.

78

<u>Table I</u>

Ultimate tensile strength (in newton/mm^2) and strain (dimension-
less) at that point for various human tissues (from Yamada [7])
and materials (from Swanson [13]).

	Strength	Strain
Skeletal muscle[1]	0.3	1.4
Spongious bone	1.2	0.006
Aorta (abdominal)[2]	1.2	1.14
Ligamentum nuchae[3]	2.4	1.25
Skin (forehead)	4	0.6
Skin (thoracal)[2]	15	1.1
Muscle fascia[4]	15	0.17
Tendon	60	0.10
Compact bone	150	0.015
Limestone	4	?
Aluminium alloy	210	0.1
Medium alloy steel	600	0.12

[1] "Fresh" value, approximated according to Yamada ([7]) from
experiments 48 hrs. post mortem.
[2] Tested in transversal direction.
[3] From cattle. Mean value for strongest (3.2) and weakest (1.6)
parts (the corresponding strains are 1.6 and 0.9 respectively).
[4] Tested along the main fiber direction.

2.1. Tensile strength characteristics

A parallel-fibred tendon (or ligament) is highly anisotropic and
its function is confined to transmit (or resist) forces along the
direction of the fibers. It is therefore sufficient to submit it
to only uniaxial tension testing, and thus refrain from investi-
gating the compressive and shearing properties as well as multi-
axial testing, when characterizing its properties.

The ultimate tensile strength and strain at that point for
various connective and supportive tissues are tabulated in Table
I. The data are derived from the reports of one research team to
enable comparisons between the different tissues without bias of
sampling and technique variations. It should, however, be emphasized that the data presented are not necessarily more "true" than
those of other investigators. From this table it is evident that
dense parallel-fibred collagenous tissue (tendons and ligaments)
is the strongest of the soft tissues and has the least extensibility as well. Of the organic materials only compact bone is stronger and stiffer; spongious bone never functions without a frame of
compact bone and is seldom subjected to only tensile forces. Muscle

tissue has been included for the sake of completeness; it is doubtful, whether these figures, extrapolated from tests performed two
days post-mortem, have any significance. They indicate that the
connective tissues, in which no autolytic changes have taken place,
do not contribute much to the tensile strength of live muscles.

Most investigators have found the ultimate tensile strength
of tendons to be in the range between 45 [14] and 125 [15] newton
per square millimeter. It should be added here that the data published by Wertheim in 1847 [16], showing the tensile strength of
human tendons to be 50 - 105 and that of canine tendons 50 - 60
newton per square millimeter, are in full agreement with data obtained by the most modern technology. There does not seem to be
any major inter-species variations. Tagikawa [17] tested tendons
from various mammals and found the tensile strength to be in the
same order of magnitude as that of human tendons (53 N/mm^2 for
calcaneal tendon in his study). He found the tissue of calcaneal
tendons from horses to be strongest (82 N/mm^2) and that from guinea pigs weakest (35 N/mm^2). The major inter-species variations in
tendon strength are, as the tissue differences are minor, of course,
due to variations in size. Takigawa also calculated the tensile
breaking load (in newton) of calcaneal tendons for various species:
e.g. horse 40,000, man 1,900 and guinea pig 90. It is possible that
some small rodents, especially rats, in young adult stages have
comparatively weaker tissue in their tendons. This assumption is
based on two observations. (i) The retarded maturation pattern of
the collagen in the rat, especially of that in its tail tendons
(on the relation between molecular structure and tensile strength
vide infra). (ii) The calcaneal tendon, when tested in the femur-
muscle-tendon-calcaneus unit, is prone to rupture in the rat [18]
but not in other animals e.g. [19,20,21]. The same pattern is seen
in most tests on the tensile properties of bone-ligament-bone specimens, the rupture occurring as an avulsion of bone [22,23,24,25],
the only exception being a study on primates [26], where the rupture most frequently occurred in the anterior cruciate ligament.
Here, however, the tensile testing was performed on specimens with
the knee joint in 45° flexion and it is therefore possible that the
loading was distributed unevenly between the various ligament fiber
bundles.

It is usually found that the tensile strength of whole tendons is lower than for single fibers or fiber bundles. Harkness
[2] calculated the ultimate tensile strength of single collagen
fiber bundles to reach up to 500 newton per square millimeter pure
collagen (using the collagen content of the wet tissue and assuming
the density of collagen to be 1.4) while the figures for whole tendons were limited to a maximum of 300. Similar size-related differences were reported by Chvapil et al. [27], Elden [28] and Millington et al. [29]. There are in principle two possible explana-
tions to this difference. The first one is associated with the prob-

lem of fixing a tendon into clamps without producing artificial
breaks due to stress concentrations at jaw edges (<u>vide infra</u> remarks on experimental techniques); it is a general experience that
it is more difficult to fix thick tendons safely into clamps avoiding slipping as well as jaw breaks. The second one is that the
larger the diameter of the tendon and thereby the number of fiber
bundles is the greater is the chance that the tensile stress is
distributed unevenly. Some of the bundles take then most of the
stress, which causes them to break, whereafter the stress is redistributed to the next group of bundles and so forth until the
whole tendon has ruptured. Then a maximum stress value considerably lower than the sum of the tensile strength of the various
bundles constituting the tendon is recorded. (Cf. Viidik & Ekholm
[30], Viidik [31].

The parameter which is usually measured together with the ultimate tensile strength of a material, is the strain, at which this
strength is reached. This parameter varies considerably between different investigations and for tendons the strain is reported to be
in the range between 0.08 and 0.35. Here several factors may influence the results of the testing. The crucial one here is the definition of original length as strain is defined as deformation
per unit original length. This length should be defined in a safely reproducible way. When comparing the results of different investigators it should be kept in mind that various portions of the
beginning of the toe part of the stress-strain curve may have been
included into it (<u>vide infra</u> discussion on definition on the starting point of the stress-strain curve). Also other, technical as
well as physiological, factors may influence the results of the
measurements significantly. If the specimen is not quite parallel-
fibred, the re-arrangement of elements to be aligned along the line
of stress application adds to the strain values recorded (cf. <u>infra</u>
the influence of fiber geometry on stress-strain behavior). Also
a decreased water content tends to make a specimen stiffer. A jaw
break "cuts off" the stress-strain curve prematurely, although with
this type of bias also the measurement of tensile strength itself
is affected. The same is the case with a variety of physiological
factors such as age, hormonal balance and state of physical training or immobilization, which may influence the results.

2.2. Stress-strain relationship

The stress-strain curves for mammalian tissues always start with
a toe part. Fig. 1 compares such curves for the strongest and stif-
fest tissues. Although it is not evident from this figure, also
the curve for compact bone has a toe part, which can be demonstrated when the recording is made with high enough a resolution. The
toe part, which is convex towards the strain axis, starts more insidiously the more extensible the tissue is.

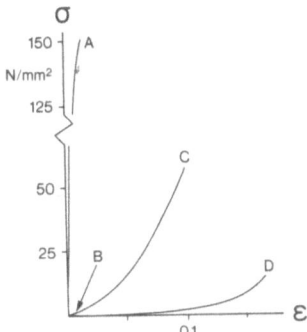

Fig. 1. Stress (σ) – strain (ε) curves for compact bone (A), spongious bone (following curve C up to the tip of arrow B), tendon
(C) and tigh fascia (D). (Adapted from Yamada [7]).

The anterior cruciate ligament in the rabbit knee joint is
a convenient specimen for demonstrating qualitative biomechanical
properties as the femur and tibia can be used as secure clamping
sites. The constant geometry from one specimen to another permits
further the use of these load-deformation curves as "stress-strain"
curves as long as quantitative comparisons between tissues with
substantial geometrical variations are not required (for discussion see Viidik et al. [22]). Such a curve is shown in Fig. 2.
This type of specimen will also be used in subsequent illustrations and the curves referred to as stress-strain curves.

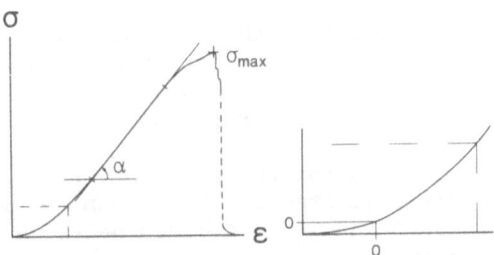

Fig. 2. (Left) Stress-strain curve for an anterior cruciate ligament from a rabbit knee joint. The elastic stiffness of the linear
segment is tan α. The specimen breaks with a tear-off fracture from
the tibial condyle at σ_{max}.

Fig. 3. (Right) A magnification of the initial part of the curve
in Fig. 2. The coordinates for the start of the stress-strain curve
($\sigma=0$, $\varepsilon=0$) are placed at the point of minimum recordable load.

The curve starts more or less insidiously with a toe part. This is shown more in detail in Fig. 3. The starting point can be defined in different ways:

(i) The point reached on the deformation axis when it is possible to record the smallest load the measuring system and recorder can disciminate from zero load. As the start of the toe part is insidious, considerable differences can arise when various equipments or degrees of magnification on the same equipment are used. Care should be taken to use the same absolute load value or, when there are considerable specimen size variations, stress value for this point throughout the series compared. Such a point is shown in Fig. 3.

(ii) The point where the morphological appearance of the specimen starts to change, e.g. the waviness in the relaxed fiber bundles seen with simultaneous incidental light microscopy starts to straighten out. Also this process starts gradually and the point is difficult to define with a high degree of reproducibility (cf. Viidik [31]).

(iii) The level of stress, "prestress", that is present in the in vivo resting state. From a theoretical point of view this is the logical definition. However, the in vivo existig "prestress" is difficult to measure and is presently not determined for most connective tissues. The tension in muscles varies and the resting tension in tendons is probably also dependent on the degree of flexion in the adjacent joints. Further, there probably does not exist a physiological "prestress" in ligaments. It depends entirely on the position of the joint whether they are relaxed or not.

It must therefore be concluded that the most satisfactory method available to define the original length of these tissues is the procedure of setting the beginning of the stress-strain curve at the point of minimum recordable load (or stress).

A fairly linear part follows after the toe part. For this segment of the curve the elastic stiffness, tan α, can be measured. The term "modulus of elasticity" should be avoided here, as it is a well defined engineering term, which implies that the material is elastic. This is not the case with tendons and ligaments, which have viscous as well as some plastic properties well before the end of the linear part of the curve (vide infra). During the course of the linear segment of the curve there are sometimes seen small "dips", i.e. sharp drops in the stress, up to 2 - 4 per cent of the maximum stress value, after which the curve is resumed with the same steepness as before. They are seen mostly in bone-ligament-bone specimens and have been interpreted as failures of small fiber bundles due to unequal loading (Viidik et al. [22], Viidik

& Levin [32]). This is supported by the observation that these dips are only seen in the first cycle of cyclic loading-unloading experiments. They are very seldom seen in specimens of isolated tendons and are, when present, most probably due to preparation injuries.

The specimen may break directly at the end of the linear segment of the curve or, which is more common, the curve bends off somewhat towards the strain axis. The curve may decrease below the point of maximum stress before the specimen breaks completely. The breaking occurs at times in a few steps and shows then as a few large dips.

The parameters usually calculated from stress-strain curves are: The coordinates for stress and strain at (i) the beginning of the linear segment, (ii) the end of it, and (iii) the point of maximum stress. Also (iv) the elastic stiffness of the linear segment as its inclination, tan α, is measured. It can be of value to calculate an additional parameter, (v) the failure energy, from the area between the curve and the strain axis. In some cases, as when testing complete functional units, a considerable intragroup variation is seen and the value of this parameter can be questioned. However, in other cases, especially when testing the functional properties of healing incisional wounds, this parameter gives a precise and useful estimate of how much energy the healing tissue can absorb without breaking. With this type of specimens the intragroup variance is about the same as for the other parameters measured.

A number of factors can influence the characteristics of the stress-strain curve. Some are physiological changes in the organism, which alter the inherent tissue properties. Others are in vitro artifacts originating in the experimental techniques used. Some of them have been discussed in connection with the tensile strength characteristics (vide supra 2.1) and they will be discussed further in the section on experimental techniques. It should, however, be noted here that the stress-strain behavior of collagenous tissue is strain rate dependent and variations in the curves can be produced by testing specimens of different lengths with the same deformation speed. Fig. 4 demonstrates the first third of two curves from one specimen (in the rheologically stationary phase). The first test was performed at a very low deformation speed and the second one at a moderately high speed. This increase of speed shifted the curve significantly to the left. Here the difference between the strain rates is about 4 orders of magnitude but also decreasing the strain rate 0.5 times achieved by using specimens of double lengths is sufficient to produce differences. The viscous components in tissue behavior are not so pronounced for tendons and ligaments as they are for tissues, which contain less collagen and more ground substance. Decreasing the strain rate to

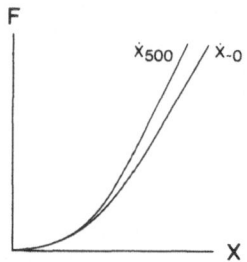

Fig. 4. Load (F) - deformation (X) curves for subsequent tests on the same specimen with speeds $\dot{x} \backsim 0$ and $\dot{x} = 500$ mm/min.

low levels probably changes the stress-strain curve more by the influence of the creep phenomenon than increasing speed to "lock" the viscous components. There are no explicit data available for this aspect tendons and ligaments. Glaser et al. [33] analysed this for skin and found the creep phenomenon to influence the stress-strain curves at strain rates lower than 0.4 per minute. Probably this "safety limit" is somewhat lower for tendons and ligaments.

2.3. Visco-elasticity and plasticity

When performing testing by cyclic loading and unloading of specimens both the visco-elastic, viscous and plastic components show already within the toe part of the stress-strain curves. The curve successively shifts to the right [34,35,36]. Some of this change is recoverable and due to visco-elasticity, earlier called elastic aftereffect [37,38]. Another part of it is not and remains as irreversible viscosity and plasticity [39]. Earlier reports that rather low loads or loads of short duration [38,40] did not cause any permanent deformation in vitro have not been reproducible later and may be based on insufficient resolution in the measuring equipment used.

It is useful to visualize the elastic, viscous and plastic components with a rheological analogy when evaluating the interaction between them. Such an analogy can be constituted of electrical or mechanical components. An electrical analogy can, when an analog computer is used, directly generate the appropriate curves e.g. [41,42]. The "meaning" of the various components and their interaction is, however, not so easily visualized. Also mechanical analogies have been used for such purposes. The behavior of the wall of the sea anemone has thus been described by a Kelvin element [43]. Also the mechanical properties of synthetic high polymers have been characterized by combinations of such elements [44].

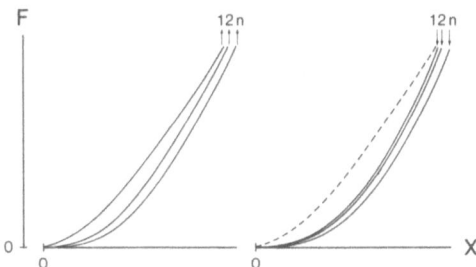

Fig. 5. Initial load-deformation curves for rabbit anterior cruciate ligament preparation up to "100%" in Figs. 6-7, which is one third of failure load. The curves to the left show the loading segments and those to the right the unloading ones (the dashed curve is for the 1st loading cycle). The 1st, 2nd and the stationary phase curve (n:th) are shown.

It has further been applied to describe qualitatively complex biological tissues such as the arterial wall [45, 46] and bone tissue [47]. This approach seems appropriate to approximate the behavior of biological tissues as the elements and their interaction are easy to visualize and reasonably simple mathematical analysis can be used for verification. The present author has therefore chosen to use mechanical analogies to analyse the rheological behavior of parallel-fibred dense collagenous tissue [23,39,48,49,50]. For review of this topic see [5]. We have attempted to reproduce the essential features of the experimental observations with the minimum of components required. With this approach "ideal" springs, dashpots and dry friction elements are used to visualize elasticity, viscosity and plasticity respectively. For the analysis of these properties of these "ideal" elements and their interactions relatively simple mathematical expressions can be used. It should, however, be remembered that these idealized elements do not necessarily correspond to physical events in the real tissues.

One of the basic rheological features, an increased viscous damping with increased strain rate, was demonstrated by a shift of the stress-strain curve to the left in Fig. 4. The characteristic toe part of the stress-strain curve, however, is present even at very high strain rates [51], which means that all the elastic components are not parallel to viscous dampers. On the other hand, a substantial part of the viscosity is recoverable, which indicates that it is present in visco-elastic (Kelvin element) form, besides the irreversible (Newton element) part of it. When repeating loading-unloading cycles the curve shift to the right and becomes steeper in its loading segments but not in the unloading ones. This indicates the presence of a strain-hardening element (a combination of dry friction elements), cf. [39,49]. These features

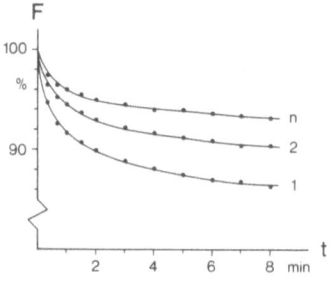

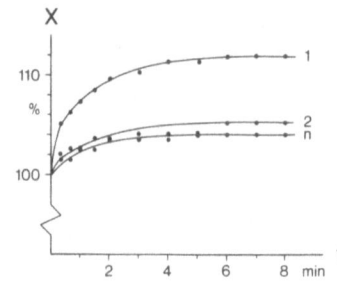

Fig. 6. (Left) Same as Fig. 5, but load-relaxation at the deformation reached at "100%" load.

Fig. 7. (Right) Same as Fig. 5, but creep phenomena at the "100%"
load level.

are shown for an anterior cruciate ligament preparation in Fig. 5.
By the n:th cycle the stress-strain curve does not shift any further to the right and the stationary phase has thus been reached.
The corresponding shift in the visco-elastic and viscous behavior
are demonstrated by stress-relaxation (Fig. 6) and creep phenomenon (Fig. 7). Here stress and strain values respectively reach
constant levels asymptotically.

The mechanical analogy satisfying these characteristics is
shown in Fig. 8. K_i and ΣY_i are the irreversible viscous and strain-
hardening elements respectively, and act only in the initial loading-unloading cycles until the n:th one. They come, of course, into action again if the load is brought to a higher level than during
the previous cycles. The remaining part of the analogy belongs to
the stationary phase behavior. The elastic element here, C_H, is
non-linear. It can be represented by an array of springs that come
into action successively with increased strain (as suggested by

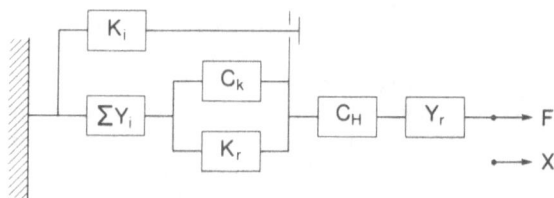

Fig. 8. Rheological model for the tissue behavior in Fig. 5-7
(adapted from Viidik [39]. For explanation of symbols see text.

Viidik & Mägi [48] and later elaborated [39,49,50]). Here a sufficient number of steps can be included to approximate specimen
behavior satisfactorily. It can also be symbolized by a "non-ideal"
spring, the coils of which are straightened out, whereafter the
wire itself is strained. This gives a continuous non-linear elasticity, although the mathematical expression of it is not easy
visualized [49]. This model for the stationary phase was verified
experimentally with other sets of experiments than used to compose the analogy by Frisén et al. [50] using the array of springs
coming stepwise into action as model for the non-linear elasticity.

The constitutive equation for this model can be written as

$$\dot{F} + F(\phi+C_K)/K_K = \dot{X}\phi + XC_K\phi/K_K - C_K\psi/K_K$$

The following nomenclature is used: X is deformation (strain in
the general case), F load (stress), C_K stiffness for the Kelvin
element spring, ϕ step function spring stiffness, K_K dashpot constant (in the Kelvin element), ψ another step function, and a dot
above a symbol indicates time derivative. In the subsequent equations subscript 0 indicates the starting level and A the asympto-
tic one.

The constitutive equation can be written for the special case
of stress-relaxation (Fig. 6) as

$$F = (F_0-F_A)^{\delta_1 t} + F_A$$

and provided ϕ is constant in the region studied (it is for the
examples given, as the tests were run at the level of the linear
part of the curve) the curve can be plotted in a linear-logarithmic diagram as a straight line with the slope

$$\delta_1 = -(C_K+\phi)/K_K$$

The corresponding equation for the case of creep phenomenon is

$$X = X_A - (X_A-X_0)^{\delta_2 t}$$

Also this is a straight line linear-logarithmic split and has the
slope

$$\delta_2 = -C_K/K_K$$

Further special cases can be expressed. The equation for very low
speeds is

$$F = (\phi X-\psi) \cdot C_K/(\phi+C_K)$$

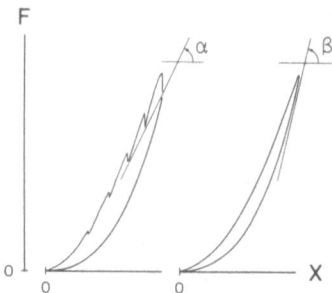

Fig. 9. The curve to the left shows the procedure for "extremely low" deformation rate. Each dip is load-relaxation for 2 min. tan α is the elasticity of C_K and C_H of Fig. 8 acting in series. The curve to the right shows a load-deformation cycle at finite speed, where tan β is the elasticity of the spring array C_H at the reversion point.

and here the elastic stiffness (within one step of the step function, in this case the linear part, where all steps are in action)

$$\tan \alpha = \phi C_K / (\phi + C_K)$$

This can achieved in the experimental situation by exhausting the stress-relaxation at stepwise higher and higher levels and then plot the curve from the "bottom points" with the stiffness of the linear part being tan α (Fig. 9). On the other hand, at very high speeds the Kelvin element is "locked" and deformation occurs only in the spring array. The stiffness of the whole system is then

$$\tan \zeta = \phi$$

and constant throughout the linear region. The Kelvin element does not influence the curve just after reversion from loading to unloading. The stiffness of the beginning of the unloading curve is thus that of the spring array (cf. Fig. 9)

$$\tan \beta = \phi$$

This set of equations gives a possibility to verify each constant from two different equations and experimental situations (cf. discussion on the verification of the model [50]). A suitable set of these experimental procedures can be used to investigate changes in the tissue (e.g. enzymatic removal of certain tissue components, influence of pharmacological therapy, physiological changes in the organism).

Another type of model has also been proposed for parallel-

fibred collagenous tissue. Zeck & Arnold [42] assembled a combination of an elastic element in parallel with a series of a viscous
and an elastic element. All three components were non-linear and
they derived analog computer curves simulating stress-relaxation
but did not proceed further with their analysis. Their model is
therefore difficult to evaluate at the present time. It seems to
have the same draw-back as some mathematical models, which can describe certain experimental conditions but lack versatility and
can not therefore satisfy other types of testing procedures.

3. INTERRELATION BETWEEN STRUCTURE AND FUNCTION OF COLLAGEN

The collagen molecule is a triple helix, which is 300 nm long
(4.4D) and with a diameter of 1.5 nm. Each chain of about 1000
amino acid residues is coiled into a left-hand helix (pitch 0.87
nm) and the three of them are wound together into a right-hand
superhelix (cf. [11]). There are non-coiled telopeptides with 15-
30 residues each at the amino- and carboxyterminal ends. The hydroxyproline residue is of importance for the stability of the
collagen molecule. It probably forms intra-molecular hydrogen
bonds or hydrogen-bonded water bridges. This stabilizing effect
can be demonstrated by preventing the hydroxylation of proline.
"Protocollagen", a molecule which is unstable already at physiological temperatures, is then formed. The molecular stability of
collagen can be assessed by measuring its shrinkage temperature
(i.e. when its strict structural arrangement is converted to the
random coiled one of gelatin). It has been found that the skin collagen in cod has 155 imino acid residues per 1000 residues and a
shrinkage temperature of 40 degrees centigrade. The corresponding
figures for shark are 191 and 53 and for calf skin 232 and 65
[52]. The protofibril is aggregated of five rows of molecules,
each row quarter-staggered with one D in relation to the previous
row (Fig. 10). These five rows are wound together into a cylindrical rope. There is also on this level of organisation a rotatory

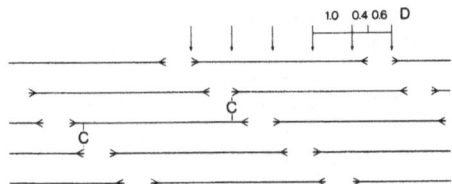

Fig. 10. The quarter-stagger arrangement of collagen molecules. D
is 68 nm. Two cross-links (-C-) between the helical region of one
molecule and the telopeptides of two adjacent molecules are indicated.

elements in the geometry as the five strands are wound together with a long pitch [53,54]. The molecules are held together by a variety of intermolecular bonds. The most important of them are the cross-links between a (hydroxy)allysine in a telopeptide and a (hydroxy)lysine residue in position 87 or 927 in the helical part of an adjacent molecule. These sites are marked by -C- in Fig. 10. Heat and acid labile borohydride reducible aldimine cross-links (dehydro-hydroxylysinonorleucine) as well as physio-chemically stable but reducible ketoimines (hydroxylysino-5-keto-norleucine, lysino-5-keto-norleucine) exist in vivo, while there is so far no evidence that three-chain cross-links (e.g. histidino-hydroxymero-desmosine) do so [55-57]. The cross-links have probably their greatest importance on the organisational level of the five-stranded rope. There are indications that on higher levels structural glycoproteins play a major role [58,59].

The protofibrils are aggregated into fibrils, seen in the electron microscope with diameters of 50-100 nm [2] and are of unknown lengths. They have a characteristic banding with a periodicity of 68 nm (1.0 D), which was shown with negative staining [60] to be caused by the gap and overlap regions in the molecular arrangement (0.6 and 0.4 D respectively in Fig. 10). The same periodicity is seen in low-angle x-ray diffraction [61]. On the other hand a periodicity of 0.286 nm is seen in wide-angle x-ray diffraction [62] and reflects the molecular coiling. The fibrils are assembled into fibers with diameters of mostly 1-12 µm and constitute in turn fiber bundles about 300 µm thick. On the light microscopic level the fiber bundles of relaxed parallel-fibred tissue have in polarized light a dark-light banding, which is due to a planar waviness and the birefringence of collagen (for discussion of this topic see Viidik [6]).

It has been calculated that a force of about 3000 newton per square millimeter collagen would be required to break the -C-N-bond in a molecular chain [63], while collagen fibers break at a stress level of at most 500 [2]. It is therefore justifyable to assume that the breaking of a parallel-oriented aggregate of collagen occurs by failure of lateral intermolecular bonds. It can be shown that the tensile strength of collagen decreases when the intermolecular cross-linking is prevented e.g. by β-aminopropionitrile [64,65]. On the other hand it is not very probable that the lability of cross-links to physical or chemical means is reflected in a lower mechanical strength [66].

Some information is available on the correlation between these structural characteristics and the stress-strain behavior of the parallel-fibred collagenous tissue. During the toe part of the stress-strain curve the waviness seen in the light microscope is straightened out [30,31,67] gradually, beginning earlier in some fiber bundles than in others [31]. This is also anticipated as

parallel-fibred tissue even in vivo seldom is loaded evenly [68].
It is reasonable to assume that most of the stiffness increase during the toe part is due to the straightening out of the fiber bundles and fibers so that the fibrils can start to resist stress and
thereby be strained themselves. However, some of the stiffness increase is probably due to a geometrical alignment of the fibers
along the line of stress application (vide infra influence of geometrical configuration of fibers in relation to stress application).
After the end of the toe part no further changes can be observed
on the light microscopical level. However, after the end of the
linear region reappearance of waviness can be seen in some of the
fiber bundles as a result of partial ruptures [31]. Some of the
minor ruptures occur already in the upper part of the linear region. They have been observed at strain levels of 0.05 - 0.06 [67]
and 0.08 - 0.10 [30,31].

On the electron microscopical level the periodicity of 68 nm
is gradually increased during the linear part of the curve up to
about 72.5 nm, i.e. about 6 per cent [30]. A similar increase of
the wide angle x-ray diffraction pattern from 0.286 to 3.1 nm
(about 8%) has been recorded [62]. Recently an investigation into
this matter has been published by Riedl & Nemetschek [69]. By
using synchrotron x-ray emission they were able to shorten the exposure time significantly. They showed that the elongation of the
fibril periodicity of 68 nm [30] had a corresponding change in the
low angle x-ray diffraction pattern and confirmed the observation
[62] of the change in the wide angle pattern of 0.286 nm. The reason for, why the changes they found are only 1.5 and 0.5 per cent
respectively and thus considerably less than those previously reported, is not obvious. It can be concluded that there are changes
in the structure on several levels that are related to the stress-
strain behavior. The physiological range of tendon function, i.e.
up to about one fourth or one third of stress value [12], corresponds mostly to the disappearence of the waviness of fiber bundles during the toe part. It is supplemented by some of the changes
in the molecular configuration, probably the changes in the 68 nm
pattern, which mostly reflect small intermolecular movements. The
tissue properties include for the linear segment of the stress-
strain curve also a certain change in the pitch of the intramole-
cular helices, although it is uncertain whether these changes can
be elicited by physiological stress levels.

With increased molecular stability also the tensile strength
of the tissue increases. However, this is true only up to a certain degree of structural rigidity. When additional artificial
cross-links are introduced thereafter, the strength instead decreases [70]. There is with maturation and aging an increase of
cross-linking in vivo and thereby structural stability. A corresponding decrease in tensile strength is observed also in this
case after a certain point [71]. This is accompanied by a decrease

of the plasticity [37,71] and of the visco-elasticity [37,69,71].
These effects can be explained by two changes: (i) the increased
cross-linking and rigidity prevents movements in and between the
collagen molecules, and (ii) the interfibrillar substance is decreased and/or has changed its characteristics. Data from biochemical analyses support both possible mechanisms. Riedl & Nemetschek
[69] also studied the visco-elasticity after introducing artificial
cross-links with glutaraldehyde as well as formaldehyde and found
both the stress-relaxation and creep phenomenon to decrease, as
with aging but more pronouncedly. Viidik [72] found formaldehyde
to influence only the elastic part of the Kelvin element in the
rheological model. It could be suggested that these changes are
due mostly to increased structural stability of the collagen. However, it cannot be ruled out at present that the inter-fibrillar
material plays a role here, as the artificial cross-linking agents
might alter also the properties of glycosaminoglycans and structural glycoproteins.

Not much information is available on the mechanism of fibril-
lar rupture. It is probable that this occurs as breaking of intermolecular bonds in a rather diffuse part of the fibril and that
the pattern depend on how the stress is redistributed among the
remaining subunits of the fibril. Steven et al. [73] studied in
the scanning electron microscope ruptured bundles of tendon fibrils and found the ruptured ends coiled or knotted. They were
able to remove the tapering of the collagen fiber ends by trypsin
incubation and concluded that the collagen at the failure site was
denatured. The recoiling part of the mechanism is supported by the
observation of Viidik & Ekholm [30] that at high strain level some
fibrils had periodicities shorter than 64 nm, which is suggestive
for a recoiling mechanism. The samples of Steven et al. [73] were,
however, pretreated with crude bacterial α-amylase. It has recently been shown [74] that α-amylase, which in purified form should
have no effect on any of the components in connective tissue, affects the tensile strength of films polymerized from purified collagen. It can therefore at present not be excluded that the tapering of the collagen fiber ends after rupture are related to changes introduced by the α-amylase treatment.

4. REMARKS ON EXPERIMENTAL TECHNIQUES

A number of factors can influence the results of biomechanical testing. Some of them have already been discussed, e.g. the definition of original length of specimen. A method that enables to measure this parameter reproducibly augments the precision of the
strain data obtained. In a similar way the measurement of specimen
cross-sectional area affects the stress data. There are methodological problems also with the measurement of cross-sectional areas
of fresh tendons: (i) the geometrical shape of the cross-section

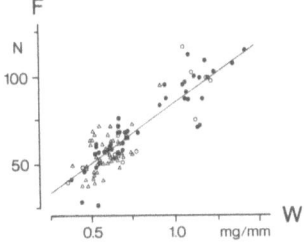
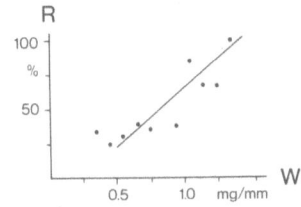

Fig. 11. (Left) Correlation between maximum load (F) and per unit tendon wet weight for rabbit hind limb tendons. Open symbols denote clamp jaw breaks. (Adapted from [76]).

Fig. 12. (Right) Correlation between per unit tendon wet weight (W) and per cent of ruptures in the free space between clamp jaws (R). (Adapted from [76]).

and (ii) the size of the area are not uniform along the tendon from the muscle junction to the insertion into bone, and (iii) the fresh tissue is somewhat deformable and compressible. Several methods have been used to measure the "real" cross-sectional area: planimetry of enlarged images of cross-sections (e.g. [15]), the principle of Archimedes [37]) and a double-caliper to compress a segment of the tendon into rectangular shape [75]). With these methods the magnitude of error in the measurement is inversely related to the size of the cross-section. Other methods have been sought for more exact measurement of small specimens, e.g. limb muscle tendons of laboratory animals. For such specimens indirect measures of "functional" cross-sectional areas have been found useful and employed on the assumptions that all collagen fibers participate fairly equally in the tensile load-bearing function and (for the methods measuring weights) that a constant fraction of the weight per unit length is collagen. One of these methods [76] is illustrated in Fig. 11, which shows the correlation between wet weight per unit tendon length and failure load for four different hind limb tendons from thirteen male rabbits of equal age. The correlation was highly significant (r = 0.87) and the coefficient of variance for this group of tendons (n = 101) decreased from 31.4 for failure load to 17.0 for this "functional" tensile strength (expressed in newton per milligram weight per millimeter length). However, when the specimens in the groups are of similar size, e.g. one type of tendons from a homogenous group of animals, nothing in precision is gained by transforming failure load to "functional" tensile strength. This can be shown by calculating the coefficient of variance for failure load and "functional" tensile strength for one type of tendons from the abovementioned animals. They are 13.2 and 14.4 respectively. This method required precisely standardized procedures with regard to prevention of drying out as well as overhydration.

Similar methods to estimate "functional" cross-sectional area, which, however, are not influenced by fluctuations in water content, are the use of dry weight [12] and amount of collagen [77] per unit specimen length. The last-mentioned method should be chosen when it is not possible to measure the "real" cross-sectional area with accuracy and when a reliable method to measure collagen content by colorimetric assessment of hydroxyproline is available.

Another problem that should be considered with tensile testing of soft connective tissues, especially parallel-fibred tendons, is the possible error the method of clamping introduces. There is a multitude of clamp designs described in the literature. The ideal clamp should fix the tendon firmly without permitting any slipping and at the same time it should not create any stress concentrations at the jaw edges, which would produce artificial premature failure sites. The type of clamps, which is most efficient in preventing slipping, is the one with serrated jaws. It is advantageous to use this type when studying the stress-strain curve into its linear part and when studying the visco-elastic and plastic properties well below the failure point. In tensile strength testing, on the other hand, it is quite obvious that the serrated jaws produce premature failure at the edges. This can be illustrated by citing a report [78], where the tensile strength was found to be only 21 - 28 newton per mm^2 and all the specimens had failed as jaw breaks. This methodological bias or error can be avoided by analysing the experimental design carefully. Compton [79] used clamps with flat surfaces and found no differences in tensile strength between the specimens failing in the free space and those breaking at a jaw edge. The lack of such a difference indicates that deleterious stress concentrations at the jaw edges are of negligible influence if present at all and that the failure occurs at a random point. However, the specimens Compton used were dried and subsequently pre-treated tendons and therefore rather rigid and without the pronounced tendency to "flow" when clamped that fresh tendons have. This problem with fastening fresh tissue into clamps with flat surfaces can be illustrated with another study [75], where out of 30 specimens 16 slipped from the clamps, 2 ruptured at the jaw edges, 1 broke at a previously damaged point and only 11 ruptured in the free space.

It is the experience of the present author that the clamps should be designed or appropriately modified for each size or type of tendon and that the optimal compression applied (i.e. for the ideal "mid-position" between slipping and jaw break) should be found empirically. This will be examplified by clamps we developed for testing rabbit hind limb tendons with wet weights between 0.3 and 1.5 mg per mm tendon length [76]. The contact surfaces were smooth and with rounded edges towards the inter-clamp "free space". A few layers of thin cotton cloth were glued to the surfaces so that the thickness towards the "free space" gradually

diminished and the last millimeter of the surface was covered only
by one layer. Waterproof abrasive paper was glued on the top of the
cloth. The tendon was compressed between these two surfaces when
the clamp halves were joined with screws and a torque wrench was
used to regulate and determine the forces applied and thereby the
resulting compression of the tendon. The "ideal" level of torque
was determined empirically. No differences in tensile strength was
found between the specimens that failed in the "free space" and
those breaking at jaw edges. (Cf. the fairly even distribution of
the different types of rupture along the failure load vs. weight
per unit length correlation line in Fig. 11). A further analysis
showed that with this method (i.e. type of clamps and level of
compressive force applied) there was a significant correlation between the weight per unit length and the percentage of tendons
failing in the "free space" (Fig. 12).

The problems of determining the original length and the cross-
sectional areas of specimens and the fastening of them by clamps
into the materials testing machine are directly related to the methodology of testing. There is, however, also a set of more general
problems, which must be considered when a series of experiments is
designed: (i) storage of the specimens, and (ii) environment during
testing, especially when the programme is time-consuming

Most biomechanical testing is performed under in vitro conditions. It is doubtful whether there are biologically significant
changes in collagenous tissue, when care is taken to avoid changes
in the water content of it. Tipton et al. [25] compared in vitro
and in situ testing of rat tibia - medial collateral ligament - femur preparations. They found that the junction strength and ligament
stiffness were slightly but significantly increased and ligament
elongation decreased when tested in vitro. This change seems to be
systematic and compatible with straining of the specimens during
handling (introducing strain-hardening and a slight residual deformation). There are no reasons to believe that the measurement of
physiological changes would be distorted by in vitro testing as
such. Care should, however, be taken especially of "fragile" specimens to avoid straining before the testing starts (cf. the rheological model). Further, for most types of experiments here is no
possibility to perform in situ and in vivo testing without too time-
consuming procedures, if at all.

Most investigators agree that collagenous tissues can be stored
for at least 24 hours without any other precautions than keeping
the water content unchanged [22,32,80,81]. For longer time periods
storage in the frozen state is advisable. The main stress-strain parameters are not influenced significantly by this procedure [32,34,
80-82]. There are, however, no comparative studies available on
whether any changes occur in the detailed rheological properties.
We feel that the possible hazard lies in protracted freezing and

thawing times, as ice crystallization and high concentrations of electrolytes (in comparision to the amount of liquid available) may harm the more sensitive tissue components. Embalming, on the other hand, changes the tissue properties considerably in most cases as artificial cross-linking is introduced [14,32,83-85]. As this change is not systematic [14], testing of embalmed tissues should be avoided. Independent of what mode is chosen for storing the specimens before testing, they should be stored as tissue blocks of such a size that the specimens are well protected by the surrounding tissues. They should be dissected out from the tissue blocks just before the testing.

The environment, in which the "naked" specimen is stored and tested, may influence the results significantly. Collagenous tissue swells in water, least at physiological pH. It swells more markedly in acid solutions, whereby the stiffness of the tissue decreases markedly [86]. It should be noted that the tissue swells also in physiological saline, which results in larger maximum strain values (and thereof higher failure energy values) while in loading--unloading experiments a larger residual deformation is found [32, 81]. Also storing in dextran solution (10%) and blood plasma increase the water content of the tissue [81]. On the other hand, exposure to air causes loss of water, which stiffens the specimen [14,16,86] and may in time-consuming testing sequences introduce a systematic bias. This can be avoided by keeping the relative humidity higher than 65 per cent (at 21 ^{o}C) [81], while it is sufficient to provide a cover of saline-moistened gauze for small specimens [23]. It should be concluded on the basis of these data that it is not possible to formulate general rules of procedure. The experimental conditions and their possible effects on the results must be evaluated for every testing programme. This can be examplified by the observation that tissue from aorta can, contrary to tissue from tendons, be stored overnight (at +4 ^{o}C) in buffered Ringer-Krebs-glucose solution without any changes in the mechanical properties of its connective tissues [87].

The temperature during the testing does not seem to be of any greater importance. Rigby et al. [34] found no changes in the mechanical properties of rat tail tendons in the temperature range 0 - - 37 ^{o}C. Others have arrived at similar conclusions [45,46,69,87]. Temperatures above 39 ^{o}C, on the other hand, may influence the mechanical properties of collagen and show as lowering of the stress--strain curve as well as changes in the visco-elastic properties, cf. [88,89]. Such a change at about 40 - 45 ^{o}C is anticipated as it has beeen shown that there is a transition zone for the molecular behavior of collagen in that region [89]. It should be remembered, when a temperature different from the room temperature is chosen, that the in vivo temperature for most tendons is around 28 - 32 ^{o}C, and that only the connective tissues in e.g. blood vessels, liver and spleen have the same temperature as the body core.

Previous stress-strain history of the specimen to be tested
is related to the methodology of testing a specific series as well
as to the general principles of biomechanical testing. The importance of taking previous stress-strain history into account is obvious, when the character of soft connective tissues is considered;
the tissue properties include besides elastic components also viscous ones, some of which are irreversible, as well as plastic ones,
which are always irreversible. Here also minute manipulations of
the specimen may influence the results, provided the resolution of
the measuring equipment is high enough, cf. the data of Tipton et
al. [25] on in situ and in vitro testing differences discussed
above. For a number of experimental programs the specimen is
usually "preconditioned"; this means that by a number of preliminary test cycles the irreversible viscous and plastic components
are eliminated (cf. K_i and ΣY_i in Fig. 8). This is both useful and
necessary, when a number of consecutive tests are to be performed
on the same specimen, as there is a continuous change of specimen
behavior during the initial testing cycles. "Preconditioning"
brings the specimen into the stationary phase of rheological behavior. On the other hand, testing to failure recording of the
stress-strain curve should be performed on "virginal" specimens.
Although the tensile strength of a specimen most probably is not
altered by "preconditioning", the original length is increased and
the strain measurements are thereby affected; probably also the
shape of the toe part of the stress-strain curve is altered, even
when the change in original length is disregarded.

When considering the possible errors in the experimental techniques used, also the characteristics of the testing and measuring
equipment should be evaluated. Most force and displacement transducers are linear within their appropriate ranges of measurement.
It should, however, be remembered that the error of measurement in
transducers as well as in electronic units coupled to them often
is expressed in per cent of maximum ranges. Therefore, when only
a small part of the range is used, the error may become considerable and should always be taken into account. The most often neglected aspect in the evaluation of measurement errors is that introduced by force transducers. From an engineering point of view
the most appropriate mode to measure deformations is to apply the
displacement transducer to the relevant portion of the specimen
in the space between the fixing clamps. This is feasible with
specimens of hard tissues, e.g. bone, but seldom with those of soft
tissues, as safe clamping of the transducer to the specimen is difficult if not impossible. Therefore, in most instances the relevant
portion of the specimen is delineated directly with the fixing
clamps and the deformation of the specimen is measured as the displacement between the stationary and movable ends of the test rig.
The deformations in other parts of the test set-up than the specimen must therefore also be evaluated. Here the deformation in the
force transducer is usually the most important one, as pointed out

by Viidik [90] and discussed in detail by Vrijhoef and Driessens [91]. The principle of most force transducers is to measure with strain gauges fairly small deformations in metal cylinders or rods. These deformations are included in the measurement of total displacement of the test rig. When experiments are performed near the maximum range of the force transducer or when the specimen it-self is fairly stiff such a deformation will influence the measure-ment and result in too large strain and too low elastic stiffness values. The stress-strain curves for force transducers are usually linear and can be compensated for in the analysis of test results. This is especially important when there is a considerable varia-tion in specimen original lengths as force transducer deformation contributes significantly more to the deformation measured for short specimens' than to that for longer ones.

It is the experience of the present author that chart recor-ders using potentiometer controlled chart feeding for the recor-ding of deformation, especially when the in-put system is coupled to the cog wheel system of the materials testing machine, are not reliable enough for the recording of especially loading-unloading cycles. The use of a linear voltage differential transformer, moun-ted as near the fixing clamps as possible, together with a true x-y-recorder or a two-channel strip chart recorder (chart drive as time axis) is recommended as the most reliable recording system for low speed testing. For high speed testing such systems have too low a response time; here an oscilloscope must be used. The present author has found it advantagenous to use a digital storage oscilloscope with an analogue output for replaying the signals at low speed and record the load-deformation curve on an x-y-recor-der. Such an oscilloscope can also be used to record testing at low speed to enable repeated "on-line" analyses of the stress-strain data.

For high speed testing also the performance of the transducers must be considered. While the differential transformers usually have sufficient capacity, most force transducers, based on strain gauges, are inadequate. Here transducers using piezo-electric ele-ments must be employed. It must, however, be remembered that their capacity to record a constant force is limited to short time inter-vals and they can therefore not be used for low speed and complex program testing.

5. BIOMECHANICS OF COMPLEX TISSUES

A tissue can be complex with regard to (i) its geometry, (ii) its composition, or (iii) both. In the most strict sense none of the tissues discussed so far is "simple", i.e. consisting solely of parallel-fibred collagen. Muscle tendons and joint ligaments con-tain small amounts of ground substance and there are some, mostly

minor, irregularities in their fiber arrangement. For practical
purposes they can, however, be regarded as parallel-fibred collagenous tissues, as enzymatic removal of the small amount ground
substance present does not alter their stress-strain characteristics significantly [73,74] and "preconditioning" augments the
parallel alignment of the fibers (vide supra 3). So at least data
on the stationary phase of the rheological behavior is that of
parallel-fibred collagenous tissue. When an isolated specimen is
tested the only remaining source of error, besides those discussed in the section on experimental techniques, is that the tissue
is flattened in the clamps and may have, when the inter-clamp
space is too short in relation to the diameter of the specimen,
a dumbbell shaped form to such a degree that it influences the
results of the testing. On the other hand, when bone-ligament-bone
specimens are tested the ligament is not deformed. Here, however,
the specimen is at least theoretically complex and it must be considered to what extents the recorded deformation occurs in the
ligament and the bones respectively. It is obvious from the data
on the mechanical properties of bone (as illustrated in Fig. 1)
that the deformation that occurs in mature bone is negligible compared to that in ligamentous tissue. Cartilaginous epiphyseal plates may, however, when present, influence the measurements, provided the clamps are not especially designed to counter the deformations occurring in the epiphyses, cf. [22,92,93].

Also the question whether the tensile strength recorded from
tests on bone-ligament-bone (or bone-tendon-muscle-bone) specimens
is due to the properties of bone merits attention. In the case
when most specimens fail in the ligament itself, cf. [18,26], the
evaluation may seem easy. It should, however, be questioned, whether this pattern of failure is due to uneven loading of the various fiber bundles in the ligament or to some inherent properties
of the ligamentous tissue (vide supra 2.1). In the opposite case,
i.e. when most specimens fail as tear-off fractures from one of
the bony insertions of the ligament, it is plausable to assume
that the tensile (or breaking) strength measured is that of the
bone in the ligament insertion area. Care should be taken in this
case when the results are interpreted. This can be illustrated with
results from a recent series of experiments in our laboratory [94].
It is known that systemic administration of corticosteroids stiffens
soft connective tissues [95]. Oxlund [94], however, found that,
while the tensile strength of muscle tendons increased after local
corticosteroid application, the strength of ligament insertions
decreased, due to steroid-elicited local osteoporosis. The same
type of strength decrease can be seen after immobilisation [26,96],
a condition causing osteoporosis.

100

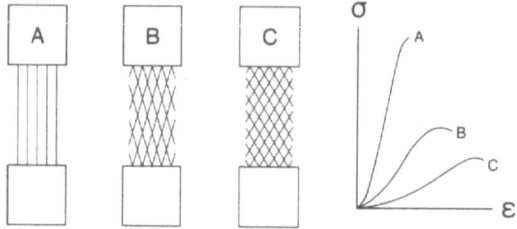

Fig. 13: Theoretical parallel-fibred (A) and meshwork-configurated tissues, of which B is strained along its "main fiber direction" and C is more "neutral". The boxes indicate clamps. To the right the corresponding stress-strain curves.

5.1. Influence of geometrical configuration

The importance of the geometry of a tissue for the mechanical be-havior of it was demonstrated in an uncomplicated way by Bull [97], who compared the elastic or reproducible load-strain behavior of nylon thread with that of nylon fabric. He found the thread to have a linear curve for loading part of the cycle and that the one for the unloading part followed the same curve down again. The curve for the loading of the fabric, on the other hand, was curved towards the strain axis and the curve for unloading was steeper and displaced to the right. A hysteresis was thus displayed by the loading-unloading cycle, probably due to dry friction between the fibers in the fabric. It should be added here that also the shape of the meshwork, i.e. whether the meshes are totally symmetrical or there is a "main fiber direction", influences the shape of the curve. Fig. 13 shows the configurations of and the stress-strain curves for theoretical parallel-fibred and meshwork-configurated tissues. Tissue "A" has a reasonably linear stress-strain curve and the small toe part is either due to alignment of the fibers (assuming the clamping was not quite perfect) or to inherent tis-sue properties. In tissue "B" there is a "main fiber direction", which is the same as that of the tensile testing. The fibers here have the same tensile properties as those in tissue "A". The lower elastic stiffness of tissue "B" is due to the geometrical configu-ration and the lower tensile strength to the fact that when the specimen was cut out some fibers were cut and thus not clamped in both ends for proper load bearing. This is more pronounced for tissue "C", in which the "main fiber direction" is not so accen-tuated, and reflected in the stress-strain curve, which is lower, as the strength exhibited by this tissue is entirely dependent on the friction, cohesion or binding between the fibers in the mesh-work. The displacement of the curve to the right, compared to that

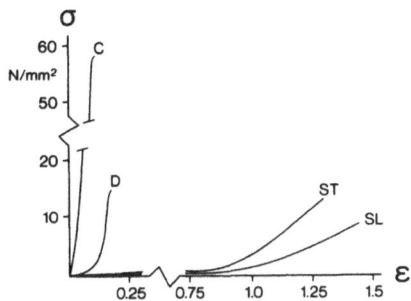

Fig. 14. Stress-strain curves for thoracal skin, tension applied transversally (ST) and longitudinally (SL), compared with tendon (C) and fascia (D). (Adapted from Yamada [7]).

for tissue "B", results from the increased rearrangement of the meshes into the direction of tension application before the fibers themselves (and the factors holding them together) begin to absorb the main part of the tension. The transition between these two processes should, however, be regarded as gradual. It can be concluded from this theoretical discussion that the cutting out of the specimen influences the results of the biomechanical testing, more pronouncedly when the line of "main fiber direction" does not coincide with the length axis of the specimen and/or when the width of the specimen is small.

The same changes in properties are encountered when connective tissues are tested. Harkness [2] found that while the tensile strength calculated in newton per square millimeter of pure collagen varied for parallel-fibred tissue from 150-300 (for tendon) up to 500 (for isolated fibres), that for skin was only 100; for a discussion of mathematical analysis of these differences see Tregear [99]. Galante [81] analysed systematically the influence of fiber direction on specimens from the annulus fibrosus of lumbar intervertebral discs. Here the fibers are arranged in lamellae with their main axes at angles of about 30 degrees to the horizontal plane. He found the tensile strength of specimens with their axes of testing horizontally to be about 3.5 N/mm^2 and that of those with axes along the main fiber direction to be about 9.0 N/mm^2. Galante recalculated his results to pure collagen and arrived at figures in agreement with those of Harkness [2]. Galante further studied elongation, energy absorption and residual deformation parameters and found also these parameters to be highly dependent on the geometrical configuration.

The curve for muscle tendon in Fig. 14 is comparatively steep

102

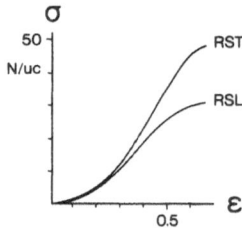

Fig. 15. Stress-strain curves for rat skin, tension applied transversally (RST) and longitudinally (RSL) to strip specimens of dorsal skin. The stress is expressed in newton/mg collagen/mm specimen length. (Adapted from Viidik [6]).

and the toe part inconspicuous, as the strain axis is extended (cf.
Fig. 1). The curve for muscle fascia is less steep and lower; here
the fiber bundles are less parallel-aligned in the direction of
testing. The tissue with most pronounced extensibility in Fig. 14
is skin; when the tension is applied transversally, it is along the
axis of main fiber direction, and when longitudinally at a right
angle to it (cf. [98]). The curve for the latter is, as expected,
lower and more to the right. It should be pointed out here that
the data published on in vitro extensibility of skin vary considerably. Yamada [7] reports the breaking strain for that from the
parietal part of head to be 0.57 and that from axillary fossa to
be 1.44. Here is also variation between different investigators;
the mean value for skin from upper abdomen is according to Yamada
[7] 1.26 and Rollhäuser [100] 0.34. They agree, however, somewhat
better on the tensile strength of skin from this locus, reporting
values of 11.3 and 16.1 N/mm^2 respectively. The determination of
the original length of the strip specimen in vitro is probably the
crucial point; the very long and low toe parts of the curves of
Yamada compared to those of Rollhäuser can well explain a major
part of the difference between their results. Fig. 15 shows stress-
strain curves for rat skin, tested in longitudinal and transversal
directions; the method to determine specimen original length described above in section 2.2.(i) has been used. The breaking strain
of rat skin is here about 0.65, while Yamada [7] reports a figure
of 0.92.

So far the influence of the fiber geometry on the mechanical
behavior of tissues with meshwork geometry has been discussed on
the basis of uniaxial testing of strip specimens. These tissues
are, however, two- or three-dimensional in their fiber arrangements
and uniaxial stress application of them, which never occurs in
vivo, results in compression along the two axes at right angles to
the stress direction. A number of methods to measure two-dimensional tensile properties of skin have been designed. Most of these
methods are based on cups applying negative or positive pressure

to a diaphragm of skin and measured the resulting distension. The reports of Dick [101] and Grahame & Holt [102] should be mentioned here; for review and discussion see Viidik [5, 98]. In all these methods the stress application is actually three-dimensional, while the analysis is one-dimensional; this complicates the analysis of experimental results considerably. From a tissue biomechanical point of view the best two-dimensional analysis should use two-axial stress application, as three-axial application is technically impossible because of the small thickness of skin. Such a method was developed by Lanir & Fung [103,104] in spite of considerable technical difficulties. They found that rabbit skin was aniso-tropic in its mechanical properties, as could be expected, but that it probably possesses orthotropic symmetry. A "preconditio-ning" procedure was required but in spite of it the equilibrium was difficult to obtain. Constant strain-rate tests showed the biaxial stress-strain relationship to be non-linear and to have a considerable hysteresis, which is in full agreement with the conceivable behavior of a three-dimensional meshwork of collagen, to which a considerable amount of ground substance (and some ela-stic fibers) are added. Lanir & Fung further demonstrated that similar uniaxial testing resulted in lower stress values and that uniaxial relaxation tests were not true relaxation tests; both phenomena can be attributed to considerable changes in the cross-section dimensions, as compression and release of compression re-spectively are permitted.

Skin is the only connective tissue, which is available for biomechanical investigation with non-invasive techniques. A num-ber of methods have therefore been devised for such in vivo inve-stigations. The main principles have been distension into suction cups, compression of skinfolds or skin against bone surfaces and torque measurement by devices glued to the epidermal surface. There are some limitations inherent in all these methods, since the sub-cutaneous tissue can interfere with the measurements and it is dif-ficult to delineate the area investigated; for review of this to-pic see Viidik [98]. Most of these limitations are seen when quan-tification is attempted. The methods are, however, useful tools for semi-quantitative evaluation of some physical properties, espe-cially from a clinical point of view, i.e. "elasticity", exten-sibility and turgor of the complex of epidermis, dermis and sub-cutaneous tissue. Also some quantity-independent properties and rheological analyses can be performed and some of these methods have been refined in recent years, see Suominen [105] and Wijn [106]

5.2 Influence of non-collagenous tissue components

While about 75 per cent of the dry weight of skin is constituted of collagen, elastin accounts for 2-4 per cent and plays a role

104

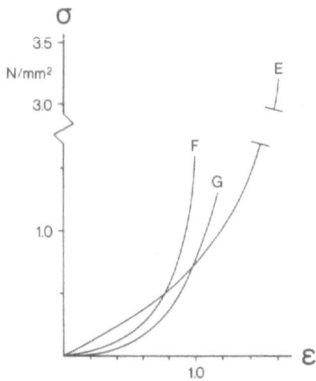

Fig. 16. Stress-strain curves for the rectiform (E) and conjunct
(F) parts of ligamentum nuchae, and abdominal aorta (G), tension
in transverse direction). (Adapted from Yamada [7].

in its biomechanical properties. Studies with enzymatic removal of
elastin [107] suggests that elastic fibers contribute mostly to the
toe part of the stress-strain curve, although it is difficult to
determine to what extent. Crude elastase was used in the above-mentioned study and it has been shown [108,109] that even purified
elastase affects also collagen. It is therefore necessary for the
elucidation of the role of elastin in complex tissues to remove
in successive steps other structures than the highly resistant
elastin and evaluate the changes in the mechanical properties
after each step [110,111]. Ground substance can be removed enzymatically from skin without changes in the stress-strain behavior
[108,109] but the structure is disintegrated when collagen is removed. The role of elastin in complex tissues has therefore been
studied most extensively in elastic ligaments and arteries.

The mechanical properties of ligamentum nuchae, an elastic
ligament, are markedly different from those of a collagenous ligament or tendon (Fig. 16, cf. Fig. 1). The tensile strength is in
the range of 1.6 - 3.2 N/mm^2 compared to 50 - 80 N/mm^2 and the
breaking strain is 0.99 - 1.60 compared to about 0.10 (according
to Yamada [7]). Fig. 16 also shows for strip specimens from aorta
a static stress-strain curve, which is similar. These curves do
not show the mechanical properties of elastin per se as both tissues contain considerable amounts of collagen (Table II). In spite
of this it seems that the tissue from ligamentum nuchae is more
elastic (i.e. containing less viscous and plastic components) than
collagenous tissue as Wood [114] found consecutive stress-strain
curves to follow the same line up to a strain level of 0.30 - 0.40.
Carton et al. [115] tested single fibers from ligamentum nuchae in
an attempt to minimize the influence of collagen as well as the

Table II

Fiber content in per cent of dry weight

	collagen	elastin	
Human aorta	12-24	28-32	[2,112]
Lig. nuchae	16.3	71.3	[113]

position of the elastic fibers in the meshwork. They found the
stress-strain curve to have an exponential form and the maximum
strain to be about 1.20, somewhat more·for larger and more colla-
gen-containing specimens. They could not, however, eliminate the
influence of collagen completely, as also single fibers contain
some collagen. Several methods to purify collagen have been developed. It seems that from biochemical and morphological (evaluated by scanning electron microscopy) points of view a combined
guanidine and collagenase treatment is both mild and efficient
[116]. Hot alkali yielded almost as good results but may have caused a slight disturbance of the amino acid sequences in the terminal groups. Formic acid treatment, on the other hand, was less
efficient for purification and disturbed the molecular structure
significantly. Mechanical tests on strips from ligamentum nuchae
[116] showed that the breaking str·in was reduced from over 0.80
to about 0.60 with the three abovementioned purification procedures and that formic acid treatment reduced the stress levels reached to about half of those recorded after the hot alkali and com-
binded guanidine-collagenase treatments. Fig. 17 shows the curve
for formic acid treated specimens compared with native ones. It

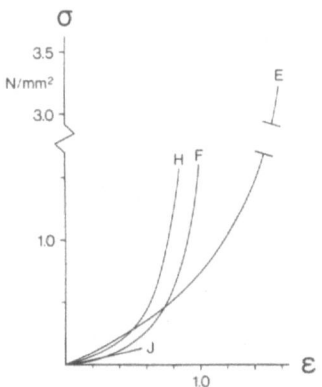

Fig. 17. Stress-strain curves for the two parts (E,F) of ligamentum nuchae (from Fig. 16) together with curves for untreated (H)
and formic acid incubated (J) ligamentum nuchae specimens (adapted from Minns et al. [117]).

106

Tabel III

Elastic stiffness at ε = 0.2. (Data from Minns et al. [117]).

"Pure" elastin (aorta)   0.081 N/mm^2

"Pure" elastin (lig. nuchae)   0.069 N/mm^2

Elastic fiber (Carton)   0.045 N/mm^2

is worthwhile to note that the stiffness of isolated elastic fibers
is reported to be lower than that of biochemically purified elastic
tissue (Table III), which is contrary to the properties of collagen
(the fibers being stronger than larger structural units). The significance of this observation is at present not clear.

    Elaborate methods to remove one component at a time from aor-
tic tissue have been developed by Hoffman and co-workers [110,111,
118]. They removed the ground substance by incubating the specimens
in hyaluronidase or hyaluronidase and β-glucuronidase and found the
stress in the initial part of the stress-strain curve increased,
which suggests that the ground substance has a lubricating effect.
After treatment with bacterial collagenase the tensile strength
was drastically reduced (Figs. 18-19) while the stress in the initial part of the curve was only slightly reduced, i.e. by 13 per
cent at the strain of 0.15. It is interesting to note here that
stress-relaxation at this strain level was absent after the collagenase treatment, while it was increased after removal of the ground

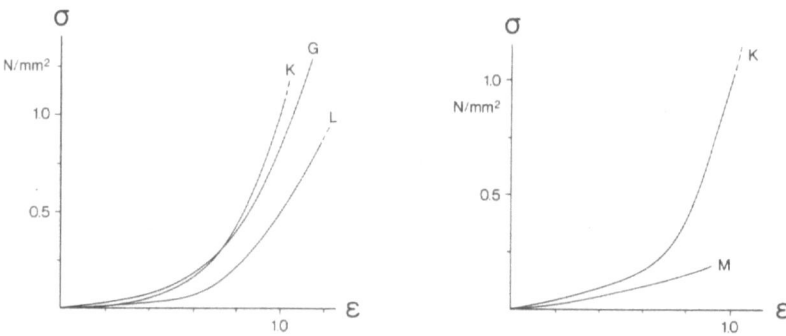

Fig. 18. (Left) Stress-strain curve for aorta (G) from Fig. 16 together with curves for untreated specimens of aorta (K, L) (adapted from Hoffman et al. [110]).

Fig. 19. (Right) Stress-strain curves for aorta. An untreated specimen (K) is compared with one incubated in collagenase (M) (From
Hoffman et al. [110]).

107

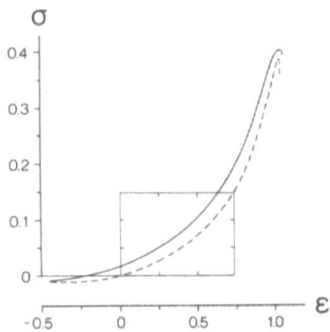

Fig. 20. Stress-strain curves for ring-shaped specimens from rabbit aorta. The solid curve is from a specimen stimulated by 0.1 mM norepinephrine added to the buffered Ringer-Krebs-glucose solution. The dashed curve is after paralysis by 0.2 mM papaverine sulphate.. "Stress" is expressed in load (newton) per unit specimen width. The normal blood pressure of 100 mm Hg would create a force of 0.06 newton in this specimen. (From Viidik et al. [87]).

substance. It seems therefore that the stress-relaxation to a large extent can be attributed to the collagen fibers or meshwork. The collagen contributes thus successively more to the stress-strain curve with increasing strain level. In these series of experiments the breaking strain after collagenase treatment was about 0.90, while that of native samples reached about 1.20. Hoffman et al. [111] suggests that collagen and elastin networks are "interweaving" so that the elastin network is forced to stretch around crimped collagen fibers. This would result in a higher stress also at low strain levels; a decrease can be seen when collagen is removed enzymatically. This concept is supported by the observations that tissues, from which collagen is removed not only break at considerably lower stress values but also at strain values, which are significantly lower than those found for native tissues as well as those for single elastic fibers [108,109,111,116,117]. It is also supported by the observation that collagen seems necessary to maintain and restore the geometrical configuration of the elastic network in tissues [119].

There is one further component with biomechanical implications in the arterial wall, the system of smooth muscle cells. They are intricately interrelated with the elastin and collagen networks from a morphological point of view (for review see Milch [120]). Their function from a mechanical point of view seems to be purely regulatory within rather small margins. This is illustrated in Fig. 20, which compares the stress-strain curves after stimulation by norepinephrine and after paralysis by papaverine.

It is beyond the scope of this chapter to discuss the mechanical properties of arteries comprehensively, see e.g. [121-124], and the background for and details of the properties of elastin, see e.g. [125-127].

6. CONCLUDING REMARKS

We have to-day a good and reasonably detailed knowledge of the biomechanics of mature collagenous tissues, especially regarding tendons, ligaments and skin. In these tissues the collagen is of Type I and extensively cross-linked. The correlation between the function and molecular structure of these tissues starts to emerge. An important question here is how changes in the cross-linking is related to the increasing strength and stiffness, which occurs with maturation and aging. The correlation between function and structure on supramolecular level is understood but the role of the elastic fibers in skin warrants further investigations. The difficulty here is obvious: the elastic fibers are very resistant and other tissue components are harmed, when the removal of them is attempted and at the same time the elastic network is too fragile, when collagen is removed.

There are also other types of collagen with important mechanical functions. Type II is that of cartilage and nothing is known about the mechanical characteristics of its fibers per se. Type III is important in embryonic skin and in the arteries. Physico-chemical data show that this collagen is very stable and resistant. Also for this type of collagen we lack knowledge of the mechanical properties, as it is found in the tissues mixed with Type I. It is possible to extract, purify and reconstitute it for mechanical testing. It is, however, very stable and its cross-linking includes disulphide and ketoimine bonds. It has been purified only after pepsin digestion, a procedure, which removed the telopeptides and thereby the cross-linking sites. Consequently the reconstituted fibers would have characteristics profoundly different from those of native fibers.

Information on the properties of elastin increases steadily and sequential removal of tissue components has proved to be a valuable tool in this type of research. Investigations on the correlation of function and structural properties are hampered by our limited knowledge of its structural organisation. At present it is not possible to make such correlations for the molecular structure level. For such investigations prevention of cross-linking by lathyrogenic agents may well prove to become a useful tool. Also for higher levels of structural organisation further data on the correlation between morphology and function are needed. Here, however, the necessary tools of investigation are available.

There remain thus questions to be answered before a comprehensive picture on the biomechanical properties of the various connective tissues is completed. It must not be forgotten that connective tissues are present thorughout the body except the central nervous system. They are important mechanically in most tissues and organs. For some of them data are already emerging, i.e. the lung [128-130]. Others, e.g. the urinary bladder and the various parts of the intestinal tract, are still virtually terrae incognitae.

REFERENCES

1. F.G. Evans, Mechanical properties of bone, Charles C Thomas, Springfield, Ill., 1973.
2. R.D. Harkness, Biol.Rev. 36: 399-463, 1961.
3. R.D. Harkness, In: Treatise on collagen, (B.S. Gould, ed.), Vol. II A, pp. 247-310. Academic Press, New York, 1968.
4. D.H. Elliott, Biol.Rev. Cambridge Phil. Soc. 40: 392-421, 1965.
5. A. Viidik, In: International review of connective tissue research, (D.A. Hall & D.S. Jackson eds.), Vol. VI, pp. 127-215. Academic Press, New York, 1973.
6. A. Viidik, Verh.Anat.Ges. 72: 75-89, 1978.
7. H. Yamada, In: Strength of biological materials, (F.G. Evans, ed.), Williams & Wilkins, Baltimore, Maryland, 1970.
8. G.N. Ramachandran (ed.), Treatise on collagen Vol. I, Academic Press, New York, 1967.
9. B.S. Gould, (ed.), Treatise on collagen Vol. II, Part A and B, Academic Press, New York, 1968a,b.
10. A. Viidik & J. Vuust, (eds.), Biology of Collagen, Academic Press, London, in press 1979.
11. G.N. Ramachandran & A.H. Reddi, (eds.), Biochemistry of collagen, Plenum Press, New York, 1976.
12. D.H. Elliott & G.N.C. Crawford, Proc.Roy.Soc.Ser. B 162: 137-146, 1965.
13. S.A.V. Swanson, In: Advances in biomedical engineering, (R.M. Kenedi, ed.), Vol. I, pp. 137-187. Academic Press, London, 1971.
14. K. Stucke, Arch.klin.Chir. 265: 579-599, 1950.
15. A.E. Cronkite, Anat.Rec. 64: 173-186, 1936
16. H.G. Wertheim, Chim.Phys. 21, 385-414, 1847.
17. M. Takigawa, cited by Yamada [7], 1953.
18. T. Barfred, Acta Pathol.Microbiol.Scand.Sec. A 79: 287-292, 1971.
19. P.E. McMaster, J. Bone Jt.Surg. 15: 705-722, 1933.
20. L. Davidsson, Ann.Chir.Gynaec.Fenn. 45: 103-113, 1956.
21. A. Viidik, Acta orthop.scand. 40: 261-272, 1969.
22. A. Viidik, L. Sandqvist & M. Mägi, Acta orthop.scand. Suppl. 79, 1965.

110

23. A. Viidik, In: Studies on the anatomy and function of bone and joints, (F.G. Evans ed.), pp. 17-39, Springer Verlag, Heidelberg, 1966.

24. C.M. Tipton, R.J. Schild & R.J. Tomanek, Amer.J.Physiol. 212: 783-787, 1967.

25. C.M. Tipton, R.D. Matthes & D.S. Sandage, J. Appl.Physiol. 37: 758-61, 1974.

26. F.R. Noyes, P.J. Torvik, W.B. Hyde & J.L. DeLucas, J. Bone Jt.Surg. 56: 1406-1418, 1974.

27. M. Chvapil, Z. Hruza & Z. Roth, Gerontologia 6: 102, 1962.

28. H.R. Elden, In: International review of connective tissue research, (D.A. Hall & D.S. Jackson eds.), Vol. IV, pp. 283-347, 1968.

29. P.F. Millington, T. Gibson, J.H. Evans & J.C. Barbenel, In: Advanc.Biomed.Eng. (R.M. Kenedi ed.), Vol. I, pp. 189-248, Academic Press, London, 1971.

30. A. Viidik & R. Ekholm, Zschr.Anat.Entw.-gesch. 127: 154-164, 1968.

31. A. Viidik, Zschr.Anat.Entw.-gesch. 136: 204-212, 1972.

32. A. Viidik & T. Lewin, Acta Orthop.Scand. 37: 141-155, 1966.

33. A.A. Glaser, R.D. Marangoni, J.S. Must, T.G. Beckwith, G.S. Brody, G.R. Walker & W.L. White, Med.Electron.Biol.Engng. 3: 411-419, 1965.

34. C.J. Rigby, N. Hirai, J.D. Spikes & H. Eyring. J.gen.Physiol. 43: 265-283, 1959.

35. M.M. LaBan, Arch.phys.Med.Rehabil. 43: 461-466, 1962.

36. J.D. Van Brocklin & D.G. Ellis, Arch.phys.Med. 46: 369-373, 1965.

37. H. Rollhäuser, Gegenbaurs morph.Jb. 90: 157-179, 1950a.

38. J.W. Smith, J.Anat. (Lond.) 88: 369-380, 1954.

39. A. Viidik, J. Biomechanics 1: 3-11, 1968.

40. G. Annovazzi, Arch.Sci.biol. (Napoli) 11: 467-502, 1928.

41. D.G. Fantuzzo & G Graziati, In: Proc. Digest 7th Intern. Conf.Med.Biol.Engng., (B. Jacobson ed.) p. 506, Stockholm, 1967.

42. M. Zech & G. Arnold, Verh.Anat.Ges. 69: 771-775, 1975.

43. R. McN. Alexander, J.exp.Biol. 39: 373-386, 1962.

44. T. Alfrey & E.F. Gurnee, In: Tissue Elasticity, (J.W. Remington ed.), pp. 12-32, Amer.Physiol.Sco., Washington, D.C., 1957.

45. J.T. Apter, Cir.Res. 19: 104, 1966.

46. J.T. Apter, In: Biomechanics: Its foundations and objectives, (Y.C. Fung, N. Perrone & M. Anliker, eds.), pp. 217-235, Prentice-Hall, Englewood Cliffs, New Jersey, 1972.

47. E.D. Sedlin, Acta orthop.scand.suppl. 83, 1965.

48. A. Viidik & M. Mägi, In: Proc. Digest 7th Intern.Conf.Med. Biol.Engng., (B. Jacobson ed.), p. 507, Stockholm 1967.

49. M. Frisén, M. Mägi, L. Sonnerup & A. Viidik, J.Biomechanics 2: 13-20, 1969.

50. M. Frisén, M. Mägi, L. Sonnerup & A. Viidik, J. Biomechanics 2: 21-28, 1969.
51. A. Viidik & J. Melvin, unpublished data.
52. L. Stryer, Biochemistry, pp. 214-215, W.H. Freeman and Company, San Francisco 1975.
53. B.L. Trus & K.A. Piez, J.Mol.Biol. 108: 705-732, 1976.
54. K.A. Piez & B.L. Trus, J.Mol.Biol. 110: 701-704, 1977.
55. A.J. Bailey, Pathol.Biol.(Paris) 22: 675-80, 1974.
56. A.J. Bailey, S.P. Robins & G. Balin, Nature 251: 105-109, 1974.
57. A.J. Bailey & S.P. Robins, Sci.Prog.Oxf. 63: 419-444, 1976.
58. J.C. Anderson, Scand.J.Clin.Lab.Invest. 29: Suppl. 123, p. 4, 1972.
59. J.C. Anderson & D.S. Jackson, Scand.J.Clin.Lab.Invest. 29: Suppl. 123, p. 4, 1972.
60. B.R. Olsen, Z.Zellforsch.Mikrosk.Anat. 59: 199-213, 1963.
61. R.S. Bear, J.Amer.chem.Soc. 66, 1297-1305, 1944.
62. P.M. Cowan, A.C.T. North & J.T. Randall, Symp.Soc.exp.Biol. 9: 115-126, 1955.
63. K.H. Gustavson, The chemistry and reactivity of collagen, Academic Press, New York, 1956.
64. A. Viidik, T. Andreassen, N. Busted & H. Oxlund, Geron, Helsinki, 21: 16-27, 1976.
65. M.L. Tanzer, In: International review of connective tissue research, (D.A. Hall ed.), Vol. III, pp. 91-112. Academic Press, New York, 1965.
66. N.D. Light & A.J. Bailey, In: Biology of Collagen, (A. Viidik & J. Vuust eds.), Academic Press, London, in press 1979.
67. M. Abrahams, Med.Biol.Eng. 5: 433-443, 1967.
68. C.H. Barnett, D.V. Davies & M.A. MacConaill, Synovial joints - their structure and mechanics, Longmans, Green, New York, 1961.
69. H. Riedl & Th. Nemetschek, Molekularstruktur und mechanisches Verhalten von Kollagen, Springer-Verlag, Berlin, 1977.
70. V. Mohanaradhakrishnan & N. Ramanathan, Leather Sci. 12: 12-20, 1965.
71. H.G. Vogel, J.Med. 7: 177-187, 1976.
72. A. Viidik, In: Thule International Symposia: Aging of connective and skeletal tissue, (A. Engel & T. Larsson eds.), pp. 125-148, Nordiska Bokhandeln, Stockholm, 1969.
73. F.S. Steven, R.J. Minns & J.B. Finlay, Injury 6: 317-319, 1975.
74. H. Oxlund & T. Andreassen, in preparation.
75. L.B. Walker, E.H. Harris & J.V. Benedict. Med.Electron.Biol. Engin. 2: 31-38, 1964.
76. A. Viidik, Biomedical Engng. 2: 64-67, 1967.
77. A. Viidik, In: Vth European Symposium on Basic Research in Gerontology, (U.J. Schmidt et al. eds.), pp. 271-284. Perimed Verlag, Erlangen, 1977.
78. D.G. Wright & D.C. Rennels, J.Bone Jt.Surg. 46: 482-492, 1964.
79. E.D. Compton, J.Amer.Leather Chem.Ass. 44: 140-151, 1949.

80. M.D. Ridge & V. Wright, In: Biomechanics and related bio-engineering topics (R.M. Kenedi ed.), pp. 165-175, Pergamon Press, Oxford, 1965.
81. J.O. Galante, Acta orthop.Scand. 38: Suppl 100, 1967.
82. A. Nachemson, Acta orthop.Scand. Suppl. 43: 1960.
83. D.H. Curtis, The effect of chemical crosslinking agents on the mechanical properties of rat-tail tendon. University Microfilms, Ann Arbor, 1963.
84. H.R. Elden, J.Gerontol. 19: 173-178, 1964.
85. P.L. Blanton & N.L. Biggs, J. Biomech. 3: 181-189, 1970.
86. H. Rollhäuser, Gegenbaurs Jahrb. 90: 180-191, 1950.
87. A. Viidik, A. Björkerud & G. Bondjers, in preparation.
88. C.G. Warren, J.F. Lehmann & J.N. Koblanski, Arch.Phys.Med. Rehabil. 52: 465-474, 1971.
89. P. Mason & B.J. Rigby, Biochim.biophys. Acta 66: 448-450, 1963.
90. A. Viidik, Acta Physiol.Scand. 74: 372-380, 1968.
91. M.M.A. Vrijhoef & F.C.M. Driessens, J. Biomech. 4: 233-238, 1971.
92. Å. Rundgren, Acta Physiol.Scand.Suppl. 417, 1974.
93. E. Morscher, Reconstruct.Surg.Traumatol.10: 1968.
94. H. Oxlund, in preparation.
95. H.G. Vogel, Connect.Tissue Res. 2: 177-182, 1974.
96. C.M. Tipton, R.D. Matthes, J.A. Maynard & R.A. Carey, Med. Sci. Sports 7: 165-175, 1975.
97. H.B. Bull, In: Tissue elasticity, pp. 33-42, American Physiological Society, Washington, 1957.
98. A. Viidik, In: Frontiers in matrix biology, (L. Robert ed.), Vol. I, pp. 157-189, Karger, Basel, 1973.
99. R.T. Tregear, Physical functions of skin, Academic Press, London, 1966.
100. H. Rollhäuser, Gegenbaurs morph.Jb. 90: 249-261, 1950.
101. J.C. Dick, J.Physiol., Lond. 112: 102-113, 1951.
102. R. Grahame & P.J.L. Holt, Gerontologia 15: 121-139, 1969.
103. Y. Lanir & Y.C. Fung, J. Biomech. 7: 29-34, 1974.
104. Y. Lanir & Y.C. Fung, J. Biomech. 7: 171-182, 1974.
105. H. Suominen, Effects of physical training in middle-aged and elderly people. University of Jyväskylä, Jyväskylä, 1978.
106. P.F.F. Wijn, A.J.M. Brakkee & A.J.H. Vendrik, In: Proc. 1st Intern.Conf. Mech.Med.Biol., Aachen, 1978
107. C.H. Daly, Proc. 8th Int. Conf. on Mech. Biol. Engng., Tokyo 1969, p. 18-7; cited by Millington et al. 1971 [29].
108. A. Viidik, H. Oxlund & T. Andreassen, In: Proc. 3rd. Intern. Cong. Biorheol., La Jolla, 187-188, 1978.
109. H. Oxlund & T. Andreassen, in preparation.
110. A.S. Hoffman, L.A. Grande & J.B. Park, Biomat., Med. Dev., Art. Org. 5: 121-145, 1977.
111. A.S. Hoffman & C.H. Daly, In: Biology of Collagen (A. Viidik & J. Vuust eds.), Academic Press, London, in press 1979.
112. E.G. Cleary, M.D. Thesis, University of Sydney, Australia, 1962.

113. D.S. Jackson, L.B. Sandberg & E.G. Cleary, Biochem. J. 96: 813, 1965.
114. G.C. Wood, Biochim.Biophys. Acta 15: 311-324, 1954.
115. R.W. Carton, J. Dainauskas & J.W. Clark, J.Appl.Physiol. 17: 547-551, 1962.
116. F.S. Steven, R.J. Minns & H. Thomas, Connect.Tissue Res. 2: 85-90, 1974.
117. R.J. Minns, P.D. Soden & D.S. Jackson, J. Biomech. 6: 153-165, 1973.
118. A.S. Hoffman, L.A. Grande, P. Gibson, J.B. Park, C.H. Daly, P. Bornstein & R. Ross, In: Perspectives in Biomed. Engng. (R.M. Kenedi ed.) pp. 173-176, The Macmillan Press Ltd, London, 1973.
119. R.J. Minns & F.S. Steven, Micron. 5: 127-133, 1974.
120. R.A. Milch, Monogr.Surg.Sci. 2: 261-341, 1965.
121. D.H. Bergel & D.L. Schultz, Progr.Biophys.Mol.Biol. 22: 1-36, 1971.
122. M.G. Sharma & T.M. Hollis, J. Biomech. 9: 293-300, 1976.
123. S.C. Ling & C.H. Chow, J. Biomech. 10: 71-77, 1977.
124. K. Fronek & Y.C. Fung, In: CRC Handbook of Engineering in Medicine and Biology Sec. B Instruments and Measurements (B.N. Feinberg & D.G. Fleming eds.) Vol I, pp. 195-200, CRC Press Inc., Palm Beach, Fl. 1978.
125. J.M. Grosline, In: International review of connective tissue research, (D.A. Hall & D.S. Jackson eds.), Vol VII, pp. 211-249, Academic Press, New York, 1976.
126. C.A.J. Hoeve & P.J. Flory, Biopolymers 13: 677-686, 1974.
127. L. Gotte, M. Mammi & G. Pezzin, In: Symposium on fibrous proteins, (W.G. Crewther ed.), pp. 236-245, Butterworths, Australia, 1968.
128. T. Sugihara, J. Hildebrandt & C.J. Martin, J.Appl.Physiol. 33: 93-98, 1972.
129. R.M. Senior, D.R. Bielefeld & M.K. Abensohn, Am.Rev.Respir. Dis.111: 184-188, 1975.
130. G.L. Snider & J.B. Karlinsky, Pathobiol.Annu. 7: 115-142, 1977.

BIOMECHANICAL ASPECTS OF PLASTIC SURGERY

Professor Tom Gibson

Regional Director, Glasgow and West of
Scotland Regional Plastic and Maxillofacial
Surgery Service, Canniesburn Hospital,
Bearsden, Glasgow, and Visiting Professor of
Bioengineering, University of Strathclyde,
Glasgow, Scotland.

Plastic surgery is a rather ill-defined specialty
concerned with the reconstruction and transplantation
not only of skin and subcutaneous tissue but also of
the supporting tissues, cartilage, bone, fascia and
fat and the activating structures, muscle and tendon.
It is indeed a somewhat specialised brand of
structural engineering in which the materials possess
certain unique properties. They are self-reparative,
self-generating and self-adhering. These biological
characteristics are well known, relatively well
understood and put to good use in every surgical
operation. Biological properties are however in a
sense four-dimensional; they require time in which
to occur. At any instant of time and often indeed
during short intervals, the biological activities
of the body tissues may be ignored and it is then
perfectly justifiable to regard them purely as
materials with precisely measurable structural
engineering characteristics. However, a surgeon's
training today will hardly enable him to read an
elementary electronic circuit or understand the
simplest mechanical analysis. Excisional ablative
surgery does not ask that he should; a competent
technique and the vis medicatrix naturae are all
that are required for "successful" results. On
the other hand, reconstructive surgery, while it
has made striking advances by trial and error alone,

has now reached the stage where far more precise
information of many factors - structural,
mechanical and biological - must be gained before
further progress is made. With long experience
a plastic surgeon develops an instinctive
appreciation of the material characteristics of
the tissues he handles. The amount that skin
will "stretch" for example, the design of flaps,
or the line in which the central limb of a
Z-plasty will finally lie, become intuitive if
occasionally inaccurate and unreliable. But an
engineer would consider it absurd to design a
structure without full knowledge of the mechanical
behaviour of the materials he was about to use; yet
reconstructive surgery is still based on empirical
and imprecise data. It is facile to describe and
excuse this as being "art" rather than "science";
the highest artistry demands a complete understanding
of the materials employed.

Every plastic surgical operation involves the
manipulation of skin and most of the lecture will
deal with the mechanical and related characteristics
of skin. A final section will be devoted to
cartilage which is a useful skeletal support and
has quite different characteristics.

THE TENSIONS NORMALLY PRESENT IN THE SKIN

The various degrees of tension which are present in
the skin at the site of a plastic surgical operation
are important not only in so far as they permit or
prevent the manipulation of the skin, but also in
the type of scarring which results. Most - but not
all - of the body skin exists in tension; when cut,
the wound edges retract. There are, however,
enormous individual variations: between youth and
age; between the slim and the corpulent; and
between the slim who has always been slim and the
slim who once was fat. It is the variations in
skin tension in the same individual, however,
which are of most interest to the plastic surgeon:
those which occur in different directions at the
same site, and the wide range of tensions in
different sites.

The directional quality of skin tension is well
known, and the importance of siting incisions along
lines of maximum tension, well recognised. The
lines of maximum tension parallel the crease lines

of the body since a crease will only form if the tension at right angles to it is minimal. Wounds made across these tension lines are much more likely to produce a stretched or hypertrophic scar than those which parallel them.

In 1861 Karl Langer, an anatomist in Vienna, published some research in which he stabbed cadavers all over the body with a sharp pointed, round bodied instrument. In most places this produced a cleft in the skin and the clefts formed themselves into lines running in various but predictable directions. These cleavage lines lie in the directions of minimum extensibility. At first there was doubt if they were also lines of tension. This was because Langer's original paper could not be found because the reference copied from paper to paper was wrong. The "lines" had also been redrawn many times and some had come to cross crease lines and thus could not be tension lines. However, Langer's paper was finally discovered in a library in Prague and in addition, others of his works, which proved conclusively that the cleavage lines were also tension lines. While such information is valuable it is but qualitative; we have yet to find a technique for measuring precisely the amount of tension at any point on the surface of the body.

The variation in tension in different sites of the body is striking. On the face, areas of taut skin and lax skin alternate in a fairly characteristic way. The skin is lax, for example, between the eyebrows and just below the temple lateral to the eye; it is taut on the cheek and in a horizontal direction on the forehead. The size of a skin defect which can be closed directly therefore varies from site to site. One of the refinements of the art of plastic surgery has been the design of local flaps which will transfer a skin defect uncloseable in an area of taut skin to an area of lax skin where it may be sutured directly. Alexander A. Limberg of Leningrad analysed certain mathematical and mechanical aspects of such local flaps which demonstrate the forces involved in the manipulation and many of the factors on which successful design depends. The basis of his study, however, has been paper models and the results obtained on such a nonextensile material are not exactly transferable to skin, which, in addition to the varying tensions,

118

also possesses varying degrees of "rigidity" or
"extensibility". Similar criticisms apply to
formulae for the Z-plasty which depend on the
mathematics of plane rigid surfaces.

THE EFFECT OF INCREASED TENSION ON SKIN

Clinically one can distinguish four quite different
effects on skin subjected to increased tension.

1.   Blanching and subsequent necrosis. When
increasing tension is applied to skin there comes
a point at which the skin blanches as the capillary
patency is obliterated. This blanching tension is
fairly precisely measurable; it varies with the
blood pressure and with the vascularity of the part.
It is familiar to all and if allowed to persist
will produce necrosis. In a skin flap the blood
supply is already impaired and quite a small amount
of increased tension may lead to a zone of blanching
across the flap and necrosis of all the distal area.

2.   Rupture of the dermis. Tensions which are not
great enough to cause blanching may, if long
continued, rupture the dermis causing the striae
which occur in the abdominal skin of many women
during pregnancy. Striae are seen elsewhere on
rapidly enlarging breasts and over the buttocks,
thighs and shoulders in the increasing adiposity
of Cushing's disease. It has been suggested that
they are in part due to adrenal cortical hyper-
activity even in pregnancy. This may be so but
they still occur in skin subjected to increased
tension and striae have been reported in patients
with normal adrenal cortical activity, e.g. over
the muscles of young men taking "body building"
exercises. Langer showed that his cleavage lines
were imposed on the body by the infants' movements
during its first year and the only factor which
will change them is a rapid increase in the volume
of the contents enclosed by the skin, e.g. in
pregnancy. Of course not all parous women have
striae; in some the extensibility of their
abdominal skin seems adequate for the emergency.

3.   Permanent stretching of skin. At tensions
insufficient to produce striae, skin will stretch
permanently and often to three or four times its
normal length. This lateral extension is a feature
of slowly increasing adiposity or oedema and is a

fascinating phemonenon since if it could be
accomplished artificially, much of the need for
skin grafting would disappear.

4. Persisting increased tension with no effect on
    normal skin. If increasing fat or fluid
underneath the skin can cause permanent stretching
one may well ask why scar contractures for example
do not induce the surrounding skin to stretch and
make good the defect. Most plastic surgeons who
have used the method of multiple-staged excision
of facial naevi will have noted the persistence of
increased tension in the skin; when the scar of
the previous excision is removed, the wound retracts
apparently to its original shape. We have made
measurements in one such case in a four-year-old
boy on three occasions at yearly intervals; while
the tension persisting in the skin was still above
normal, a certain amount of relaxation and stretch
had occurred.

THE EXTENSIBILITY OF SKIN

When skin is increasingly stretched the extension
curve which results may be considered to have three
parts, an initial flat portion in which considerable
extension occurs from the application of very little
force, an intermediate portion or elbow where the
direction is changing rapidly, and a terminal almost
vertical portion where very little extension occurs
even with great increase in load. There are many
variations in this basic curve: e.g. at different
sites on the same body; at the same site on
different bodies; in different directions at the
same site. The directional variations are to allow
joint movements without resistance within the normal
range of the joint. Skin extensibility is greatest
in infancy; as the individual ages it is replaced
by laxity which of course still allows free joint
movements but is much less attractive.

THE MOBILE FIBROUS NETWORK OF THE DERMIS

From an engineering point of view, skin does not
behave as a homogeneous material. Rather it is to
be regarded as a series of networks, the varying
pattern of which underlies its mechanical
characteristics. There are five major network
systems in the dermis composed of collagen fibres,
elastic fibres, capillaries, lymphatics and nerve

fibrils. It is with the fibrous network that we are mainly concerned but the others are intimately entwined through it and deformation of the fibres may produce blanching, oedema, or pain. In the interstices of the various networks lies the "interstitial fluid" whose composition is constantly changing but which always contains a proportion of mucopolysaccharides.

THE COLLAGEN FIBRE NETWORK. In an ordinary section of human skin, the collagen fibres of the dermis are apparently arranged haphazardly; such skin is fully relaxed before fixation. If, however, the skin is held in a stretched position during fixation, a proportion of the fibres will be found orientated along the line of stretch; at high loads practically all the fibres are so aligned, at low loads, only a few. No matter in which direction the skin is stretched, the same orientation results. The scanning electron microscope confirms this in a much more three dimensional way.

The collagen fibres are very long structures compared to their diameter; they may be teased out of unfixed skin and show no evidence of any firm attachments between the adjacent fibre bundles which seem free to move relative to each other. The collagen fibre pattern is therefore an intertwined network of fibres so arranged that if stretched in any direction most of the fibres will eventually become parallel along the line of stretch. There are many such arrangements possible; a knitted fabric is a common example but the pattern of skin is much more complex and variable.

The collagen network behaviour explains the shape of the stress-strain curves of skin. At low loads the collagen fibres move easily relative to each other; in other words, relaxed skin can be readily stretched - so far. As more and more fibres become aligned and "take up the strain" the resistance to further extension rapidly increases. The strength and relatively inextensible nature of fully orientated collagen is well illustrated by tendons, and fully stretched skin is a structure with comparable characteristics.

One interesting discovery was that stretched

collagen fibres change their staining reaction.
Relaxed collagen fibres stain green with the
Masson-Goldner trichrome method; when stretched
they stain red. This change persists for some
time in skin after the stretching force has been
released and it is thus possible to pick out
histologically those fibres which have been
stretched.

It has been shown that the gap between the cross
striations of the collagen molecule increased
as skin is stretched and this accompanies the
change in staining.

THE ELASTIC FIBRE NETWORK. In relaxed skin, many
of the elastic fibres in the dermis are looped
spirally around collagen fibres. End-to-side
junctions of the elastic fibres are also common,
and probably provide fixed points from which the
fibres may act. When skin is stretched, elastic
fibres also become aligned in the direction of
stretch and lie sandwiched between the collagen
fibres.

Elastica fulfills the same purpose in skin as it
does elsewhere, i.e., it acts like a spring or
more precisely as an energy storage device to
return the stretched collagen to its relaxed
position. In order to fulfill this function there
must be sufficient interstitial fluid available to
refill the relaxed network since fluid is
displaced from the dermis as the fibres become
fully orientated.

THE INTERSTITIAL FLUID plays an important part in
determining the mechanical characteristics of
skin. It is the medium in which the networks
move, acting as lubricant on the one hand and
buffer against too sudden change on the other.
Time is required to move fluid from one point
to another and this is probably one reason for
the "time-dependence" (see below) of the
behaviour of skin under tension. Increase in
the amount of interstitial fluid in inflammation,
during wound healing or injection of a local
anaesthetic, increases the resistance of skin to
deformation in terms of the force required to
deform.

122

THE TIME-DEPENDENCE OF SKIN DEFORMATION

If a piece of skin in vitro is suddenly stretched
a certain amount and held in that position, it is
found that the force required to keep it there
decreases with time, a phenomenon known as stress-
relaxation. On the other hand, if a certain load
is suddenly applied to a piece of skin, and the
load maintained constant, the amount of extension
will increase with time, and the skin is said to
"creep".   Creep and stress-relaxation are viscoelastic effects and skin exhibits these to an
increasing degree, the greater the loads being
used. The reasons for them are probably multiple:
the extrusion of fluid from the network, compacting
of the stretched fibres in the deformed network and
perhaps visco-elastic properties in the aggregated
collagen bundles themselves. Visco-elastic effects
are more easily studied in vitro but can be
demonstrated in vivo.   Much more study is required
before their clinical importance can be fully
assessed; there is no doubt, however, that in a
wound or flap stitched under increased tension,
a certain amount of relaxation will occur as the
skin "creeps". Further, by applying a strong
pull to a wound margin, "creep" can again be
produced thus permitting on occasion a wound to
be closed which otherwise would be impossib⁻э.

THE EFFECT OF PRESSURE ON SCARS

In certain varieties of florid or hypertrophic
scars, continuous pressure will hasten their
regression and this is accompanied by a change in
their collagen structure from a nodular to a
laminar pattern.

SOME MECHANICAL PROPERTIES OF CARTILAGE

Cartilage is a prestressed material; in more precise
engineering terms, there exists a system of self-
locked stresses which are nicely balanced in intact
cartilage but which may be released and cause
distortion when cartilage is cut. These inbuilt
stresses have been measured accurately in human
cartilage. Throughout the thickness of costal
cartilage, areas of tension are found to alternate
with areas of compression. To avoid deformation
when carving a cartilage graft, it is obvious that
these forces must remain symmetrically balanced.
Unfortunately no two cartilaginous ribs have the
same distribution or magnitude of forces, and
measurement of the individual forces destroys the
rib. Absolute precision is therefore impossible.

The "balanced cross sections" found by trial and
error however, are a useful approximation, although
it must be stressed that, even when these principles
are strictly adhered to, a small proportion of
grafts may still show a tendency to warp, albeit
much less so than when the principles are ignored;
this is particularly so with tapering sections.

The only absolute way of preventing warping is to
carry out no trimming at all. This is rarely
feasible, but carving should always be kept to a
minimum by selecting for the graft that portion
of cartilage which most nearly approaches the
size and shape required. For example, in seeking
a costal cartilage graft to support the nasal
bridge, the lower margin of the rib cage is
explored through a rectus-splitting incision. The
free-lying cartilaginous tip of the eighth rib is
occasionally so shaped that it may be used intact;
more frequently a little trimming is needed. For
thicker grafts the lower half of the seventh
cartilage usually presents suitably straight
segments.

Like most biological tissues, cartilage also has
visco-elastic properties; time is required before
the maximum deformation occurs. Thus, a cartilage
graft whittled into shape and immediately popped
into a cavity will have warped when the dressings
are later removed. In practice the time required
for a carved piece of cartilage to reach its
maximum deformation is about 30 minutes. It is

wise to allow this period to elapse before final
insertion. Any warping which has occurred may
then be corrected by further trimming or
abolished by making small cuts along the curved
surfaces. This latter practice, however, weakens
the graft.

Of course distortion of cartilage is not always
necessarily objectionable. This property may
be exploited to obtain a suitable curve in a
cartilage graft and also forms the basis of
certain techniques for correction of prominent
ears.

The self-locked stress system of cartilage is a
vital property which disappears as the chondrocytes
die. It is this fact more than any other which has
made the use of stored, dead cartilage so
attractive to so many plastic surgeons, although
in the long term most dead cartilages are
absorbed.

SELECTED REFERENCES

Skin

GIBSON, T. and KENEDI, R.M.: Biomechanical Properties of skin. Surg. Clin. North Am. 47, 279, 1967.

GIBSON, T. and KENEDI, R.M.: Factors affecting the mechanical characteristics of human skin, In Proceedings of the Centennial Symposium on Repair and Regeneration, New York, McGraw-Hill Book Company, 1968, p. 87.

GIBSON, T. and KENEDI, R.M.: The structural components of the dermis, In Montagna, W., Bentley, J.P. and Dobson, R.L.(Eds.): The Dermis. New York, Appleton-Century-Crofts, 1970, p. 19.

GIBSON, T., STARK, H. and KENEDI, R.M.: The significance of Langer's lines, In Hueston, J.T. (Ed.): Transactions of the Fifth International Congress of Plastic and Reconstructive Surgery. Australia, Butterworths, 1971, p. 1213.

KENEDI, R.M., GIBSON, T. and DALY, C.H.: Bio-engineering studies of the human skin. I. In, Jackson, S.F., Harkness, R., Partridge, S. and Tristram, G. (Eds.): Structure and Function of Connective and Skeletal Tissues. London, Butterworths, 1965, p. 388.

Cartilage

CURRAN, R.C. and GIBSON, T.: The uptake of labelled sulphate by human cartilage cells and its use as a test of viability. Proc. R. Soc. (Biol.), 155,572, 1956.

DAVIS, W.B. and GIBSON, T.: Absorption of autogenous cartilage grafts in man. Br. J. Plast. Surg., 9, 177, 1956.

GIBSON, T.: Viability of cartilage after freezing. Proc. R. Soc. (Biol.), 147, 528, 1957.

GIBSON, T.: Cartilage grafts. Br. Med. Bull., 21, 153, 1965.

GIBSON, T.: Cartilage Grafts, In Seiffert, K.E. and Geissendorfer, R. (Eds.): Transplantation von Organen und Geweben. Stuttgart, Georg Thieme Verlag, 1967, p. 203.

GIBSON, T.: Bone and cartilage transplantation, In Rapaport, F.F. and Dausset, J. (Eds.): Human Transplantation. New York, Grune and Stratton, 1968, p. 313.

GIBSON, T. and DAVIS, W.B.: The fate of preserved bovine cartilage grafts in man. Br. J. Plast. Surg., 6, 4, 1953.

GIBSON, T. and DAVIS, W.B.: Some further observations on the use of preserved animal cartilage. Br. J. Plast. Surg., 8, 85, 1956.

GIBSON, T. and DAVIS, W.B.: The distortion of auto-genous cartilage grafts: Its cause and prevention. Br. J. Plast. Surg., 10, 527, 1958.

GIBSON, T. and DAVIS, W.B.: A bank of living homograft cartilage: A preliminary report. Trans. Int. Soc. of Plastic Surgeons, 2nd Congress, London. Edinburgh, Livingstone, 1960, p. 452.

GIBSON, T., DAVIS, W.B. and CURRAN, R.C.: The long-term survival of cartilage homografts in man. Br. J. Plast. Surg. 11, 177, 1958.

GIBSON, T., DAVIS, W.B. and GILLIES, H.D.: The encapsulation of preserved cartilage grafts with prolonged survival. Br. J. Plast. Surg., 12, 22, 1959.

KENEDI, R.M., GIBSON, T. and ABRAHAMS, M.: Mechanical characteristics of skin and cartilage. Hum. Factors, 5, 525, 1963.

GAIT ANALYSIS*

A.B. Thornton-Trump

Department of Mechanical Engineering, University of
Manitoba, Winnipeg, Canada

ABSTRACT. The general theory on which quantitative analysis of
bipedal locomotion is based is presented in detail, including the
description of the digital filter used to smooth data. The analysis
is presented in terms of the following aspects: 1. General locomotion; 2. Kinematic analysis; 3. Force and energy considerations; 4. The endo-prosthesis problem; 5. The exo-prosthesis
problem. Average data for normal subjects is given and aspects of
data on individual subjects are discussed in detail. Conclusions
are drawn regarding the use and the development of gait analysis.

1. GENERAL LOCOMOTION

Human locomotion is an apparently learned accomplishment which
requires the control and integration of the motion of the body
segments. It is the small differences in the control and integration of these body segment motions which gives us our personal
and perhaps unique gait. This uniqueness allows individuals to be
recognized from a distance long before other aspects of their person
become distinguishable. But this uniqueness of gait may be
attributed to small variations on a basic pattern of bipedal locomotion. It is one of the fundamental objectives of gait analysis
to define the characteristics of the basic pattern.

To define a basic pattern of gait becomes a question of degree
or of limits within which the variation of parameters is allowed
while the gait is described as normal. The definition of a pattern

*This work has been supported by NRC Grant No. A8920.

assumes some quantitative data, and the data normally gathered
during gait studies of normal subjects can be considered associated
with four general problems; the kinematic, the dynamic, the endo-
prosthetic and exo-prosthetic problem. If the definition of the
gait pattern is simply considered as definition of the instantaneous spatial arrangement of the body segments, then definition becomes a question of kinematics; that is, a question only of the
displacement, velocity and acceleration of the body segments without
consideration for the forces necessary to cause the motions. The
solution to the kinematic problem is, of course, where gait analysis
began.

To define the motion of the limbs, all techniques rely on an
instantaneous record of body segment displacement, both translational and rotational, taken at discrete time intervals. In the
studies by Professor E.J. Marey [1] done in 1873 he developed the
technique of chronophotography, whereby he marked the limbs with
reflective tape and used a single sheet of film, exposing it at
regular time intervals as the subject passed by. Of course, the
development of cinematography allowed H. Elftman [2, 3, 4] to employ
that technique and also allowed variable time intervals between
frames on exposures. Indeed, the high-speed movie camera is still
used quite extensively in patient evaluation during physiotherapy
since it allows the motions to be slowed for viewing thus giving
the viewer a qualitative sense of the integration of the motions
of the body segments. Though cinematography also offers much quan-
titatively in that the time interval between frames can be varied,
there are many researchers using videotape systems which allow a
more direct data conversion system [5, 6, 7]. Data is, however,
generally limited to the rate of sixty frames per second (in North
America) to simplify equipment requirements. This more direct data
conversion system as described by Winter [5] avoids the high data
reduction time required by cine film methods, as reported by Bresler
and Berry [8] and appears to allow sufficient detail to describe
the motions of the body during locomotion.

1.1 Motions during locomotion

The motions of the leg during locomotion can be ascribed to
two phases of activity. There is the stance phase or support phase
of motion which is the period from initial heel-contact to toe-off
of the same foot and represents about 60 percent of the cycle.
Following toe-off, the leg motion is that of swinging the leg segments forward, thus this phase of activity is called the swing phase
which represents the other 40 percent of the gait cycle and is the
period from toe-off to next heel-contact of the same foot. The
period from heel-contact to next heel-contact of the same foot is
considered a cycle.

Within the two phases of the cycle, there are also periods of distinct activity. In the stance phase, the periods of distinct activity are monitored by three foot switches placed at heel, ball and toe. Heel-contact is recorded by a switch on the heel and is accompanied by particular reaction force patterns. Heel-contact is followed by full contact of the sole of the foot (called 'Foot-flat') which is monitored by the heel, ball and toe foot switch. During the next 'Mid-stance' period of full foot contact the body weight is vaulted over the extended leg and the centre of force on the foot moves forward to cause the heel to lose contact as 'Heel-off occurs. The ball and toe then supply the force to vault the body over the other leg, thus giving rise to the push-off period which is terminated by toe-off.

The swing phase activity may also be characterized by three distinct periods of activity. There is an initial period of acceleration during which the leg is accelerated to swing forward faster than the mean body speed. This initial period is followed by 'mid-swing' during which the leg passes beneath the body. The final period of the swing phase is marked by the deceleration of the leg preparatory to heel contact. Figure 1 indicates the phases of the gait cycle and the periods of activity in each.

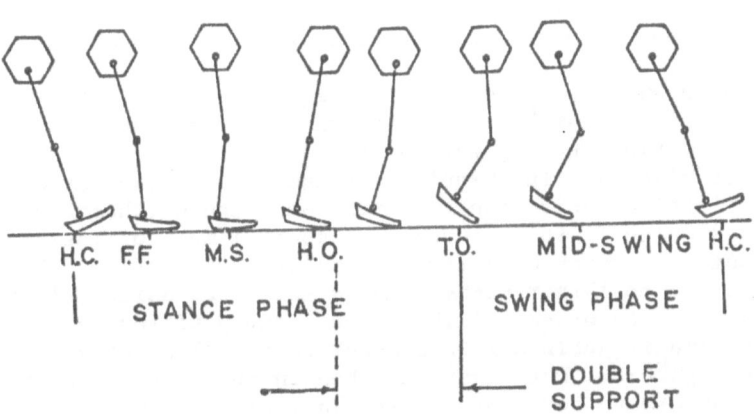

Figure 1. Phases and activities of the gait cycle.

The characterization of the gait cycle given in Figure 1 does not explicitly integrate the motion of the entire body but deals only with one leg. However, there is a period of time, called 'Double-support', when both legs are in the stance phase, since in walking toe-off on one foot does not occur until after heel-contact

of the other foot. Double-support occupies about 10 to 25 percent
of the gait cycle and decreases as walking speed increases. Running
can be characterized by the lack of the double support period and
will exhibit a period of no support.

A more detailed characterization of the general categorization
of activities during locomotion is given by Peizer and Wright [9].
The analytical techniques will be considered in greater detail
here.

2.   KINEMATIC ANALYSIS

Since before the dynamics problem of locomotion can be properly
considered the kinematics must be defined, the techniques used for
kinematic data reduction and the interpretation of such data must
be dealt with first. There are two basic systems of data acquisition. One system measures displacement at discrete time intervals
and then, using appropriate data smoothing techniques, twice differentiates to obtain accelerations. The other technique employs
accelerometers to directly measure the accelerations of the body
segments. The accelerations can then be twice integrated to predict
displacement as shown by Gage [10] and Smidt et al [11]. The latter
technique is less developed at present but offers the advantage of
acceleration data smoothed only by instrument response and directional sensitivity. Unfortunately the accelerometers will respond to
skin and muscular activity if not mounted with special care, thus
data taken may not be considered absolute.

All displacement techniques first require a means of defining
the limb segment. Marey [1] used tape on the limbs, but it is
sufficient to define the segments using point markers as was done
by Bresler et al [12]. The Winnipeg system as described by Winter
[5] uses reflective markers on the limbs and records their motions
on video tape which is then played to a special monitor interfaced
with a computer in which data from a sampling grid defines the limb
markers relative to larger background markers. By using a limb
marker near each end of each limb segment, the position and alignment of the limb is defined with respect to the plane of viewing,
as shown in Figure 2. Data must be taken in two or three projections
if all motions are to be recorded with sufficient accuracy. Most
studies have been confined to data acquisition in the sagittal plane,
which reduces the mathematical complexity of data abstraction and
reduction. However, since the principles of data abstraction are
similar in each plane, the process need be described for one plane
only.

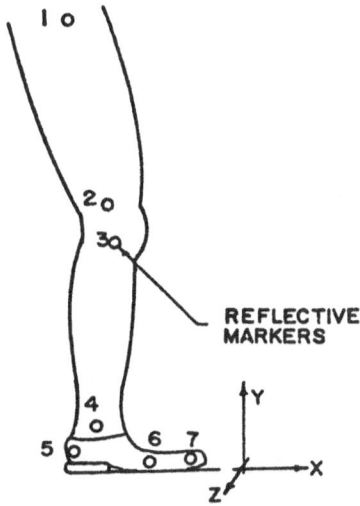

Figure 2. Lower limb marked for video gait analysis.

When taking data using the video system, it is necessary to have a reference for the alignment of the limbs since the anatomical sights for the marks will not be defined very accurately. The procedure followed is to record the subject in a normal standing position prior to the locomotion run, thus defining the angular alignment of the limbs in stance. This stance alignment then becomes a reference position for interpretation of angular movement of the thigh and shank-foot segments.

Assuming that a subject is suitably marked as in Figure 2, the positions of the markers may be stored as arrays X1(I), Y1(I) for one cycle or more, usually defining the cycle as occurring from heel contact to next heel contact of the same heel. The projected angular line segment between the two markers on the segment, which gives the acute angle to the vertical of

$$\theta_1(I) = \sin^{-1}[X2(I) - X1(I)]/[(X2(I) - X1(I))^2 + (Y2(I) - Y1(I))^2]^{1/2}$$

Using this system for each limb segment, the absolute angles θ_i for each of i limb segments are defined and the internal angles for flexion-extension evaluation are available.

Joint velocities can be computed in several ways, but perhaps the least complex approach is to locate the anatomical joint relative to the markers then define the velocity components of the marker in the i and j direction by subtracting the positions $X_i(I)$ and $Y_i(I)$ between two frames and dividing each by the time interval T as is shown,

$$V1X(I) = (X1(I + 1) - X1(I))/T \quad \text{i}$$

$$V1Y(I) = (Y1(I + 1) - Y1(I))/T \quad \text{j}$$

and from the alignment angles, the angular rotation of a limb segment is defined by:

$$\Omega 1(I) = (\theta 1(I + 1) - \theta 1(I))/T \quad \text{k}$$

The joint velocity can therefore be calculated since for any point B on the limb segment the velocity may be given by the sum of the velocity of the marker point 1 plus the cross-product of the rate of rotation and the displacement vector from the marker to the joint position. If the displacement vector components are XP_i and XP_j, then the joint velocity VP(I) is defined as

$$VP(I) = VM1(I) + \Omega 1(I) \text{ x } (XP_i + YP_j)$$

where VM1(I) is the marker velocity.

The relationship of the vector directions to the anatomical directions is arbitrary. In Figure 2, the directions are given for the vector quantities used here. Figure 3 defines the anatomical direction relationships which are more commonly used to describe the relative motion of the body segments since active muscle groups can be related more directly to the relative motions of the body segments in terms of extension, flexion, adduction and abduction.

Regardless of how the data is taken, if velocities and accelerations are to be related to the integration of the body motions it is the motion of one body segment with respect to another which is of the prime importance. The relative motions are in turn caused by the muscular activity and the muscle groups are grouped according to their relative function. A good data abstraction system, then must be able to interpret the data in terms of the anatomical directions shown in Figure 3. If data is taken in the sagittal plane only, then abduction and adduction are particularly difficult to determine. The velocities and acceleration components in the medio-lateral directions thus must be taken from data gathered in the frontal plane in much the same way as the data was gathered in the sagittal plane. Rotation about the vertical axis is best seen from either above the subject or below if glass walkways are possible.

133

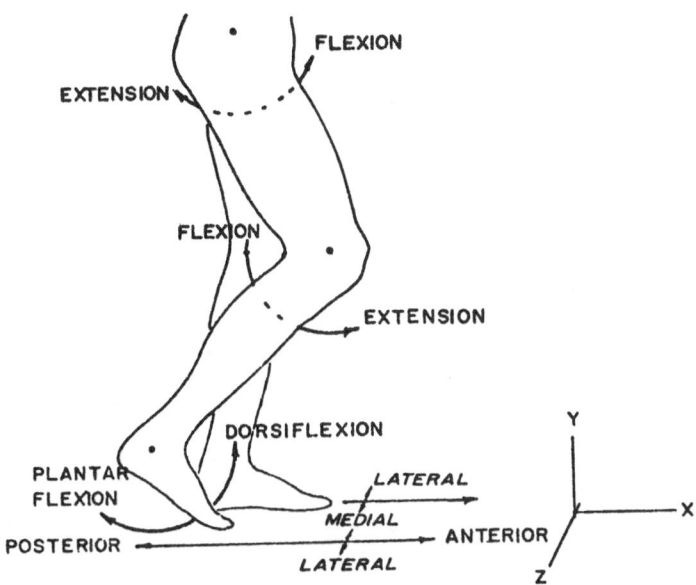

Figure 3. Anatomical direction relationships.

The definition of position is not highly accurate due to the resolution of the film or video unit, lens inaccuracies and small motions at right angles to the plane in which the data was to be taken. There is therefore 'noise' in the data. Positions in displacement data are difficult to define to much more than ± 3 mm and when the displacement data is differentiated the variations are magnified. The displacement data thus requires smoothing and although many techniques are available, digital filtering using a Butterworth filter appears to be most appropriate as pointed out by Pezzack, Norman and Winter [13]. The velocity data must also be filtered before further differentiation.

Accelerations are calculated from the velocity data in the same way as velocities were calculated from displacement data, giving the acceleration components:

$$A1X(I) = (V1X(I + 1) - V1S(I))/T \quad i$$

$$A1Y(I) = (V1Y(I + 1) - V1Y(I))/T \quad j$$

and the angular accelerations:

$$\alpha1(I) = (\Omega1(I + 1) - \Omega1(I))/T \quad k$$

134

which are again filtered to give acceleration curves of the type shown in Figure 4.

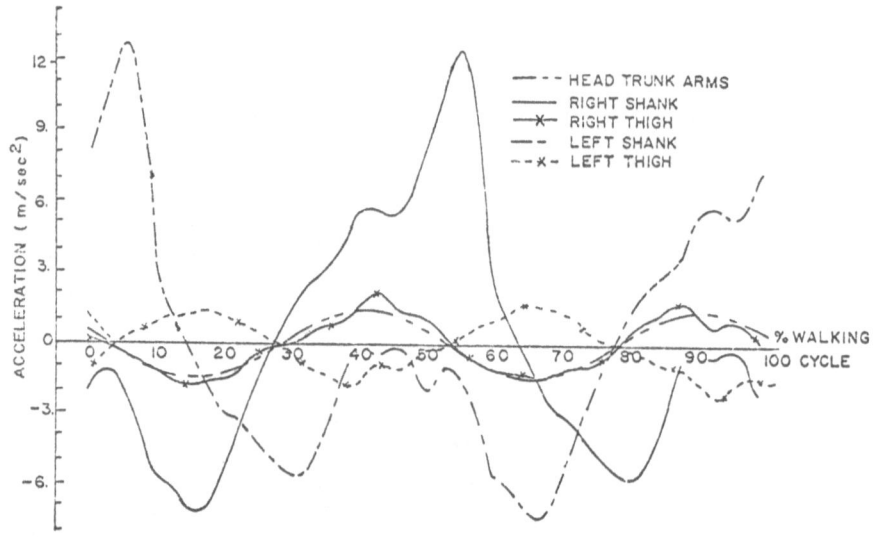

Figure 4. Accelerations of the centres of mass of body segments.

As was stated previously, the smooth curve shown in Figure 5 is accomplished by processing the data using a digital, three-pole Butterworth filter such as is given in Gold and Rader [14]. The filter when applied to digital data has the form:

$$H(z) = \frac{CZ^{-1} + DZ^{-2}}{(1 - e^{-\omega_c T} z^{-1})\{1 - 2e^{-\omega_c T/2}[\cos(\frac{\sqrt{3}}{2})\omega_c T] z^{-1} + e^{-\omega_c T} z^{-2}\}}$$

where

$$C = \omega_c [e^{-\omega_c T} + e^{-\omega_c T/2} (\frac{1}{\sqrt{3}}) \sin(\frac{\sqrt{3}}{2}\omega_c T) - \cos(\frac{\sqrt{3}}{2}\omega_c T)]$$

and

$$D = \omega_c [e^{-\omega_c T} - e^{-3\omega_c T/2} (\frac{1}{\sqrt{3}} \sin\frac{\sqrt{3}}{2}\omega_c T + \cos\frac{\sqrt{3}}{2}\omega_c T)]$$

and the output smoothed data YS(nT) is related to the input data
YI(nT) through

$$YS(nT) = C \cdot YI(nT-T) + D \cdot YI(nT-2T) + A \cdot YS(nT-T) + B \cdot YS(nT-2T)$$

$$+ E \cdot YS(nT-3T)$$

The values of A, B and E can be calculated from the expansion of
H(z), which gives:

$$A = \{e^{-\omega_c T} + 2e^{-\omega_c T/2} [\cos (\frac{\sqrt{3}}{2})\omega_c T]\}$$

$$B = \{e^{-\omega_c T} + 2e^{-3\omega_c T/2} [\cos (\frac{\sqrt{3}}{2})\omega_c T]\}$$

$$E = e^{-2\omega_c T}$$

In order to use the filter, a cut-off frequency ω_c must be selected,
and this cut-off frequency essentially limits the reaction time of
the filter and thus the maximum rate of change of acceleration that
can be considered. Presently a cut-off frequency of six to nine
radians per second appears to serve well for normal walking.

    Both a forward and a backward pass of the data must be made
and the average taken of the results in order to remove any frequency
shift, thus a few frames more data than those required for a single
cycle must be taken, since smoothed values are not defined until the
third data frame. Of course, the system which is given here defines
velocities at the mid-interval while displacement and acceleration
are defined at initiation of the interval. Interpolation could be
used to avoid this should it be perceived as a problem. The improvement in the data is remarkable, as is shown in Figure 5. Although
the data has been smoothed, little information was a result of noise
in the velocity data prior to differentiation. However any smoothing technique will increase the effective time period over which an
event takes place, thus accelerometers may be more appropriate for
studies of non-cyclic phenomena.

136

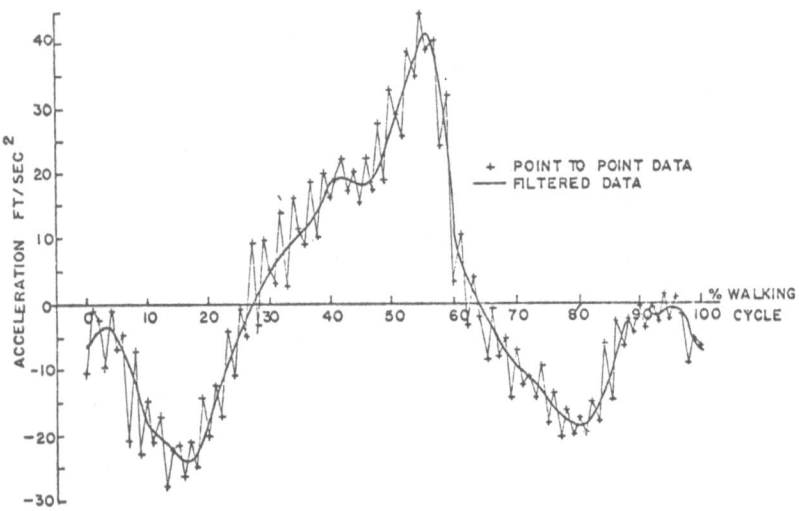

Figure 5. Acceleration of the centre of mass of the shank foot
segment computed by point-to-point differentiation of
the smoothed velocity curve and filtered using the
three-pole digital Butterworth filter.

Using suitable synchronizing pulses, the data from two planes
can be used to define the limb segments as vectors $\bar{\rho}_i$, the rotations
as rotational vectors $\bar{\Omega}_i$, velocities $\bar{v}_i$, angular accelerations $\dot{\bar{\Omega}}_i$
and linear accelerations $\bar{a}_i$. Thus the velocity and acceleration of
any point on any limb segment is available as was described by previous work [15] and are given by the general equations for velocity

$$\bar{V}_p = \bar{V}_o + \sum_{i=1}^{n} \bar{\Omega}_i \times \bar{\rho}_i + \sum_{i=1}^{n} \hat{\rho}_i \cdot \dot{\rho}_i$$

and for acceleration

$$\bar{a}_p = \bar{a}_o + \sum_{i=1}^{n} \bar{\Omega}_i \times (\bar{\Omega}_i \times \bar{\rho}_i) + \sum_{i=1}^{n} \dot{\bar{\Omega}} \times \bar{\rho}_i$$

$$+ 2 \sum_{i=1}^{n} \bar{\Omega}_i \times \dot{\bar{\rho}}_i + \sum_{i=1}^{n} \hat{\rho}_i \cdot \ddot{\rho}_i$$

where

$\overline{V}_o$ = velocity vector of the initial floating reference system

$\hat{\rho}_i$ = unit vector

$\overline{\rho}_i$ = vectors representing the limb segments or portions thereof

$\dot{\rho}_i$ = rate of extension of $|\overline{\rho}_i|$

$\dot{\overline{\rho}}_i$ = rate of change of the vector

$\ddot{\overline{\rho}}_i$ = rate of change of $\dot{\overline{\rho}}_i$

$\dot{\overline{\Omega}}_i$ = angular acceleration of the ith segment

i = subscript denoting the limb segments.

When absolute rates of rotation are used, the acceleration
expressions are considerably reduced in complexity. However, any
analysis of limb displacement done by placing markers on the limb
does not locate the joints particularly accurately. Small variations in marker positions can change the point of intersection of
the lines representing the limbs. Thus the true centre of rotation
of, say, the knee joint is not particularly apparent. The knee
joint is a good case in point because the centre of rotation between
shank and thigh is a function of the included angle between the two
limb segments. This polycentric aspect of the knee joint lends
stability to bipedal locomotion but also requires great sophistica-
tion in the design of a prosthetic replacement. Since the centres
of rotation are not known to great accuracy, then the results from
equations describing joint accelerations are going to be slightly
in error although of the correct order of magnitude.

In gait analysis the greatest emphasis has been placed on the
lower limbs since their motion is of fundamental importance in the
design of prostheses for amputees. To allow a person to walk again
is certainly the highest priority, but other aspects of kinematic
analysis are used daily in physiotherapy clinics. In the attempt to
redevelop the proper function of joints, the normal range of motion
of the joints must be known, thus the data shown in Table 1 is of
particular interest. Of course, the detailed curve of angle vs. %
gait cycle may be of greater use once the range of motion is available
Such curves are given in [9].

Table 1
Usual Range of Angular Motions

Motion	Range
Vertical Torso Displacement	±5 cm (sinusoid)
Lateral Torso Displacement	±5 cm (sinusoid)
Pelvic obliquity	±4° irregular
Pelvic rotation	±8° irregular
Hip joint rotation	±3° irregular
Femoral-Tibial rotation	int. 6° ext. 10°
Tibial rotation	int. 3° ext. 8°
Foot rotation	8°
Hip-flexion-extension	from 1° to 45°
Knee flexion-extension	from 4° to 62°
Plantar flexion-extension	Dors. 5° plant. 22°

The angle data in Table 1 is often collected through the use of goniometers which may be mounted on joint centers as is used clinically by Foort [16]. Relative rotation between the body segments on either side of the goniometer causes the output voltage from the goniometer to change in proportion to the included angle. However, it is more difficult to use goniometer data for velocity and acceleration analysis since relative data only is produced.

The display of angle data developed from gait analysis is of particular interest since much can be determined from the phase relationship between the angles at the joints. Dr. Milner [17] developed such a plot which is reproduced here in Figure 6. The subject was suffering from osteoarthritis of the right hip. The plot of knee flexion (vertical axis) against hip flexion shows a large open diagram for the least affected side (left side) which would be the more normal pattern. The plot for the affected side exhibits a very narrow figure in which the excursions of angle are naturally very much smaller. However, the fact that the diagrams are different in general shape indicates that the phase relationship of the angles has been changed. The main significance of the diagram is that it dramatically separates the abnormal from the normal behaviour, thus allowing better evaluation of the subject both before and during treatment.

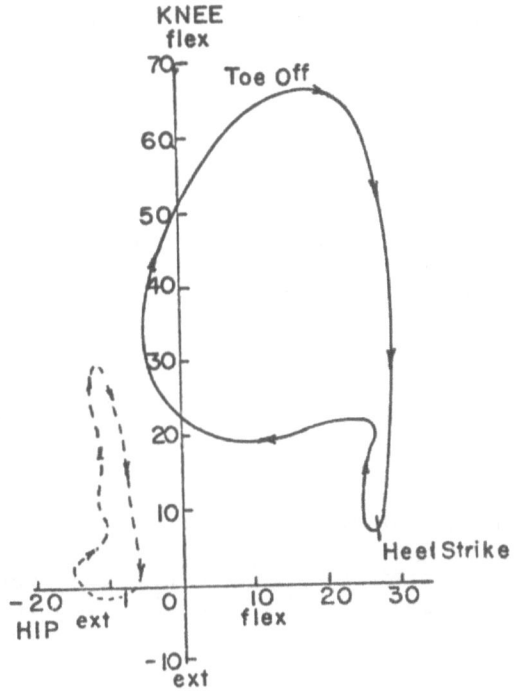

Figure 6. Angle diagram for a patient with osteoarthritis of the
          right hip. Knee flexion angle (degrees) is the vertical
          axis and hip flexion is the horizontal axis.

    The data shown thus far refers to the lower limbs in detail
and classifies the head, arms and trunk as a single segment. While
this classification may be acceptable if the lower limbs are the
prime consideration it could lead to difficulty when more refined
analysis is required for the comparison of prosthetic knee joint or
prosthetic foot alignment. It is quite possible that, in the effort
to control the lower limbs in a pattern close to normal a subject
may require considerably greater motions of the upper body. Fewer
studies have been done of upper body motions, though the Berkley
studies [12] and that of Elftman [3] are generally available.

    The range motions of the body segments and the phase relation-
ship between these motions are thus a major concern of gait analysis.
A kinematic study of gait is thus a study of the motions integrated
to accomplish locomotion and these motions consist of the medio-
lateral pelvic tilt, flexion of the knee, horizontal rotation of

the pelvis, plantar flexion of the ankle and foot, lateral displacement of the torso, rotation of the shoulder girdle in two planes and swinging of the arms. In studies of abnormal gait, some of these motions will be exaggerated while others will be much reduced. The effect of these differences can be quantified to some extent by the study of the variations of forces and energies involved.

3.   FORCES AND ENERGY

Having defined the motions, the next problem is the determination of the forces that produce these motions. This is what was referred to as the dynamics problem and was first investigated by the brothers Weber [18] in 1836. Unfortunately the body segment masses and moments of inertia were not well defined. Fischer [19] developed caucasian data between 1894 and 1904 and Continii's results [20] have been programmed for use in gait evaluation performed in the Manitoba Health System by A. Quanbury. Methods of accurately determining the masses and mass moments of inertia of individual subjects in gait studies have not yet been developed to a high accuracy, through studies by J.P. Earl [21] show promise.

The relationships for the determination of the mass and inertial properties of some of the body segments can be taken from Continii [20] and written into the form dependent on a body index BI, whole body density WBD, and whole body volume WBV, which are in turn functions of the height to weight ratio of the subject. The relationships for the three parameters are as follows:

$$BI = (height/weight)^{1/3} \times 30.2$$
$$WBD = 0.690 + 0.0295 \times BI$$
$$WBV = weight/WBD$$

The coefficients in the formulae for the length, mass and radius of gyration of the lower limb segments depend on whether the subject is male or female. The coefficients are given in Tables 2 and 3 and are functions of the segment densities. These densities follow the relationships:

Foot Density = 0.04 + WBD
Shank Density = 0.38 + 0.667 x WBD
Thigh Density = 0.35 + 0.667 x WBD

Table 2

Volume Coefficients of Lower Limb Segments

Segment	Coefficient	
	Male	Female
Foot Volume	0.0124	0.0131
Shank Volume	0.0464	0.0518
Thigh Volume	0.0922	0.0987

The values in Table 2 are used to find the effective volume of the body part in question simply by multiplying the whole body volume by the appropriate coefficient. The mass of the segments is found by multiplying the effective segment volume by the segment density.

In order to calculate the centers of mass and radii of gyration, the length of the body segment must be known. These lengths again depend on whether the subject is male or female. The coefficients in Table 3 multiplied by the height of the subject give the length of the body segment.

Table 3

Body Segment	Coefficient for segment length	
	Male	Female
Foot length	0.043	0.048
Shank length	0.242	0.234
Thigh length	0.245	0.222

The centers of mass C.M. are given by the relationships:

C.M. Shank Foot = 0.45 x (Foot length + Shank length)
C.M. Thigh   = 0.41 x (Thigh length)

and the radii of gyration by

radius of gyration of shank foot = 0.29 x (Foot length + Shank length)
radius of gyration of thigh   = 0.23 x (Thigh length)

The polar mass moment of inertia about the center of mass in the sagittal plane is given by the mass of the segment multiplied by the square of the radius of gyration. The parallel axis theorem must be used if the mass moment of inertia around another position is desired.

The above definitions of the parameters of some of the body segments were developed on the basis of data for statistically

142

average subjects. Many individuals may differ significantly from
the relationships given and statistical confidence limits could be
used to indicate what particular error may be incurred by use of
average data. The methods to experimentally determine the parameters for each individual subject were investigated by J.P. Earl
[21] and it was concluded that shape data on the body segment and
bone, coupled with density for bone and flesh is at present the
most accurate method to use. The mass and inertia parameters are
calculated on an element basis using a computer.

Assuming that the masses and mass moments of inertia of the
limb segments are determined, the net joint torques and forces
required to cause the accelerations of the limb segments can be
calculated assuming the accelerations are known from the kinematic
study. Figure 7 is a free body diagram of the leg. The general
equation for the force balance on a single body segment is

$$\Sigma(\text{applied forces}) = (\text{effective force } \overline{m}\overline{a})$$

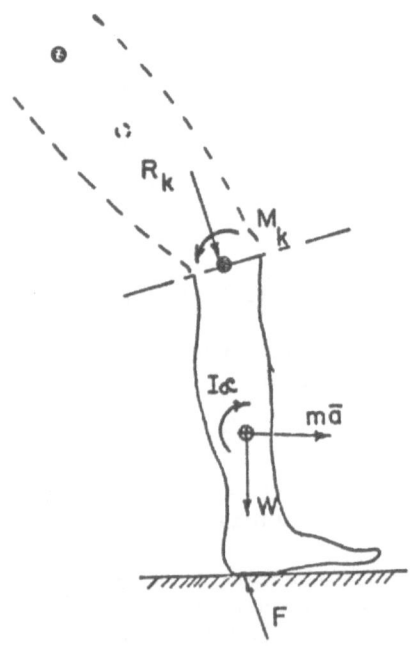

Figure 7. Free body diagram showing net knee moments and forces
due to ground reaction force and acceleration of the
shank-foot segment.

and since both the mass m of the body segment and the acceleration a of its center of mass are known, the effective force ma is known. However, if the applied forces at the proximal end of the freebody diagram are to be discovered, then the applied forces at the distal end (at the foot in this case) must be measured. In order to allow the calculation of the applied torque at the proximal end, all force components must be measured at the foot, since the effective moment is calculated according to the equation:

$$\Sigma(\text{moments of applied forces}) + \Sigma(\text{applied couples})$$
$$= (\text{moment of effective force}) + (\text{effective couple } \dot{\bar{h}}_c)$$

where $\dot{\bar{h}}_c$ is the rate of change of the relative angular momemtum $\bar{h}_c$ defined relative to the mass center.

It is in the consideration of the moments that the difference between a three-dimensional study and a two-dimensional approximation is greatest because the value of $\bar{h}_c$ is given (for principal axes) as

$$\bar{h}_c = I_{xx} \, \Omega_x \, i + I_{yy} \, \Omega_y \, j + I_{zz} \, \Omega_z \, k$$

and

$$\dot{\bar{h}}_c = \frac{\partial \bar{h}_c}{\partial t} + \bar{\Omega} \times \bar{h}_c$$

Thus the rates of rotation measured in each plane during the kinematic study will interact as a result of the calculation of $\dot{\bar{h}}_c$. This difficulty is often left hidden in the term 'inertial torque' but must be dealt with in detail for any three-dimensional analysis although the effect appears to be in the order of 10% of the major moment.

Having determined the forces and torques at one joint, the forces and torques at the next joint can be calculated by considering the reaction forces at the previous joint as the known applied forces and moments and using the accelerations and limb segment data to compute the effective forces and torques. In each case, of course, the weight of the limb segment must be included.

The patterns or force curves of an analysis such as described above will follow a reasonably regular pattern but will show variation from individual to individual. The variations from individual to individual can be seen in Paul [22]. The general force pattern for the vertical force measured for a single foot is shown in Figure 8 and the data taken by Balakrishnan and the author [23] for various normal subjects is shown as well. The most notable feature of the vertical component of the ground reaction is the double hump. The size of the first hump is a measure of the hardness of the heel strike and from the data on the individual subject it can be seen to be small in some normal cases. A subject who walks with the knees flexed will have a tendency to soften the heel strike, as will a person walking in bare feet. At heel contact the centre of mass of the body is moving downward and the force transmitted from the heel must not only bear the weight of the body but supply the force necessary to accelerate the mass of the body upward again. During mid stance the center of mass of the body is reaching its maximum height and therefore the foot need only transmit a force equal to the body weight less the force required to accelerate the centre of mass back downward. The second hump is the result of the acceleration of the body mass upward again to allow the body to climb over the extended leg, thus the toe supplied a 'push-off'.

The force curve for both feet includes the double support phase of the gait cycle and exhibits the extra peak combining the push-off to heel contact peak as load is transferred from one foot to the other. The general aspects of the curve are indicated in Figure 9. The magnitude of the inertial contribution is a measure of the amplitude over which the centre of mass of the body moves while the narrowness of the peaks represents the sharpness of the centre of mass trajectory.

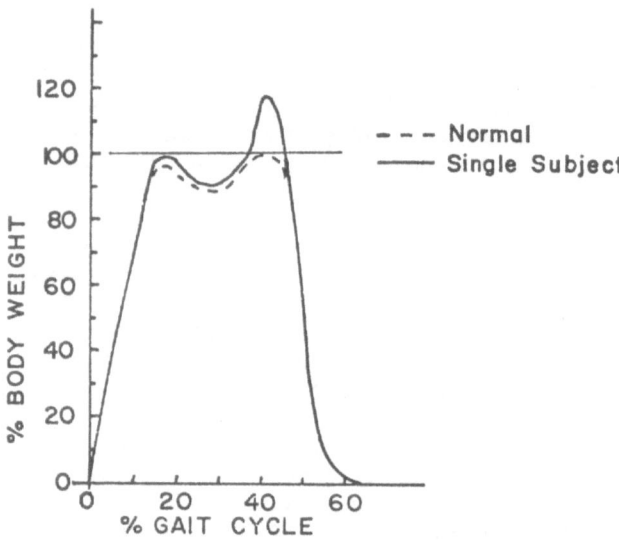

Figure 8. Floor reaction force pattern for a single foot.

The single subject curve is again for an apparently normal subject. The high centre peak has been associated with age by some but the subject was under forty. What the peak may represent is a combination of very soft heel strike and spring in the toe-off. The curve suggests that the single subject is not using the most efficient stride, but may have adapted his walk to other conditions in his past.

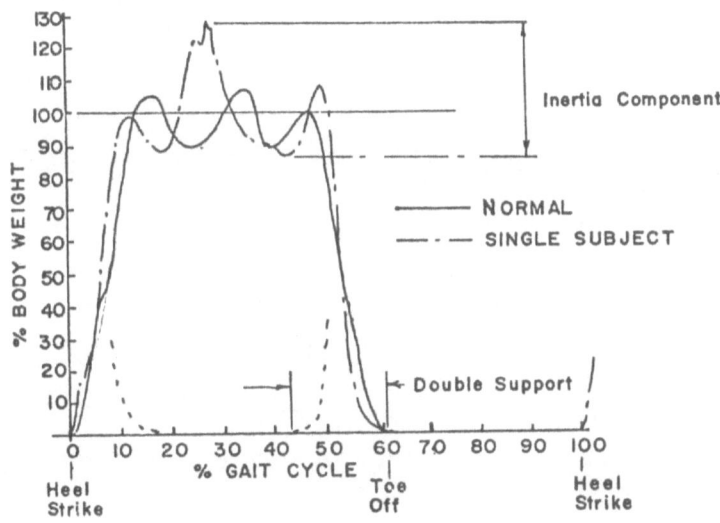

Figure 9. Floor reaction force for two foot cycle.

Using the freebody diagram and solving the equations for known motion, the net forces at the joints can be calculated and have been reported by Paul [24] but are within about 15% of the floor reaction force. Such net forces do not take muscle forces into consideration and thus are only a fraction of the total joint force.

Of greater concern in gait analysis are the moments generated
at the joints. Given the reaction forces, the joint moments can be
calculated using the relationships developed from the free body
diagram. The significance of the moments lies in their relationship
to the muscle forces required to generate them. The muscle force
generates a moment about the joint which is given by the force
multiplied by the perpendicular distance between the force vector
and the instantaneous joint center. Since the distance from the
joint centre cannot be large, then large moments require large
muscle forces. The average curves for such moments at hip, knee and
ankle are shown in Figure 10 taken from Bresler and Frankel [25].
In general, the maximum moment would be used for the design of prostheses, but since the relationship between muscle force and body
segment angle are not constant, maximum forces could occur at other
than the maximum moment position, particularly if the gait pattern
is abnormal.

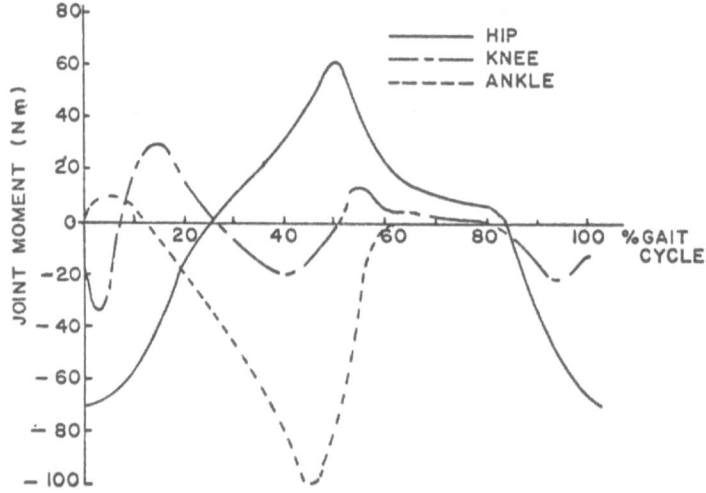

Figure 10.   Joint moments in the sagittal plane.

The foregoing analysis of the dynamics of locomotion may be
referred to as a momentum based analysis of gait. There are, of
course, two aspects of energy. The first aspect is the physiological
energy expended during normal bipedal locomotion and this has been
measured using oxygen uptake measurements by Bard and Ralston [25]
and the relative energy requirements for walking are shown as a
function of speed. An abstraction of their work is shown in
Figure 11.

The changes in energy requirements are remarkable enough that
Andriacchi et al [27] have suggested walking speed as a basis gait

evaluation. However, if gait speed is above 50 m/min (.9 m/sec) then their data suggests that time of support and time of swing vary linearly with forward velocity. The slope of the linear variation changes depending on the condition of the subject. These changes in gait are reflected in the original curve shown in Figure 11.

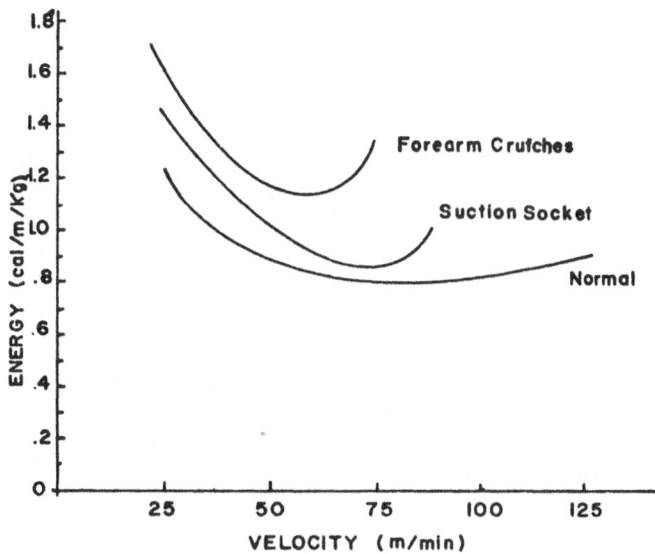

Figure 11.   Energy expenditure in normal walking for normal
            subjects and subjects with various styles of pros-
            theses.

Energy, however, may also refer to the mechanical potential and kinetic energy of the body. The energy expression for a body segment i may be written:

$$E_i = \frac{1}{2} m_i v_i^2 + \frac{1}{2} I_i \Omega_i^2 + m_i g h_i$$

where E_i is the total instantaneous energy of the body segment;

m_i is the mass of the segment;

v_i is the velocity of the centre of mass of the segment;

I_i is the polar mass moment of inertia taken about the centre of mass at right angles to the ω vector;

Ω_i is the absolute rate of rotation of the body segment;

h_i is the height of the centre of mass of the body segment above datum;

g is the acceleration due to gravity.

148

Again, if the analysis is done for the sagittal plane only, then I, which is in reality a second order tensor, can be reduced to a scalar. For three-dimensional work all the appropriate terms of $I_{k\ell}$ must be employed. However, even for the sagittal plane only the energy flows across joints can be considered. This principle has been employed in the analysis by the Winnipeg group by Winter, Quanbury and Reimer [6] and by work done by Cappozzo, Figura, Marchetti and Pedotti [28]. Cappozzo et al [28] go considerably farther than Winter et al [6] in that they also examine the accompanying electromygraphic data.

Of first interest, however, is the interpretation of the mechanical energy data. Consider Figure 12, the total energy. The magnitude of the total energy change is the energy demand of the system and thus should be related to fatigue. However, Figure 10 does not include the energy of the arms or of the rotation of the torso about a vertical axis, thus it is not truly total mechanical energy. If the total energy curve were available, it may be an aid in the development of prostheses for above-knee amputees in order to approach minimum energy gait. Quanbury et al [29] employed energy analysis in an attempt to evaluate polycentric knee joint designs for prostheses for above-knee amputees. The basis of the analysis is that energy flow into or out of a limb segment must be accomplished by muscle action. Unfortunately, the muscles need not be only those operating across the joints of the body segment in question, as is illustrated by the peg leg which lacks a knee joint altogether but energy changes still occur in the shank-foot section of the leg.

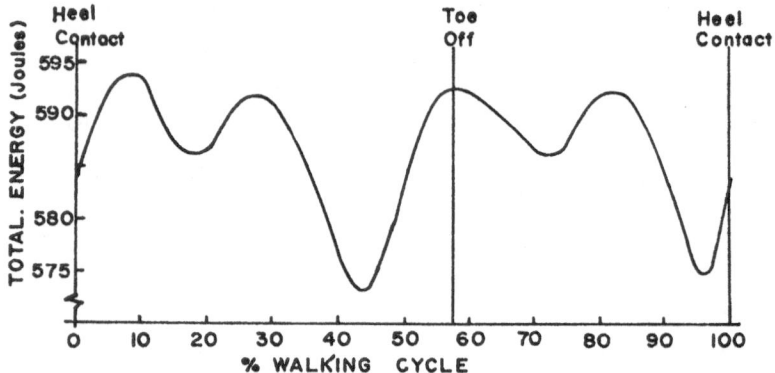

Figure 12.   Total mechanical energy of the body during normal locomotion.

As gait analysis methods develop faster turnaround, it may be possible to evaluate prostheses performance and alignment on the basis of the segmental energies. Data from at least two planes,

the sagittal plane and the frontal plane would appear necessary
since upper body motion appears very significant.

4.   THE ENDO-PROSTHETICS PROBLEM

Any implanted prosthesis which bears load must be designed to
carry the loads to which it will be subjected both from a structural
point of view and from a fixation point of view. In the previous
section, the importance of joint moments was considered in terms of
the muscle forces which were necessary to cause them. The compressive muscle force must have an equal and opposite joint reaction
force. Thus by considering the geometry of the muscle and attachment to the bone, the forces required to create the appropriate
moment can be calculated. These joint forces have been reported by
Paul [23].

In order to consider the muscle forces, the muscles actively
contributing to the moment must be determined. Thus the endo-
prosthetics problem requires a third fundamental measurement, that
of muscle activity related to the phases of the motions of the body
segments during locomotion. Electromyographic activity of muscle
groups during locomotion has been reported [22] and is commonly
gathered in clinical evaluations.

However, there is not yet a unique relationship between EMG
activity level and force. The variables such as tissue conductivity,
enervation patterns and tissue layer thickness do not allow surface
electrode signals to be interpreted on the same basis from subject
to subject. Thus, the EMG patterns reported can be used as a guide
to the active muscle groups but the joint moments and geometry must
still be defined to predict forces.

A record of the EMG activity of a normal subject taken by
Quanbury at the Winnipeg Rehabilitation Centre for Children is shown
in Figure 13. This activity is then drawn on the EMG chart in
Figure 14 employed by the Shriner's Hospital system. The unusually
low activity of the hamstring group may be a result of the fact that
the subject does not normally lock the knee during walking. This
EMG pattern is for the same subject who exhibits the very soft heel
contact shown in Figure 8.

Having defined the muscle groups involved in the periods of the
gait cycle, the joint forces are then calculated. These joint forces
are found to be approximately four times larger than the net reaction
forces at the joints. The joint force and the net reaction forces
are shown in Figure 9. Fatigue of endo-prostheses and bearing design
must thus be calculated on the basis of much greater loads than
would otherwise be anticipated.

150

The EMG signals alone are often taken in a clinic since the degree of muscle activity itself is of interest in physiotherapy programs in that the ability of the muscle to be controlled is necessary for a useful program to be initiated. A gait study with the EMG signals of particular groups monitored is often done prior to surgery in order to ensure that a muscle is still active. In many cases, the subject may have to learn to alter the phase of the activity of a particular muscle or group. Certainly the powered prosthesis can be controlled by the voluntary EMG signal of certain muscle groups indicating that single motor units are retrainable.

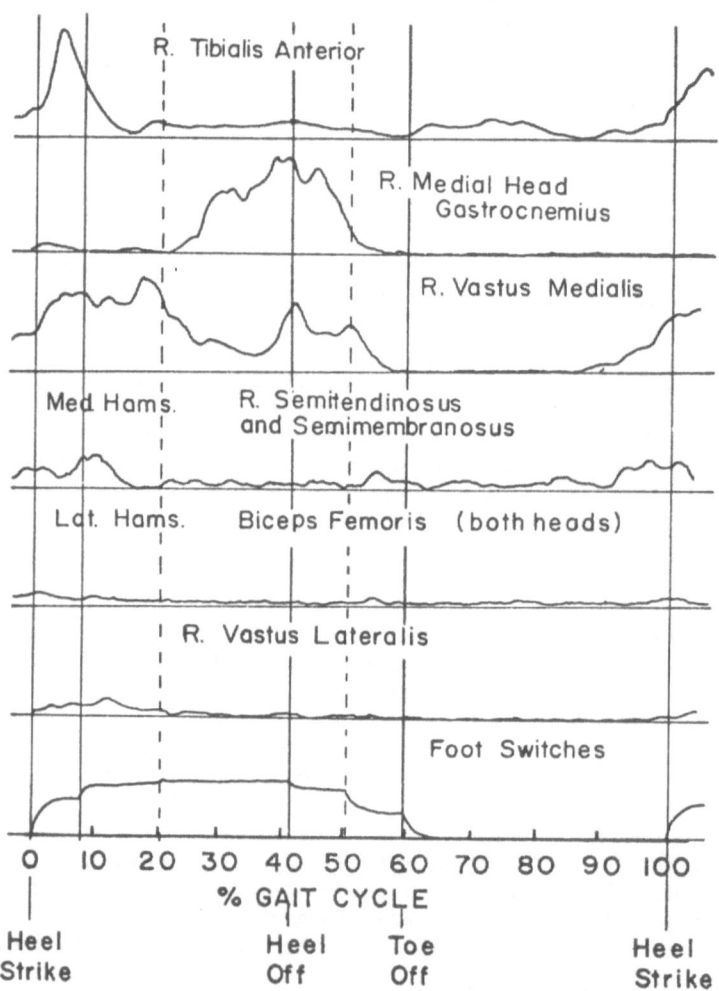

Figure 13. EMG record of selected muscle groups during normal walking.

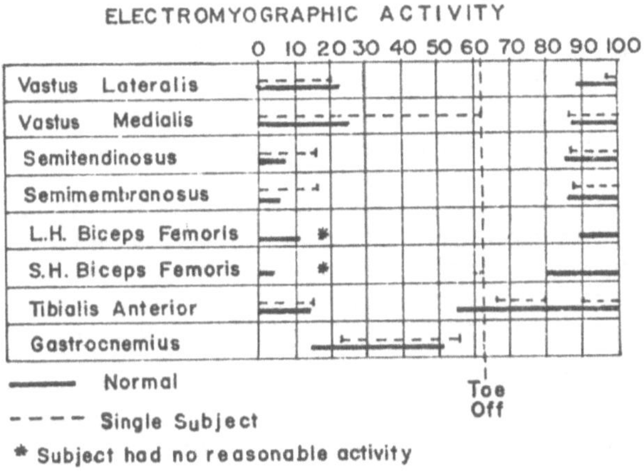

ELECTROMYOGRAPHIC ACTIVITY

0 10 20 30 40 50 60 70 80 90 100

Vastus Lateralis	
Vastus Medialis	
Semitendinosus	
Semimembranosus	
L.H. Biceps Femoris	
S.H. Biceps Femoris	
Tibialis Anterior	
Gastrocnemius	

—————— Normal

— — — — Single Subject

* Subject had no reasonable activity

Toe Off

Figure 14.   EMG data of a normal single subject compared to
average data.

5.   THE EXO-PROSTHETICS PROBLEM

Though the estimates of loading are not as difficult for the
design of an artificial limb, the duplication of the motion of the
natural limb becomes much more difficult since the shank and foot
generally have no independent power source. The motion of the
natural shank foot system is also very difficult to duplicate for
several reasons. The lack of musculature across the knee requires
that the prosthetic knee be stable at heel contact and remain
stable during the single support period of the gait cycle. The
normal knee will be flexed during much of the single support period,
thus the gait of the amputee must be somewhat altered from normal.
These alterations lead to the larger energy expenditure shown in
the energy graph in Figure 11. At toe-off of the prosthesis, the
flexible foot cannot compensate for the dorsi flexion and plantar
flexion completely. The amputee must use the resilience of the
foot to accelerate the shank-foot system upward in order to allow
him to swing the leg forward as well as give the push-off force
required to move over his good leg.

Much more motion of the upper body is used to swing the prosthetic leg through since greater elevation of the pelvis is required.
The shank-foot system usually consists of a relatively rigid ankle
joint, and since the toe of the foot cannot be raised or lowered
independently greater clearance is needed to allow the foot to
swing through. The forces and motions of the prosthesis have been

reported by Cunningham [30] and in [12]. One of the more difficult problems is that the knee is not a simple pin joint. The knee joint is formed by a cupped segment rolling and sliding on a curved con-dylar surface. The condylar surface is not circular thus the centre of the joint is a complex function of the angular alignment of the thigh and shank. Attempts have been made to model the polycentric joint by using specific designs of four bar links [31] and to control the swing phase by using a pneumatic drag cylinder.

The result of the changes in the behaviour of the prosthesis is an asymmetrical gait. In order to determine the gait pattern both legs must be marked and recorded and heel strike on each recorded. Lateral movement of the upper body also tends to increase as well as an increase in amplitude of motion in the sagittal plane.

The joint moments about all three orthogonal axes are of particular concern in the design of the lower limb exo-prosthesis because the prosthesis has no musculature at the ankle or knee to control rotation about the longitudinal axis of the leg. In general if one joint out of three is missing or damaged, the remaining two joints may be able to absorb most of the missing functions. How-ever, if two out of three joints are missing then the remaining joint is too limited kinematically to be able to compensate for the missing functions. In the case of the prosthesis for the above-knee amputee, longitudinal torsion must be transmitted through the stump socket interface and absorbed in the restricted elastic media employed in the ankle joint and foot. Dorsiflexion and plantar flexion actions are lost completely and the amputee must rely on the elastic behaviour of the foot for swing phase clearance.

Considering the great number of functions lost to the above-knee amputee and the imperfection of the prosthesis, the energy requirement curve shown in Figure 11 are far more reasonable. The main point made here, however, is that the criteria for design of knee, ankle and foot mechanisms can only be arrived at from the analysis of gait and that each new design or design change must be evaluated more thoroughly in the future than they have been in the past in order to determine the most fruitful design directions in which to develop.

6.   CONCLUDING REMARKS

The first purpose of gait analysis, that of defining normal gait, has been accomplished to a large extent for the sagittal plane and lower extremities. Although the kinematic and force curves have been developed and show similar characteristics from subject to subject, methods of mathematical comparison of the existing curves should be developed to allow fast and inexpensive gait eval-uation to be done. Only after these techniques are developed can gait analysis leave the specialized laboratory and be utilized on a routine basis for clinical practice.

The motion, force and moment curves themselves yield much necessary information for the prosthetic appliance designer and for that reason alone gait analysis as it is presently done is well worthwhile. However, the development of electronics and computation facilities over the last decade and in particular the last five years puts the analysis of the whole body, upper extremities and lower, within the range of standard clinical evaluation. Such analysis leads to more curves of angle, moment and force vs. percent gait cycle and thus emphasizes the next problem of gait analysis.

Further development of data display techniques is required to find methods of display which emphasize the abnormal aspects of gait. The technique of Milner [17] shown in Figure 6 is one such display but others emphasizing force and moment phase and magnitude differences would allow much quicker patient evaluation and could perhaps aid in diagnosis when sufficient pattern identification can be developed.

In the recent past prostheses developed on the basis of better gait analysis have become quite sophisticated. It is questionable whether further organized development can take place unless a better understanding of the total body motion involved in normal and ab-normal gait is developed. It therefore seems that three-dimensional analysis of the upper body motion must be characterized to the same extent that lower extremity motion in the sagittal plane is present-ly characterized. Such a large task must be approached with the data display and end-use considerations in mind.

Gait analysis must be adapted to serve a social or health case purpose if it is to be continued to be funded, thus the techniques of gait analysis are used in a social sense in the analysis of sport and in a health care sense for patient evaluation prior to treatment, during treatment and post-treatment. In this light the need for easier definition of normal through mathematical compar-ison of parameters, better data display, total body data and in-clinic data turnaround can be easily appreciated. The costs of such a system must also be kept within reason but the cost of computational hardware has fallen by an order of magnitude in the last five years, thus data processing may not be the magnitude of problem it initially appears.

In a clinical environment the purpose of gait evaluation will guide the data called for, whether it be kinematic, dynamic, total force or mechanical energy analysis but the foundations of these analyses have been shown to be well developed. What is called for now is the general extension of the analyses to serve as the basis for further developments in the prosthetics and orthotics design field.

154

REFERENCES

1. E.J. Marey, De la Locomotion Terrestre chez les bipedes et les Quadrapeds, Journal de l'Anat. et de la Physiol., 9, 42, 1873.

2. H. Elftman, A Cinematic Study of the Distribution of the Centre of Pressure in the Human Foot, Anat. Rec., 59, 481, 1934.

3. H. Elftman, The Function of the Arms in Walking, Human Biol., 2, 524, 1939.

4. H. Elftman, Forces and Energy Changes in the Leg During Walking, Amer. J. of Physiol., 125, 357, 1939.

5. D.A. Winter, H.G. Sidwall and D.A. Hobson, Measurement and Reduction of Noise in Kinematics and Locomotion, J. Biomech., 7, 157, 1974.

6. D.A. Winter, A.O. Quanbury and G.D. Reimer, Analysis of Instantaneous Energy of Normal Gait, J. Biomech., 9, 253, 1976.

7. D.A. Winter, The Locomotion Laboratory as a Clinical Assessment System, Med. Prog. Technol., 4, 95, 1976.

8. B. Bresler and F.R. Berry, Energy and Power in the Leg During Normal Level Walking. Prosth. Devices Res. Rept., Inst. Engng. Res., University of California, Berkeley, 1951.

9. E. Peizer and D.W. Wright, Human Locomotion in Human Locomotor Engineering, Institution of Mechanical Engineers, London, 1974.

10. H. Gage, Accelerographic Analysis of Human Gait, Amer. Soc. for Mech. Eng. Paper No. 64-WA/HUF 8, 137, 1964.

11. G.L. Smidt, J.S. Arora and R.C. Johnston, Accelerographic Analysis of Several Types of Walking, Am. J. Phys. Med. 50, 285.

12. B. Bresler, C.W. Radcliffe and F.R. Berry, Energy and Power in the Legs of Above-Knee Amputees During Normal Level Walking, Lower Extremity Research Project, Inst. of Engng. Res., University of California, Berkeley, 1957.

13. J.C. Pezzack, R.W. Norman and D.A. Winter, An Assessment of Derivative Determining Techniques Used for Motion Analysis, Technical Note, J. Biomech., 10, 377, 1977.

14. B. Gold and C.M. Rader, Digital Processing of Signals, McGraw-Hill, New York, 1969.

15. A.B. Thornton-Trump and R. Daher, The Prediction of Reaction Forces from Gait Data, J. Biomech., 8, 173, 1975.

16. J. Foort, Personal Communication, Dept. of Mechanical Engineering, University of British Columbia, Vancouver, 1975.

17. M. Milner, D. Dall, A.L. Ruff and P.K. Brennan, Pre- and Post-Operative Angle Diagrams in Cases of Total Hip Reconstruction, Digest of the 5th Canadian Medical and Biological Engineering Conference, Montreal, 1974.

18. W. Weber and E. Weber, <u>Mechanik der Menschlichen Gehwertzenge</u>, Gottingen, 1936.

19. O. Fischer, <u>Der Gang des Menschen</u>, Abhandlungen der Sacchs, Gesellschaft der Wissenschaft, Vol. 21-28.

20. R. Continii, Body Segment Parameters, Part II, Artificial Limbs, <u>16</u>, 1, 1972.

21. J.P. Earl, Measuring Body Segment Parameters of the Leg, M.Sc. Thesis, Dept. of Mech. Engng., University of Manitoba, Winnipeg, 1976.

22. J.P. Paul, Comparison of EMG Signals from Leg Muscles with Corresponding Force Actions from Walkpath Measurements, <u>Human Locomotor Engineering</u>, Institution of Mechanical Engineers, London, 1974.

23. A.B. Thornton-Trump and S. Balakrishnan, Force plate development, Unpublished work, Dept. of Mech. Eng'g, University of Manitoba, Winnipeg, 1978.

24. J.P. Paul, Loading on Normal Hip and Knee Joints and on Joint Replacements, in <u>Advances in Artificial Hip and Knee Joint Technology</u>, ed. M. Schaldach and D. Hohmann, Springer-Verlag, 1976.

25. B. Bresler and J.P. Frankel, The Forces and Moments in the Leg During Level Walking, ASME Trans., <u>72</u>, 27, 1950.

26. G. Bard and H.J. Ralston, Arch. Phys. Med., <u>40</u>, 415, 1959.

27. T.P. Andriacchi, J.A., Ogle and G.O. Galante, Walking Speed as a Basis for Normal and Abnormal Gait Measurements, J. Biomech., <u>10</u>, 261, 1977.

28. A. Capozzo, F. Figura, and M. Marchetti, The Interplay of Muscular and External Forces in Human Ambulation, J. Biomech., <u>9</u>, 35, 1976.

29. A.O. Quanbury, C.D. Foley and W.D.S. Brereton, A Biomechanical Comparison of Two Above-knee Prostheses, <u>Digest of 11th International Conference on Medical and Biological Engineering</u>, Ottawa, 1976.

30. D.M. Cunningham and G.W. Brown, Two Devices for Measuring the Forces Acting on the Human Body During Walking, Biomechanics Laboratory Report, University of California, Berkeley, Calif., 1951.

31. W.D.S. Brereton, R.L. Daher and J.B. Heath, A Compact Modular Prosthetic Knee Unit with Fixed Axis Pneumatic Swing, <u>Digest of the 11th International Conference on Medical and Biological Engineering</u>, Ottawa, 1976.

ON THE BIOMECHANICS OF MAJOR ARTICULATING HUMAN JOINTS*

Ali Erkan Engin

Department of Engineering Mechanics,
The Ohio State University, Columbus, Ohio   U.S.A.

ABSTRACT. The knowledge of the kinematics of the articulating
human joints and the resistive moments associated with them is
very essential for the biodynamic modeling of the human body.
The present treatment of this subject matter includes the following sections: 1. Critique of film techniques used in kinematic
data collections; 2. Brief review of the joint models;
3. Relative motion analysis between two body segments;
4. Experimental determination of the resistive moments at the
joints.

1. INTRODUCTION

One of the approaches to determining tolerance levels of the human
body subjected to expected and/or unexpected dynamic environmental
conditions is managed via utilization of biodynamic analytical
models. The most sophisticated versions of these models are
articulated and multisegmented to simulate all the major articulating joints and segments of the human body. Effectiveness of
these theoretical models depends heavily on the proper description
of the articulating joints as well as the related biological
material properties. The primary emphasis of this presentation is
a thorough examination of the kinematics of the major articulating
joints and discussion of experimental techniques of determination
of the resistive moments at these joints. Although the shoulder
joint is taken for discussion and representative numerical results,

* This work has been supported by the 6570th Aerospace Medical
  Research Laboratory of the United States Air Force.

both the theoretical and experimental techniques which are introduced are similarly applicable to the other joints such as the
elbow, hip, knee and ankle.

The paper starts with a critique of the most widely used
kinematic data collection techniques; i.e., those involving film
and cameras. This is followed with a brief survey of the various
joint models reported in the literature. This section is concluded
with an exposé of a general joint possessing six degrees of freedom and some initial concepts for the development of an exoskeletal
device, which will be shortened to the ESD henceforth. In the
fourth section the fundamental concepts of the kinematics of the
relative motion in three dimensional space is cast into a format
which provides the prelude for the development of the theoretical
and the design aspects of the ESD. In the final section experimental determination of the passive resistive moments at the
joints is presented by considering the shoulder joint as an
example.

2. CRITIQUE OF FILM TECHNIQUES USED IN KINEMATIC DATA COLLECTION

Data collection for the kinematic and kinetic analyses of the
human motion plays a very significant role in the fields of
biomechanics and kinesiology. Among the many devices used in
understanding of the human motion are electromyographs, protractor
type goniometers, electrogoniometers, stroboscopes, still cameras,
normal-and-high-speed motion picture cameras, TV cameras, X-rays,
various force and moment transducers, and associated recording and
data reducing equipment. Our purpose here is only to examine
briefly the techniques employing film and cameras in studying
human motion.

Film and camera techniques can be most likely classified into
two categories, i.e., namely those requiring still and those
requiring motion picture cameras. Naturally, in each category
there exist sub-categories utilizing single and multiple cameras
and variations on the established techniques. In the still camera
category, the most widely used technique is chronophotography or
interrupted light photography which was developed first by Marey
[1] in 1873. Marey's method utilized a rotating disk with a
variable number of apertures placed in front of the open shutter
of a camera to take successive exposures on a single fixed piece
of film, of a walking subject who wore shiny reflecting buttons
and bands on various segments of his body which was mostly covered
by a black outfit. In 1950 Bresler and Frankel [2], in their
study of the kinematics and kinetics of walking subjects, used
continuously lighted opthalmoscope bulbs instead of shiny buttons.
By exposing a film in a darkened room to the lights 30 times a
second, they obtained a photograph containing many points of
light. With these data points they were able to calculate displacements, velocities, and accelerations of various segments

of the leg by graphic and arithmetic techniques.

The stroboscope can be used to illuminate the subject to make a composite picture of the motion by recording several instantaneous positions on a film of a still camera with open shutter. The number of positions recorded is, of course, controlled by the frequency setting of the stroboscope. If the motion is coplanar it is possible to obtain the kinematic data (i.e. displacements, velocities and accelerations) from the exposed film. However, if the motion is three-dimensional, the stroboscopic picture has the same shortcomings as chronophotography in that they cannot provide sufficient information to determine the actual kinematic data. Naturally, the biggest disadvantage of the stroboscopic photography is the overlapping images of the body segments at the boundaries of the range of motion.

Cinematography with both normal-and high speed motion picture cameras is the second category of collecting data for kinematic analysis of motion. Hyzer [3] and Mascelli and Miller [4] discuss many topics on cinematopography dealing with measurement errors due to relative movements of subject with respect to the shutter of the camera, lens aberrations, film distortions, subject-plane relation to film-plane, types of equipment, lighting, exposure, etc. Frame-by-frame analysis of the motion picture film results in composite tracings and "stick figures" showing the positions of the body segments. For the two dimensional coordinate measurements, special equipment such as a Vanguard analyzer is needed. The biggest drawback of cinematographic motion study besides its shortcomings in space and time resolution is the excessive effort requirement for frame-by-frame analysis to obtain the kinematic data.

There are two assumptions usually made in photographic data collecting: (a) the plane of photography can sufficiently approximate or model the spatial motion; (b) the spatial orientation of plane of photography is known exactly at all times. Frequently, these assumptions do not hold and are not verified experimentally. Needless to say, photographic perspective errors increase with the distance of the point of interest from the focus plane. Some investigators used telephoto lenses to minimize perspective errors by increasing camera-to-subject distances. Although there are few corrective formulas derived from trigonometric relationships between two two-dimensional perpendicular views of any position in three-dimensional space, they still depend on the measurements made on the film. Furthermore, the optical axes of multiple cameras must be perpendicular and intersect at a common point. An additional disadvantage of most multiple camera techniques is the requirement of the filming of the landmarks or targets by all cameras for determination of the three coordinates. Because of the solid, irregular, and opaque nature of the body segments, the same landmark or the target may not be seen all the time by all the cameras. Finally, it is extremely difficult to collect more than three degrees of freedom

information at a given body joint by means of film techniques.
Analyses of the complex body joints require the data collection to
be made by considering all six degrees of freedom at the joint.
In view of the above comments, it was decided to develop an exoskeletal device which is a spatial linkage system providing one
with the capability of studying the six degrees of freedom motion
between two body segments. A device such as the ESD is also
necessary since the kinematic data must be coupled with the force
data during determination of the passive moments at the joints as
will be explained in the fifth section of this paper.

3. BRIEF REVIEW OF THE JOINT MODELS

In each articulating human joint, a total of six degrees of freedom exist to some extent. We must emphasize the point that the
"degrees of freedom" used here should be understood in the sense
it is defined in mechanics, because the majority of the anatomists
and the medical people have different understanding of this concept; e.g. both Steindler [5] and MacConaill [6] imply that three
degrees of freedom is the maximum number required for anatomical
motion. In the following paragraphs a brief survey of the various
joint models reported in the literature is presented. This survey
by no means is all inclusive, but an attempt was made to include
all representative studies on joint models. The classification of
the joint models is made according to the order of increasing
complexity.

3.1 Hinge or revolute joint (Single degree of freedom joint)

This is probably the most widely used articulating joint model and
related publications are extensive. When the articulation between
two body segments is assumed to be a hinge type, the motion between
these two segments is characterized by rotation about a single
axis fixed in one of the segments. Thus, only one independent
coordinate, i.e. the angle formed between two reference lines
inscribed on the segments, is sufficient to determine the position
of one segment with respect to the other one. Some representative
publications assuming hinge joint models in the order of their
appearance in the literature, are: for the elbow by Murphy et al.
[7], Adrian [8], Ringer and Adrian [9] and by Murray et al. [10];
for the hip by Clayson et al. [11], Murphy et al. [7] and Shoup
[12]; for the knee by Saunders et al. [13], Leighton [14], Young
[15], Finley and Karpovich [16], Contini et al. [17], Lieberson
[18], Murphy et al. [7], Klissouras and Karpovich [19] and Beckett
and Chang [20]; for the ankle by Saunders [13], Finley and
Karpovich [16], Gollnick and Karpovich [21], Lieberson [18],
Murphy et al. [7], and Beckett and Chang [20]. Even the shoulder
joint has been modeled in a particular plane as a hinge joint,
Freedman and Munro [22].

3.2 Spherical joint (Limited to two degrees of freedom)

This type of joint is a special case of the three degrees of
freedom spherical or ball and socket joint. There are two
versions of this joint which received some attention in literature.
The first version differs from the three degrees of freedom
spherical joint only by the absence of the axial rotation, i.e. ψ
is equal to zero in Fig. 1; thus, the motion is determined by the
two independent coordinates ϕ and θ. Whereas, in the second
version, the axial rotation is allowed but the motion is restricted to a plane passing through the center of the sphere. In Fig. 1
this type of motion is illustrated as a slotted ball and socket
joint. The slot is defined by θ is equal to a constant and the
independent coordinates are ϕ and ψ. Some representative publications for the first version are: for the wrist by Taylor and
Blaschke [23]; for the elbow by Engen [24]; for the shoulder by
Roebuck [25]; for the hip by Paul [26]; and for the knee by

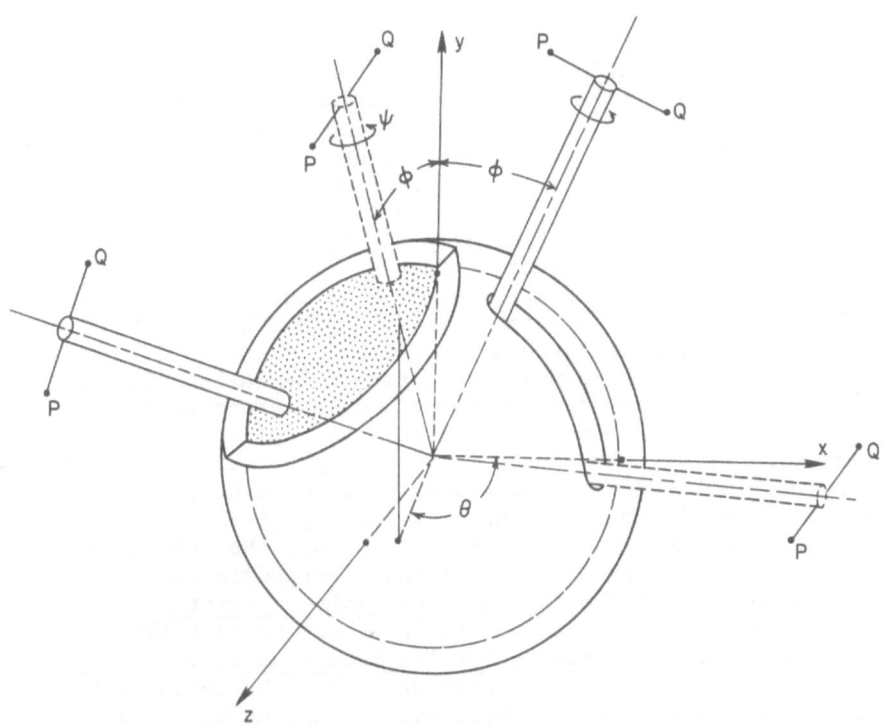

Fig. 1. Spherical or ball and socket joint is illustrated. Figure
displays both versions of the two degrees of freedom as well as
the most general three degrees of freedom spherical joint.

Bresler and Frankel [2], Eberhart and Inman [27], Hallen and
Lindahl [28] and Morrison [29]. The second version of the two
degrees of freedom spherical joint has been used primarily for
the elbow by Taylor and Blaschke [23], and by Dempster [30]; for
the knee by Dempster [30], and Lamoreux [31].

3.3 Spherical or ball and socket joint (Three degrees of freedom)

Needless to say, this type of joint is most frequently used for
the modeling of hip and shoulder joints. The motion is characterized as shown in the left hand side of Fig. 1 by the independent
coordinates ϕ, θ and ψ. For the hip we can cite the publications
by Dempster [30], McKee [32], Johnston and Smidt [33], Chao [34],
Lamoreux [31] and Smidt [35]; for the shoulder the publications
by Taylor and Blaschke [23], Dempster [30], Bahniuk and Wijnschenk
[37], Steindler [5], Bousso [38], and Risteen and Torfason [39].

3.4 Planar joint (Three degrees of freedom)

As the title suggests, this type of joint permits motion on a
single plane and allows the arbitrary location of the instantaneous axes which are always normal to the plane of motion. The
primary application of planar joint model has been the knee joint
as shown in Fig. 2. Naturally, the three independent coordinates
for determination of this type of motion are two cartesian
coordinates, i.e. the coordinates of point C, and one coordinate,
θ, defining the amount of rotation about an axis perpendicular to
the plane of motion. The rotation angle θ is equal to the angle
between P_1Q_1 and P_2Q_2. The points P_1, P_2, Q_1 and Q_2 will be
explained in the following second paragraph.
   Planar motion can be studied by a technique called "Instant
Centers", more explicitly instantaneous centers of rotation.
Dempster [30] appears to be the first one who applied this
kinematic principle to the planar motion study of the knee joint.
This principle is based upon the notion that for a body executing
a general plane motion one can show that at any given instant the
velocities of the various points of the body are the same as if
the body were rotating about a certain axis perpendicular to the
plane of motion, called the _instantaneous axis of rotation_. The
intersection of this axis with the plane of motion is called the
instantaneous center of rotation (_or instantaneous center of zero_
velocity). As the motion of the body proceeds, the instantaneous
center moves on the plane. If these centers are marked each time
on the body or on the hypothetical extension of the body, they
describe a curve on the body, called _body centrode_. If the same
thing is done with respect to a fixed reference another curve is
obtained, called _space centrode_. At any instant these two curves
are tangent at the corresponding instantaneous center and, as the

body moves, the body centrode appears to roll on the space centrode.

By the method of Rouleaux (Fig. 2) one can easily determine the instant centers in the following manner: Lateral roentgenograms of the knee are taken with 15-20° increments from full extension to 90° or more flexion. On the first x-ray film two separate points P_1, Q_1 of the femur are identified and the displacements P_1P_2 and Q_1Q_2 of these two points are determined as the femur moves from one position (1) to another (2) by viewing the two subsequent x-ray films simultaneously on top of each other and drawing lines between the successive positions of each point. These lines connecting the successive positions represent the displacement of the corresponding point. The intersection of the bisectors of the displacements of the two points will be the instant center for the displacement. The locus of these displacement centers is also the body centrode. In fact, the displacement centers for the successive positions of the femur lie between the points defining the instant centers of zero velocity. With the

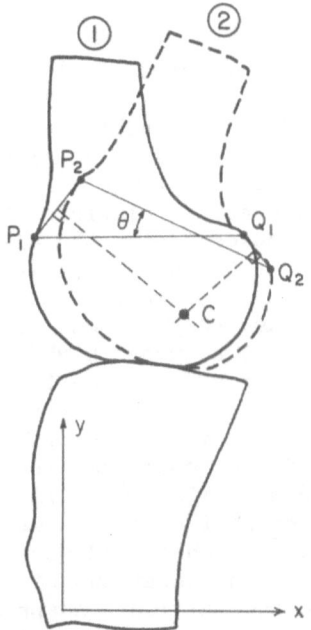

Fig. 2. Planar joint having three degrees of freedom is illustrated by the example of the knee joint. Figure also shows the application of the method of Rouleaux in determination of the instant centers.

knowledge of the location of the instant centers (of zero velocity) for the two moving bodies which are in contact, one can easily determine the type of relative motion between them since an instant center on the contact surface indicates pure rolling, while an instant center away from the surface indicates some sliding compounded with rolling.

Some notable publications for the knee joint using or accepting the planar joint model are by Barnett [40], Radcliffe [41], Burstein and Frankel [42], Shute [43], Freudenstein and Woo [44], Frankel et al. [45], Reilly and Martin [46], and Smidt [36]. Planar joint model has also been used for the shoulder and elbow by Dempster [30] and Evans [47] and for ankle by Sammarco et al. [48].

Most of the studies quoted so far have utilized protractor type goniometers, electrogoniometers, chronophotography, cinematography and sometimes simple instrumented linkages to determine the kinematics of the joint motion up to three degrees of freedom. We will next consider a joint possessing six degrees of freedom and introduce some concepts for the development of a versatile exoskeletal device.

3.5 General Joint (Six degrees of freedom)

The joint with six degrees of freedom allows all possible motions between two segments of the body. A good application of this type of a joint model is the shoulder joint where a four segment articulation between the humerus, scapula, clavicle and the rib cage exists. Of course, at the shoulder joint the six degrees of freedom refers to the motion of the humerus relative to the torso. If one considers the total number of degrees of freedom for the motions executed by the humerus, scapula, and clavicle relative to the rib cage, one can easily get a number higher than six even with the proper consideration of various constraints present in the joint complex. Most of the previous work on general joint motion have been conducted by the investigators in dentistry and prosthodontia in the study of the temporomandibular joint. Beck and Morrison [49] introduced an instrumented linkage to measure mandibular motion and later on similar system was developed by Cannon [50] and Messerman [51]. Cannon and Messerman used the instrumented linkage to define the locations of three points in the mandible with respect to the maxilla. Knapp et al. [52] studied jaw motion by relating the orientation of a coordinate system on the mandible to the one on the maxilla. Thompson [53] has developed a mechanical linkage system which consisted of monitoring the lengths of six links which are connected via ball and socket joints to the femur and the tibia for the purposes of studying the motion of the human knee. In a relatively recent study, Kinzel et al. [54] used a linkage system which was attached to the scapula and humerus of a dog by Kirschner-Ehmer

splints to determine the relative motion between the two
articulating surfaces.

The basic concept for the study of the general joint is quite
fundamental and its origin probably goes back to the classical
work by Chasles [55]. Consider the general motion of two rigid
bodies A and B in three dimensional space as shown in Fig. 3. The
relative motion of body B with respect to body A can be characterized by a unique axis called the <u>screw axis</u>. The relative
displacement of body B from position 1 to position 2 can be
defined in terms of a rotation Δα about and translation Δs along
the screw axis. For each incremental displacement of body B with
respect to body A, a new screw axis is defined. In fact, if the
increments taken by body B are made infinitesimal in size, the
collection of the screw axes will form a ruled surface called an
axode. There are two unique axodes, one associated with the
motion of body B with respect to body A, and another one is
associated with the motion of A with respect to B. During the
relative motion, the two axodes roll and slide relative to each

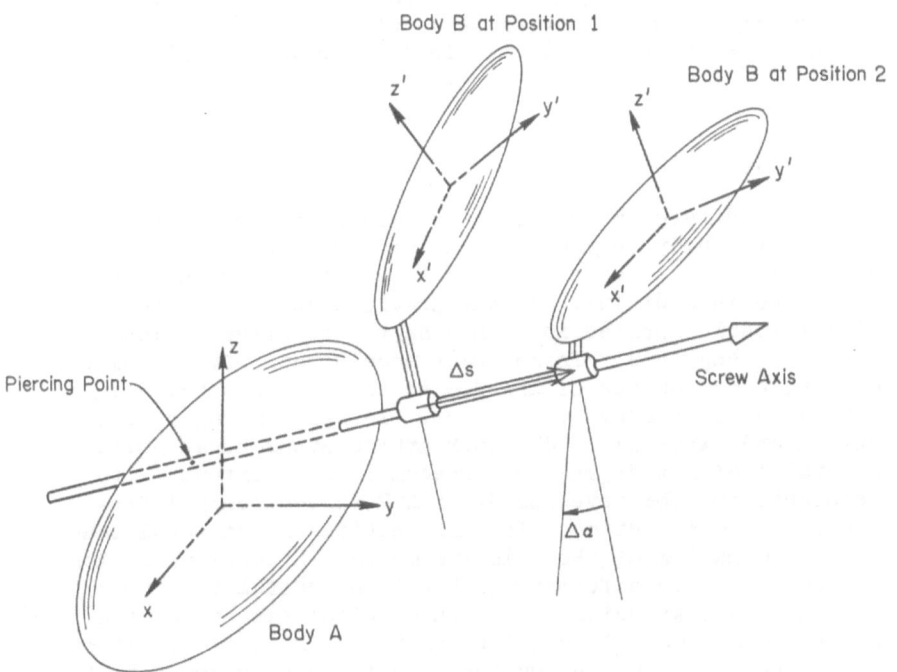

Fig. 3. General motion of two rigid bodies in three dimensional
space and the screw axis used in characterization of the relative
motion between them are illustrated.

other along a generator which is momentarily common to both axode surfaces, [56]. Incidentally, the screw axes and axodes are the generalization for spatial motion of the instant centers and centrodes associated with the general planar motion. For a planar motion, the axodes become two rolling cylinders and the curves formed by the intersection of the motion plane, i.e. the plane which is perpendicular to the generators of the two cylinders, with the cylinders are the centrodes of planar motion. For the spherical joints the axodes become two rolling cones with common apexes at the center of the sphere and for the revolute joints they simply degenerate to a single axis, i.e. the axis of the joint. Of course, in each one of these specialized cases the translation, Δs along the screw axes is zero.

In view of the above remarks, the design of ESD is governed in such a way that any instrumented linkage system must provide us with sufficient data to determine the six parameters associated with the screw axes. The six degrees of freedom between two rigid bodies are in a sense transformed to determination of following six parameters: two parameters which are the coordinates of the piercing point of the screw axes with any one of the three coordinate planes (e.g., xz plane in Fig. 3), two parameters which are the direction cosines of the screw axes, the remaining two parameters are the translations along and rotations about the screw axes.

4. RELATIVE MOTION ANALYSIS BETWEEN TWO BODY SEGMENTS

The quantitative determination of the nature of the relative motion between two body segments which are connected with a complex anatomical joint is of prime importance to biomechanicans as well as to those in medicine. In the previous section we reviewed various joint models applied in examining the relative motion between two body segments. These joint models range from a simple hinge joint with one degree of freedom to the most general joint model possessing six degrees of freedom. In reality, under both physiological and external loads, each articulating human joint displays a total of six degrees of freedom to some extent. The initial concepts for the development of ESD were already introduced in the previous section. In this section, fundamental concepts of the kinematics of the relative motion in three dimensional space will be cast into a format which will be useful for the development and understanding of the theoretical aspects of the ESD. In particular, we will examine first, the relative position of a point on the upper arm executing a motion with respect to the torso and, second, the displacement of that point during motion. We will derive matrix expressions relating the position and displacement concepts in the light of the screw axis analysis.

Let us consider the relative motion of arm designated as body segment B in Fig. 4 with respect to the torso which is designated

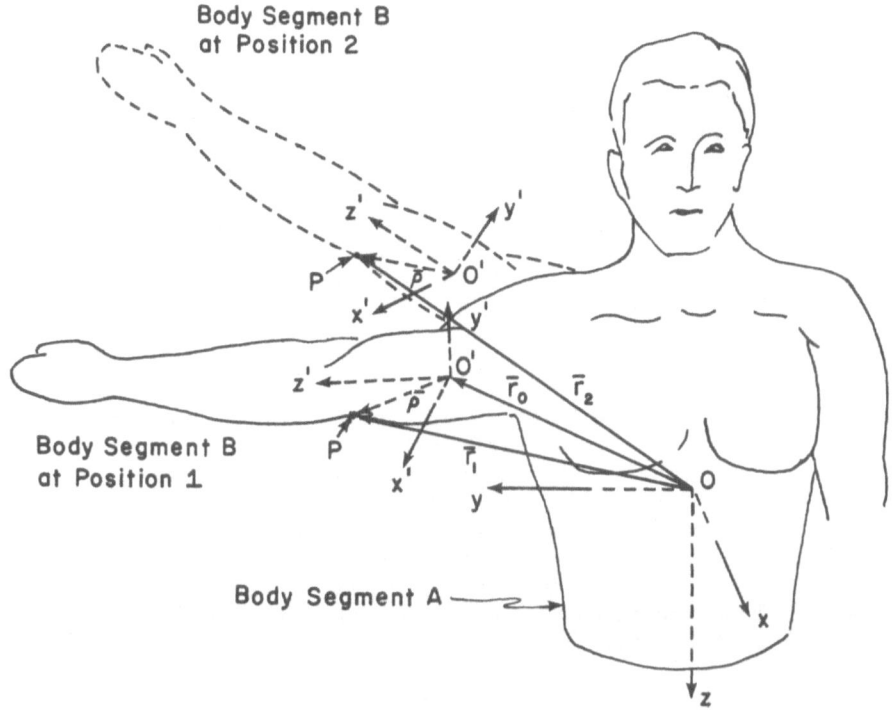

Fig. 4. Motion of body segment B with respect to body segment A in three dimensional space. Displacement of body segment B from position 1 to position 2 is illustrated.

as body segment A. For the intention of studying the relative motion between these two body segments, let us assume that one of them e.g., body segment A, be fixed and the other one, body segment B, is moving relative to body segment A. Note that the range of motion between body segments A and B is controlled by the joint anatomy and ligamentous as well as muscle forces present during motion. It is very essential to point out before we proceed further that no human body segment is a rigid body in the sense defined in mechanics. However, for the purposes of studying the nature of motion in a given anatomical joint the adjacent body segments to this joint can be assumed to be rigid bodies if certain precautions, which will be discussed in conjunction with the ESD attachment techniques to the body segments, are observed. Let the unprimed xyz and the primed x'y'z' cartesian coordinate systems be attached to the body segments A and B, respectively. These coordinate systems can be also referred to as fixed and moving coordinate systems since body segment A is assumed to be fixed and body segment B is considered to be moving.

Let P be an arbitrary point in body segment B whose position is designated by vectors $\bar{\rho}$ and $\bar{r}_1$ ($\bar{r}_1$ @ position 1; $\bar{r}_2$ @ position 2) in references x'y'z' and xyz, respectively. Since point P is fixed in a moving body segment, the components of vector $\bar{\rho}$ in reference x'y'z' will remain constant, whereas the components of vector $\bar{r}_1$ will change as the body segment B moves relative to body segment A. In fact, the relative position of the moving segment is considered completely determined with respect to the fixed segment if for every point in the moving segment and its associated local position vector $\bar{\rho}$, the corresponding $\bar{r}_1$ can be found. From Fig. 4 the relationship between vectors $\bar{r}_1$, $\bar{r}_o$ and $\bar{\rho}$ can be written in compact matrix form

$$[r_1] = [r_o] + [T][\rho] \tag{4.1}$$

where the elements of matrix T, t_{ij} are the direction cosines of the O'x', O'y' and O'z' axes relative to the axes of the xyz reference. Thus, matrix T represents rotational orientation of x'y'z', whereas matrix $[r_o]$ represents separation of x'y'z' with respect to the fixed xyz reference. It is more convenient to express Eq. (4.1) in terms of augmented vectors $\bar{r}_{1a}$, $\bar{\rho}_a$ whose first component is 1, and a single 4 x 4 matrix T_a by adding the equation $1 = 1$ to the system of equations contained in Eq. (4.1). Thus, Eq. (4.1) takes the following expanded and compact forms:

$$\begin{bmatrix} 1 \\ x_1 \\ y_1 \\ z_1 \end{bmatrix} = \begin{bmatrix} 1 & 0 & 0 & 0 \\ x_o & t_{11} & t_{12} & t_{13} \\ y_o & t_{21} & t_{22} & t_{23} \\ z_o & t_{31} & t_{32} & t_{33} \end{bmatrix} \begin{bmatrix} 1 \\ x_1' \\ y_1' \\ z_1' \end{bmatrix} \quad \text{or} \quad [r_{1a}] = [T_a][\rho_a] \tag{4.2}$$

In this paper the augmented vectors and matrices will be designated by the subscript or additional subscript "a". Note that there is a new matrix T_a for each position of body segment B, however, at a given position the matrix T_a is the same for all points of body segment B. Hence, determination of the matrix T_a is sufficient to know the position of the moving body segment relative to the fixed one. The primary goal of ESD and the related theoretical development is the determination of matrix T_a and via T_a an achievement of a unique description of the instantaneous position of the moving body relative to the fixed body.

For the total description of the relative motion between two body segments, besides the knowledge of the instantaneous positions of the one body segment relative to another, we must have a description of the nature of the displacement during the motion of the moving segment from position 1 to position 2. Needless to say, instantaneous positions and displacements are very closely related. Displacement analysis results in determination of the

set of screw axes; thus, it is essential for the accurate determination of the locations of the joint centers. As was stated in
the previous section, displacement of body segment B from position
1 to position 2 can be defined in terms of a rotation α about and
translation s along the screw axis, Fig. 5. If the two positions
considered are close enough, then the displacements are incremental and refer to a new screw axis each time.

    Let us consider a point P fixed in body segment B. As the
body segment B moves from position 1 to position 2, we can define
the position vectors $\bar{r}_1$ and $\bar{r}_2$ which are expressed in terms of
components in xyz references:

$$\bar{r}_1 = x_1\hat{i} + y_1\hat{j} + z_1\hat{k} \quad \text{and} \quad \bar{r}_2 = x_2\hat{i} + y_2\hat{j} + z_2\hat{k} \qquad (4.3)$$

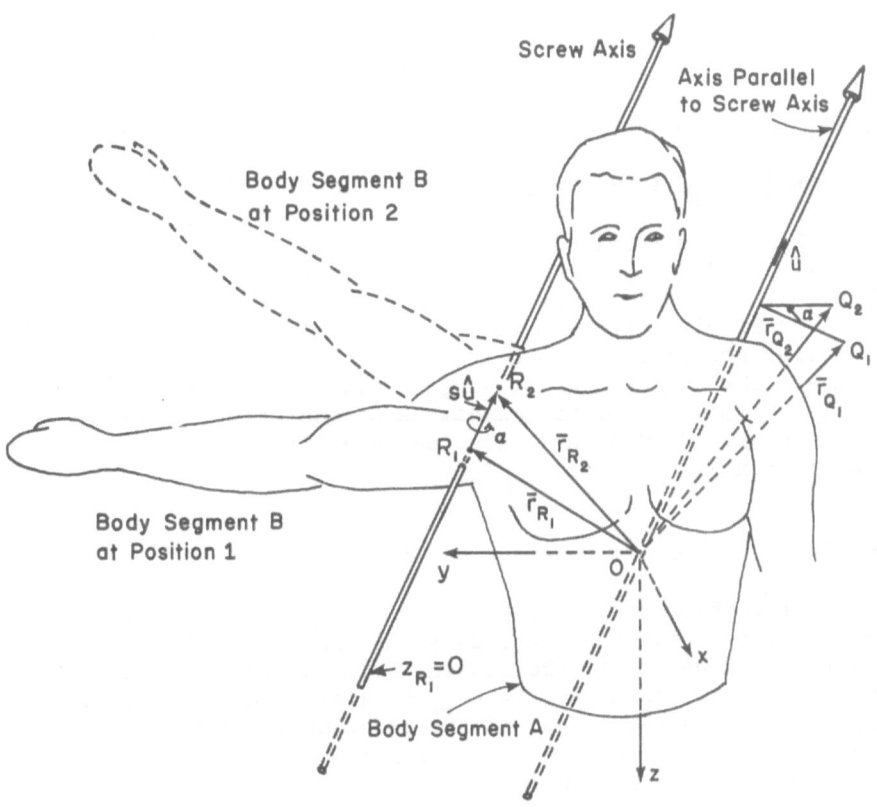

Fig. 5. Representation of the motion of body segment B from
position 1 to position 2 in terms of a rotation α about and
translation s along the screw axis. A pure rotation of magnitude
α of a point Q about an axis parallel to the screw axis is also
displayed.

170

The components of $\bar{r}_2$ will be related to the components of $\bar{r}_1$ by the following special case of an affine transformation [57]:

$$\begin{bmatrix} x_2 \\ y_2 \\ z_2 \end{bmatrix} = \begin{bmatrix} m_{11} & m_{12} & m_{13} \\ m_{21} & m_{22} & m_{23} \\ m_{31} & m_{32} & m_{33} \end{bmatrix} \begin{bmatrix} x_1 \\ y_1 \\ z_1 \end{bmatrix} + \begin{bmatrix} a_x \\ a_y \\ a_z \end{bmatrix} \tag{4.4}$$

Eq. (4.4) can be written in augmented form as

$$\begin{bmatrix} 1 \\ x_2 \\ y_2 \\ z_2 \end{bmatrix} = \begin{bmatrix} 1 & 0 & 0 & 0 \\ a_x & m_{11} & m_{12} & m_{13} \\ a_y & m_{21} & m_{22} & m_{23} \\ a_z & m_{31} & m_{32} & m_{33} \end{bmatrix} \begin{bmatrix} 1 \\ x_1 \\ y_1 \\ z_1 \end{bmatrix} \tag{4.5}$$

Eqs. (4.4) and (4.5) can be expressed in a more compact form as

$$[r_2] = [M][r_1] + [a] \quad \text{and} \quad [r_{2a}] = [M_a][r_{1a}], \tag{4.6}$$

respectively. From a mathematical point of view, the augmented form describes the motion of a three-dimensional set of points contained within body segment B relative to a hyperplane, [58]. In Eq. (4.6) matrix M represents a pure rotation about the screw axis and also contains direction cosines information for the screw axis. The augmented matrix M_a in Eqs. (4.5) and (4.6) has the total information for determination of the displacement of the moving body. We will next consider specification of the rotation matrix M.

4.1 Specification of the rotation matrix M

Since the elements of the rotation matrix M contain only the information concerning the rotation about the screw axis, the translational component of the motion, i.e. the vector whose components are a_x, a_y, a_z in Eq. (4.4), is zero. Thus, the screw axis passes through the origin of xyz reference. In Fig. 5 this is shown as an axis parallel to the original screw axis. Let S be the plane which is perpendicular to the screw axis, Fig. 6. Also, let us define $\bar{r}_1$ as the vector from the origin to a point in the moving body segment. During the motion of the moving body segment from position 1 to position 2, $\bar{r}_1$ will be rotating through an angle α about the screw axis to $\bar{r}_2$. Let $\hat{u} = u_x\hat{i} + u_y\hat{j} + u_z\hat{k}$ be the unit vector along the screw axis. Then, the projections of $\bar{r}_1$ and $\bar{r}_2$ along the screw axis are equal and given by

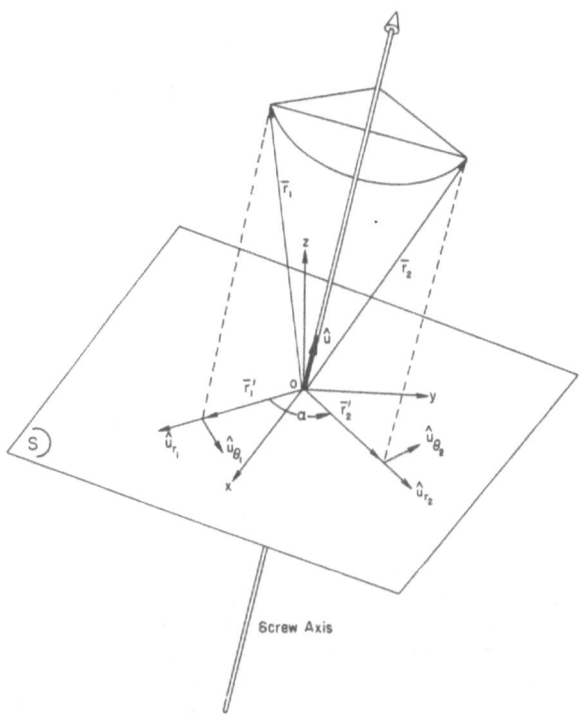

Fig. 6. Coordinate systems and the vectors used in determination of the rotation matrix M.

$$\bar{r}_{1s} = \bar{r}_{2s} = (\bar{r}_1 \cdot \hat{u})\hat{u} \tag{4.7}$$

Let $\bar{r}_1'$ and $\bar{r}_2'$ be the projections of $\bar{r}_1$ and $\bar{r}_2$ in the S-plane, respectively.

$$\text{Since } |\bar{r}_1'| = |\bar{r}_2'|, \quad \bar{r}_2' = (\bar{r}_1 \cdot \hat{u}_{r_1})\hat{u}_{r_2} \quad \text{or} \tag{4.8}$$

$$\bar{r}_2' = (\bar{r}_1 \cdot \hat{u}_{r_1})(\hat{u}_{r_1} \cos\alpha + \hat{u}_{\theta_1} \sin\alpha) \tag{4.9}$$

in view of $\hat{u}_{r2} = \hat{u}_{r1} \cos\alpha + \hat{u}_{\theta1} \sin\alpha$, where the $\hat{u}_{r1}$, $\hat{u}_{\theta1}$, $\hat{u}_{r2}$, $\hat{u}_{\theta2}$ are the unit vectors for the cylindrical coordinate systems. We can now express vector $\bar{r}_2$ as summation of $\bar{r}_{2s}$ and $\bar{r}_2'$, thus from Eqs. (4.7) and (4.9)

$$\bar{r}_2 = (\bar{r}_1 \cdot \hat{u})\hat{u} + (\bar{r}_1 \cdot \hat{u}_{r_1})\hat{u}_{r_1} \cos\alpha + (\bar{r}_1 \cdot \hat{u}_{r_1})\hat{u}_{\theta_1} \sin\alpha \tag{4.10}$$

Next let us eliminate $\hat{u}_{r1}$ and $\hat{u}_{\theta1}$ from Eq. (4.10) by recognizing equivalence of the last two terms of Eq. (4.10) to terms containing cross products of $\hat{u}$ and $\bar{r}$ in the following manner:

$$\bar{r}_2 = (\bar{r}_1 \cdot \hat{u})\hat{u} - [\hat{u} \times (\hat{u} \times \bar{r}_1)] \cos\alpha + (\hat{u} \times \bar{r}_1) \sin\alpha \qquad (4.11)$$

Since $\hat{u} \times (\hat{u} \times \bar{r}_1) = (\bar{r}_1 \cdot \hat{u})\hat{u} - \bar{r}_1$, Eq. (4.11) can be put in the form of

$$\bar{r}_2 = (1-\cos\alpha)(\bar{r}_1 \cdot \hat{u})\hat{u} + \bar{r}_1 \cos\alpha + (\hat{u} \times \bar{r}_1) \sin\alpha \qquad (4.12)$$

This is a vector relation between $\bar{r}_1$, $\bar{r}_2$; it can be cast to matrix form by substituting the components of $\bar{r}_1$, $\bar{r}_2$ and $\hat{u}$ into Eq. (4.12). Thus in the absence of translational component of the motion and in view of Eqs. (4.4) and (4.12), the desired 3x3 rotation matrix M is obtained:

$$\begin{bmatrix} u_x^2(1-\cos\alpha)+\cos\alpha & u_x u_y(1-\cos\alpha)-u_z\sin\alpha & u_x u_z(1-\cos\alpha)+u_y\sin\alpha \\ u_x u_y(1-\cos\alpha)+u_z\sin\alpha & u_y^2(1-\cos\alpha)+\cos\alpha & u_y u_z(1-\cos\alpha)u_x\sin\alpha \\ u_x u_z(1-\cos\alpha)-u_y\sin\alpha & u_y u_z(1-\cos\alpha)+u_x\sin\alpha & u_z^2(1-\cos\alpha)+\cos\alpha \end{bmatrix}$$

Note that the matrix M with elements m_{ij} is the submatrix of M_a as shown in Eq. (4.5). So far, we have determined only the rotational part of M_a. Next, we will focus our attention on the second submatrix of M_a with elements a_x, a_y and a_z to determine the instantaneous orientations of the screw axes.

4.2 Determination of the orientation of the screw axis

In general, the screw axis does not pass through the origin of xyz reference as indicated in Fig. 5. However, if we can find the direction cosines of a line, passing through the origin of xyz and parallel to the screw axis about which the actual motion takes place, we will have the direction cosines of the general screw axis. The elements, m_{ij}, of the rotation matrix M are independent of where the actual screw axis is located; the matrix M was, in fact, determined by considering a rotation about an axis passing through the origin of xyz reference.

Fig. 5 shows a pure rotation of a point Q about an axis passing through the origin. The position vectors of Q, i.e. $\bar{r}_{Q1}$ and $\bar{r}_{Q2}$ satisfy the same matrix equation given by Eq. (4.4) excluding the translational component of the motion; thus, in compact form

$$[r_{Q_2}] = [M][r_{Q_1}] \qquad (4.13)$$

Since we are looking for the components of $\hat{u}$, let us move the point Q to the axis, such that $\bar{r}_{Q1}$ and $\bar{r}_{Q2}$ are now equal and lie along the same axis. Hence,

$$[M - I][r_Q] = [0] \qquad (4.14)$$

For the nontrivial solution of $\overline{r}_Q$ the determinant of the matrix [M - I] must be zero, [59]. From Eq. (4.14) the vector $\overline{r}_Q$ can be determined only within a constant specifying the length of $\overline{r}_Q$. However, if we designate that constant as 1, then $\overline{r}_Q$ becomes $\hat{u}$ and Eq. (4.14) takes the form of

$$
\begin{bmatrix} m_{11} - 1 & m_{12} & m_{13} \\ m_{21} & m_{22} - 1 & m_{23} \\ m_{31} & m_{32} & m_{33} - 1 \end{bmatrix} \begin{bmatrix} u_x \\ u_y \\ u_z \end{bmatrix} = \begin{bmatrix} 0 \\ 0 \\ 0 \end{bmatrix} \tag{4.15}
$$

From the above equation u_y and u_z can be solved in terms of u_x

$$
u_y = \frac{m_{23}m_{31} - m_{21}(m_{33}-1)u_x}{(m_{22}-1)(m_{33}-1) - m_{23}m_{32}} \quad , \quad u_z = \frac{m_{21}m_{32} - m_{31}(m_{22}-1)u_x}{(m_{22}-1)(m_{33}-1) - m_{23}m_{32}} \tag{4.16}
$$

Substituting u_y and u_z into $u_x^2 + u_y^2 + u_z^2 = 1$ yields u_x. Thus, the direction cosines of the screw axis, i.e. the orientation of the same axis, are determined in terms of the elements of the rotation matrix M. Incidentally, once the direction cosines of the screw axis are known, the rotation angle α can be computed very easily from the m_{11} term of the matrix M

$$
\alpha = \cos^{-1} \left[\frac{m_{11} - u_x^2}{1 - u_x^2} \right] \tag{4.17}
$$

Note that both the direction cosines and the rotation angle α depend on the elements of the matrix M. Before we obtain the remaining parameters, i.e. the translation s along the screw axis and the piercing point coordinates of the screw axis, let us discuss how one can determine the matrix M_a which contains the submatrix M.

4.3 Determination of the matrix M_a

To determine the matrix M_a, it is sufficient to know the coordinates of four non-coplanar points P_1, P_2, P_3 and P_4 in the moving body segment in both positions 1 and 2. Let us designate the position vectors of these four points by $\overline{\rho}_{ij}$ and $\overline{r}_{ij}$ relative to the moving x'y'z' and the fixed xyz references, respectively. In this subscripted notation, the first subscript i (i = 1,2,3,4) is used to designate a point and the second subscript j (j = 1,2) is used for the designation of positions 1 and 2. The augmented vectors $\overline{r}_{ija}$ for each point can be related via Eq. (4.6).

$$
[r_{i2a}] = [M_a][r_{i1a}] \quad (i = 1,2,3,4) \tag{4.18}
$$

Eq. (4.18) represents four matrix equations which can be written in one equation by defining a new matrix A whose columns are the augmented vectors, $\bar{r}_{ija}$,

$$[A_j] \overset{d}{=} \begin{bmatrix} 1 & 1 & 1 & 1 \\ x_{1j} & x_{2j} & x_{3j} & x_{4j} \\ y_{1j} & y_{2j} & y_{3j} & y_{4j} \\ z_{1j} & z_{2j} & z_{3j} & z_{4j} \end{bmatrix} \quad (j = 1,2) \tag{4.19}$$

Hence, Eq. (4.18) becomes

$$[A_2] = [M_a][A_1] \tag{4.20}$$

The matrix A has a non-vanishing determinant since it is formed by the position vectors of non-coplanar points; thus, it has an inverse and the desired matrix M_a is easily obtained from Eq. (4.20),

$$[M_a] = [A_2][A_1]^{-1} \tag{4.21}$$

In theory, by means of Eq. (4.21), the matrix M_a is known and can be determined. However, Eq. (4.21) requires continuous monitoring of four non-coplanar points of the moving body segment. Thus, it does not render a convenient way of determining M_a from an experimental point of view. This situation can be circumvented by utilization of Eq. (4.2) for two instantaneous and close posi-tions of the moving body segment in determining the matrix M_a. In view of Eq. (4.2), the augmented vectors $\bar{\rho}_{ija}$ and $\bar{r}_{ija}$ for each point and position are related as

$$[r_{ija}] = [T_a][\rho_{ija}] \quad \begin{Bmatrix} i = 1,2,3,4 \\ j = 1,2 \end{Bmatrix} \tag{4.22}$$

Eq. (4.22) represents eight matrix equations or four matrix equa-tions for each position. Let us define a new matrix B whose columns are the augmented vectors $\bar{\rho}_{ija}$, i.e.

$$[B] \overset{d}{=} \begin{bmatrix} 1 & 1 & 1 & 1 \\ x_1' & x_2' & x_3' & x_4' \\ y_1' & y_2' & y_3' & y_4' \\ z_1' & z_2' & z_3' & z_4' \end{bmatrix} \tag{4.23}$$

Then, in view of Eqs. (4.2), (4.19), and (4.23) we have

$$[A_j] = [T_{ja}][B] \qquad (j = 1,2) \qquad (4.24)$$

Substituting A_1 and A_2 obtained from Eq. (4.24) into Eq. (4.20) gives

$$[T_{2a}][B] = [M_a][T_{1a}][B]$$

which yields after postmultiplication by $[B]^{-1}[T_{1a}]^{-1}$

$$[M_a] = [T_{2a}][T_{1a}]^{-1} \qquad (4.25)$$

where T_{1a} and T_{2a} are the coordinate transformation matrices between xyz and x'y'z' references for positions 1 and 2. The main task of ESD is indeed the continuous monitoring of the necessary parameters for the evaluation of T_a matrices. More will be said on this topic in the last section of this paper. We now turn back to the discussion of the parameter s, which is the translation along the screw axis, and the piercing point coordinates.

4.4 Determination of screw displacement and piercing point coordinates

To find the translational component of the motion along the screw axis, let us consider a point R_1 belonging to the moving body segment or belonging to the hypothetical extension of the moving body segment as shown in Fig. 5. The translation of this point along the screw axis from R_1 to R_2 is designated as su and the corresponding position vectors, $\bar{r}_{R_1}$ and $\bar{r}_{R_2}$, satisfy:

$$[r_{R_{2a}}] = [M_a][r_{R_{1a}}] \quad \text{or} \quad [r_{R_2}] = [M][r_{R_1}] + \begin{bmatrix} a_x \\ a_y \\ a_z \end{bmatrix} \qquad (4.26)$$

Translation along the screw axis is given as:

$$s[u] = [r_{R_2}] - [r_{R_1}] \qquad (4.27)$$

From Eqs. (4.26) and (4.27) we obtain

$$\begin{bmatrix} m_{11}-1 & m_{12} & m_{13} \\ m_{21} & m_{22}-1 & m_{23} \\ m_{31} & m_{32} & m_{33}-1 \end{bmatrix} \begin{bmatrix} x_{R_1} \\ y_{R_1} \\ z_{R_1} \end{bmatrix} = \begin{bmatrix} su_x - a_x \\ su_y - a_y \\ su_z - a_z \end{bmatrix} \qquad (4.28)$$

The coordinates of the piercing point of the screw axis and the value of s are found by setting, one at a time, x_{R_1}, y_{R_1} and z_{R_1} equal to zero. For example, the screw axis will intersect x-y plane of the xyz reference when $z_{R_1} = 0$. For this case it can be shown that Eq. (4.28) reduces to:

$$
\begin{bmatrix} x_{R_1} \\ y_{R_1} \\ s \end{bmatrix} = \begin{bmatrix} m_{11}-1 & m_{12} & -u_x \\ m_{21} & m_{22}-1 & -u_y \\ m_{31} & m_{32} & -u_z \end{bmatrix}^{-1} \begin{bmatrix} -a_x \\ -a_y \\ -a_z \end{bmatrix} \tag{4.29}
$$

Similarly, the intersections of the screw axis with x-z and y-z planes and the screw displacement s are found. With determination of screw displacement and piercing point coordinates of the screw axis we have completed the theoretical groundwork for the development of the ESD which will be one of the essential components of the experimental apparatus for determination of the passive moments at the major articulating human joints.

5. EXPERIMENTAL DETERMINATION OF THE RESISTIVE MOMENTS AT THE JOINTS

There is no doubt that biodynamic models play a very important role in understanding the behavior of the human body subjected to biodynamic conditions. Small time response of these models requires proper characterization of the passive resistive moments in articulating joints. The rest of this paper is devoted to a brief treatment of determination of these passive resistive moments. Due to drastic postmortem changes of the biomechanical properties of the body tissues, the resistive moments should be determined with some obvious limitations on live human subjects. In the following section descriptions of specially designed experimental apparatus and the experimental procedure are presented.

5.1 Major components of the experimental setup

The major components of the experimental apparatus are a subject restraint system (Fig. 7), a global force applicator, GFA (Figs. 8 & 9) and the ESD (Fig. 10). The subject restraint system with its pitch, roll and yaw capabilities can orient the subject to any desired position. This is an important feature of the subject restraint system which assists in the mobilization of subject's appropriate body segment at a constant elevation while the experimentor moves the body segment by means of the GFA throughout its entire range of motion. To eliminate the gravitational component

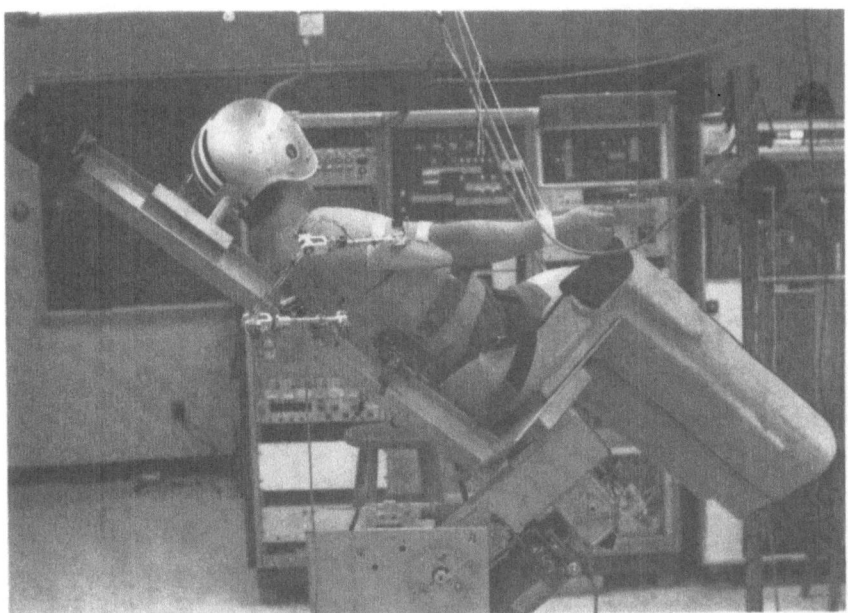

Fig. 7. Overall view of the subject restraint system and data
collection equipment. Subject is prepared for the shoulder force
data acquirement.

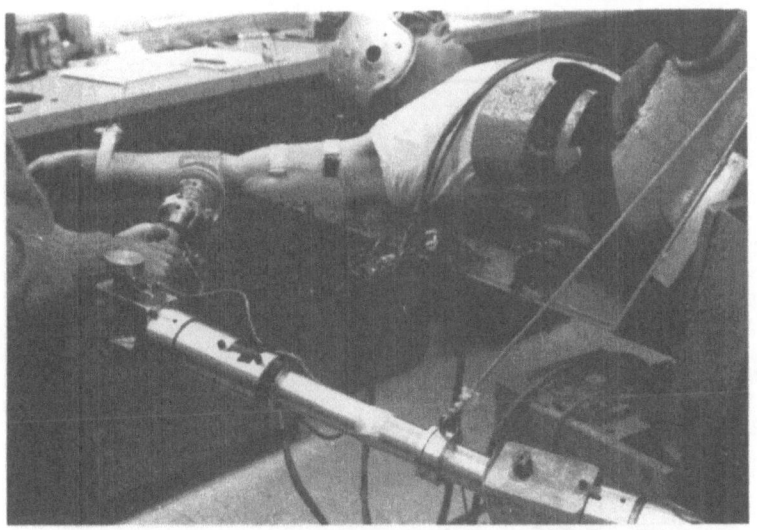

Fig. 8. Force is being applied by means of the GFA on the
subject's arm.

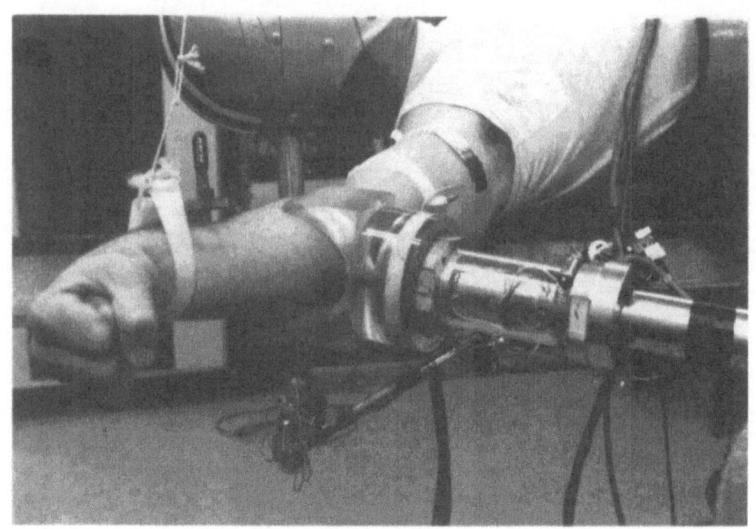

Fig. 9. Close-up view of the force transducer and the force cuff.

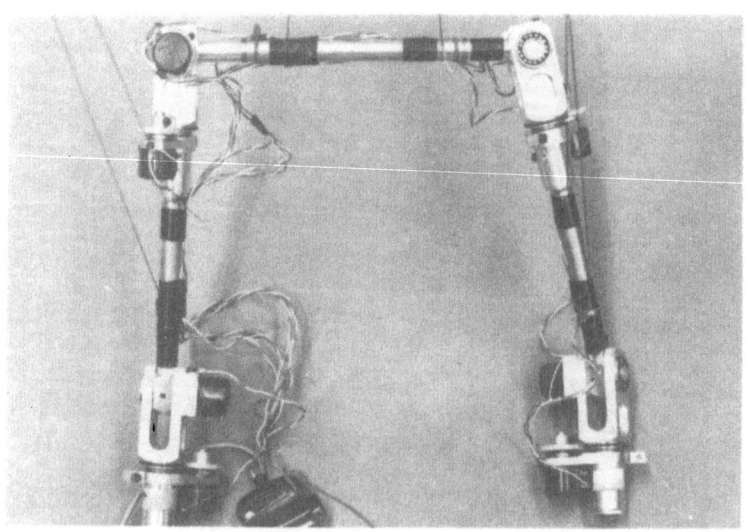

Fig. 10. Close-up view of the exoskeletal device (ESD).

of the moment values at the joint centers, the force application
to the moving body segment is made in a horizontal plane while
the elevation of the moving body segment is maintained by a
support line in such a way that in the direction of the force
application a relaxed floating type of motion of the moving body
segment is achieved. Both the security and the support characteristics of the restraint system allow total relaxation, thus
minimizing active muscle effects during the experiment.

   Forces are applied to the moving body segments by means of
the GFA (Fig. 8) which consists of four links and eight revolute
joints containing high precision potentiometers. The outputs of
the potentiometers and the length dimensions of the links are
utilized to obtain the direction as well as the point of application of the force vector. Note that in Fig. 8 the last two links
of the GFA are shown. The GFA is terminated by a force transducer
and a force cuff which is free to rotate about its axis. The
force transducer is designed and built to measure all three components of the force and moment vectors. Of course, the
predominant force component is the one along the direction of the
last link of the GFA and all the other force as well as the moment
components are relatively small in magnitude if one maintains
approximately perpendicular force application on the moving body
segment.

   The third major component of the experimental apparatus is
the ESD as shown in Fig. 10. The ESD is designed with a capability suitable to study the most complex joint, i.e. the shoulder
joint; it also consists of eight revolute joints whose rotations
are monitored by means of high precision potentiometers. Although
there are major design differences between the ESD and the GFA,
from the kinematics point of view the ESD can be considered as a
miniaturized version of the GFA. Fundamental design requirements
of the ESD are (a) capability of providing complete freedom of
motion between two adjacent body segments and (b) capability of
providing sufficient data to determine the values of the T_a
matrices defined by Eq. (4.2) for all possible motions at the
joints. According to the theoretical presentation given in
section 4 once the T_a matrices are known, the nature of the motion
at the joint of interest is completely determined. Incidentally,
any endeavor to measure directly the so-called rigid-body characteristics of two body segments must include an understanding of
certain factors such as: (a) the human body segments have no
definite physical demarcation points; (b) no human body segment
is a rigid body; (c) the physical structure of these body segments
varies from one individual to another. The treatment of these
factors varies with respect to the particular joint under study.
However, common to the study of all joints is utilization of the
principles of orthopedic bracing in attaching the ends of the ESD
to the moving and the fixed body segments. Thus, heat formable
plastic material is used in forming individually fitted shells
for the body segments. Special care is given to locate the bony

landmarks of the body segments to minimize relative soft tissue motion. This is also achieved by the light weight and very low friction construction of the ESD. In fact, the ESD is balanced by means of pulleys and small weights in such a way that the subject does not feel its presence or, stated differently, the ESD creates only very negligible resistance to the motion of the moving body segment. In the case of the shoulder joint study, the shell which is attached to the upper arm as shown in Fig. 8 makes close contacts with the medial and lateral epicondyles of the humerus; the torso shell is in contact with pelvis, the rib cage and indirectly with the cranium via a helmet.

5.2 Some representative numerical results

The development of the ESD, the GFA, the restraint system, and the associated theoretical concepts which have been presented in the previous sections were made to achieve at least three major tasks. The first one is the quantitative determination of the joint centers with respect to the adjacent body segments; the second one is determination of the joint stop envelopes which define the range of motion in all directions; the third task is quantitative determination of resistive forces and moments at the joints. Accomplishment of these tasks and the knowledge gained from them is extremely important in increasing the validity of the multi-segmented biodynamic models of the human body. We will next present some recently obtained numerical results in regard to these three tasks by considering the shoulder joint as an example.

The first of such presentations is on the topic of joint centers. Fig. 11 shows a centrode path for the shoulder joint when the arm is elevated in the frontal plane. In this and the subsequent figures, θ and ϕ angles define the orientation of the upper arm with respect to the torso. Thus, $\phi = 90°$ corresponds to the motion in the frontal plane. The points of this particular centrode path are obtained by the intersection of the screw axes with the frontal plane. Similar centrode paths can be obtained for various values of constant ϕ, each defining a plane passing through a point such as S in Fig. 11. The significance of the shape of the centrode path can be examined in the light of the anatomical structure of the shoulder joint complex. The most striking feature of the shoulder joint is the presence of four independent articulations. These are: 1. The glenohumeral joint which is a ball and socket joint where the humerus mates with the glenoid cavity of the scapula. 2. The acromioclavicular joint where the clavicle meets the acromion process of the scapula. 3. The sternoclavicular joint where the clavicle meets the manubrium of sternum. 4. The scapulothoracic joint where the scapula rotates on the thorax. In the true sense, the scapulo-thoracic articulation is not a joint, but this definition is of

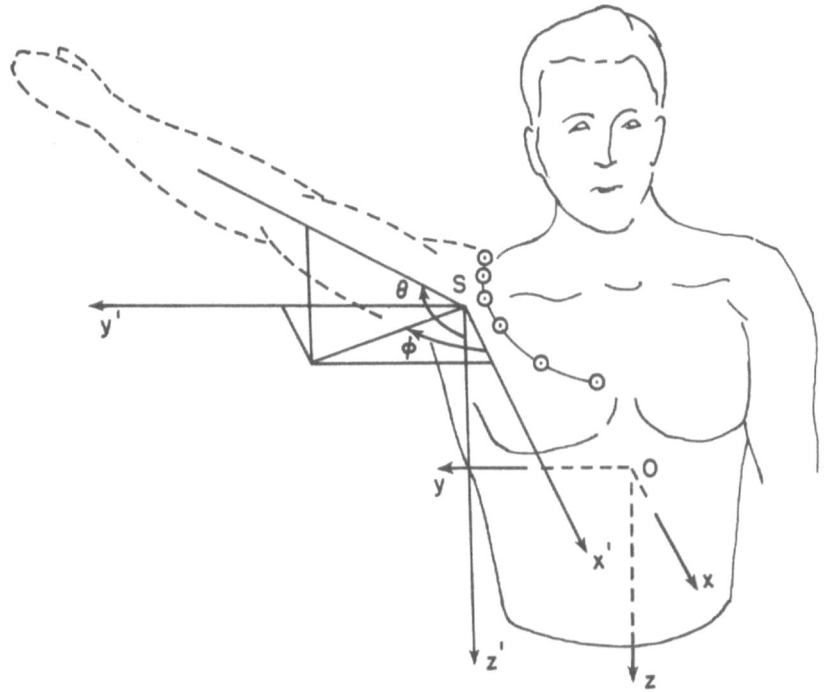

Fig. 11. Centrode curve for the shoulder joint for a motion corresponding to the elevation of the arm in the frontal plane.

value when describing the movements of the scapula over the thorax. There are numerous ligaments connecting various components of the shoulder joint. In Fig. 11 the point closest to the origin of the xyz coordinate system corresponds to the initial phase of the arm elevation ($\theta \cong 25°$). As the angle of elevation increases, the centrode path curves upward, indicating dependence of the joint motion on the glenohumeral and acromioclavicular joints, whereas the initial phases of the arm extension utilizes primarily sternoclavicular and scapulothoracic articulations.

The next item of interest is the joint stop envelopes which define the range of motion. In Fig. 12 and the subsequent figures the values of θ and ϕ are given with respect to an initial condition for which the subject is in a seated configuration with arm positioned as if the lower arm were supported by an armrest. In other words, the θ and ϕ values are obtained by subtracting the initial θ and ϕ values from those obtained by the ESD analysis. In Fig. 12 voluntary range of motion is plotted on θ-ϕ plane for three tests in which the subject, by maintaining approximately 90° between the lower and upper arm, sweeps all possible θ and ϕ angles for the shoulder joint. In addition to

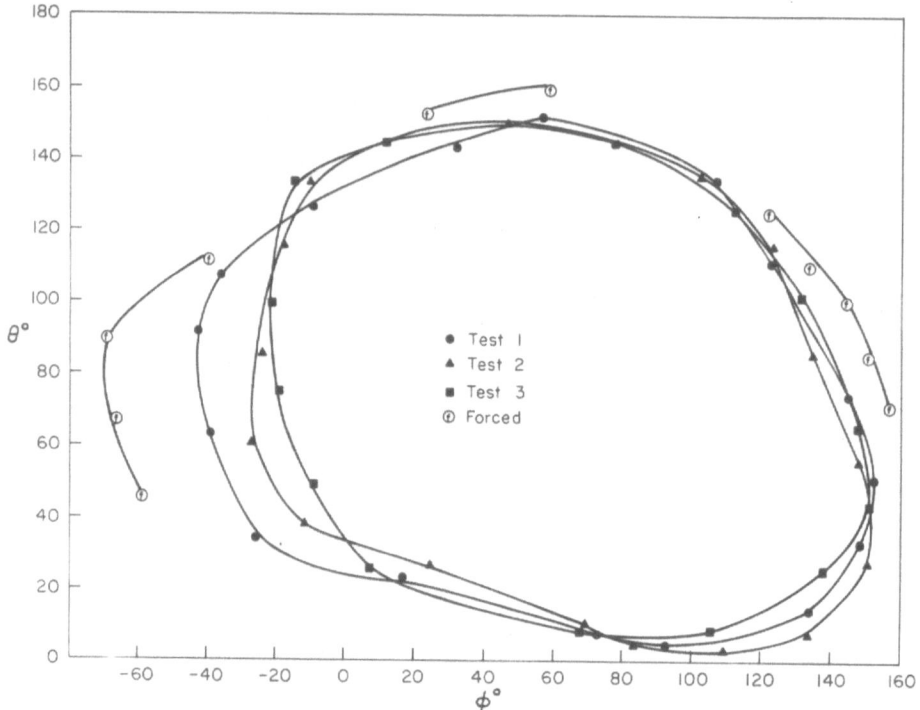

Fig. 12. Voluntary range of motion for a shoulder joint of a test subject.

this voluntary range of motion envelopes, Fig. 12 contains a limited amount of data corresponding to the tolerable levels of range of motion obtained from various forced sweep tests.

Finally, in Figs. 13-16 various aspects of resistive forces and moments at the shoulder joint of a test subject are presented. In particular, Fig. 13 contains plots of the magnitudes of the passive resistive force and moment vectors during forced sweep of the subject's arm by means of the GFA in lateral and medial directions. Components of the passive resistive moment vector calculated at a point S (Fig. 11) with coordinates x = 0, y = 0.186m, z = -0.156m with respect to the thorax coordinate system, are displayed in Fig. 14. The choice of point S is arbitrary; since for any other point in the shoulder joint complex the corresponding moment vector is addition of the moment vector given at point S and the vector obtained by the cross product of the position vector, which extends from that point to point S, and the force vector itself. Results which are displayed in Figs. 13 and 14 represent a very small portion of the data obtained for the shoulder joint of a subject; in fact they only represent the data collected for θ values ranging between approximately 60° thru 85°. By positioning subject's torso in various orientations and repeating

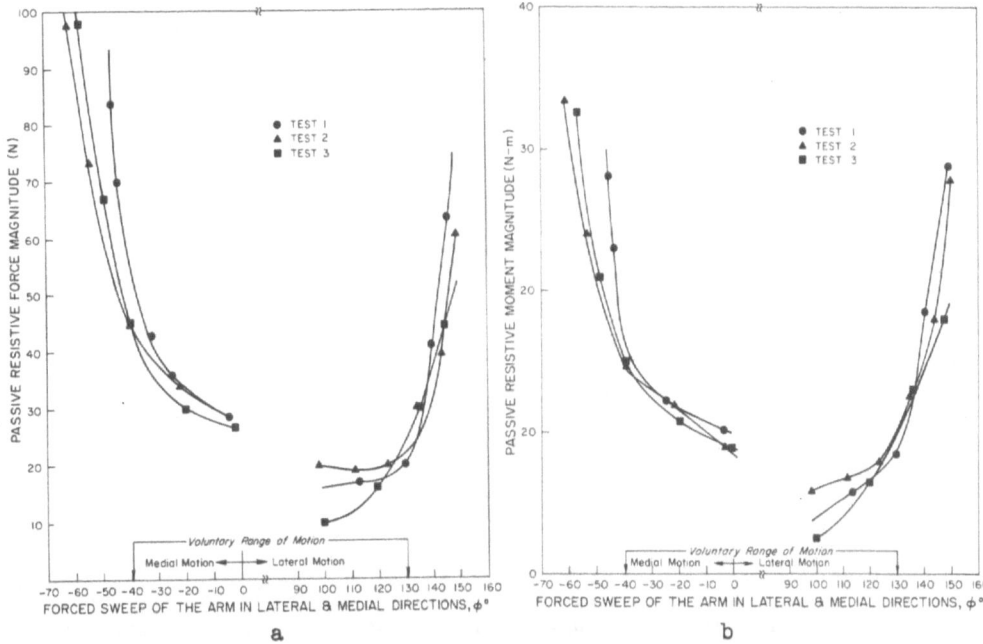

Fig. 13. Magnitudes of the passive resistive force (a) and moment
(b) vectors at the shoulder joint during forced sweep of the arm.

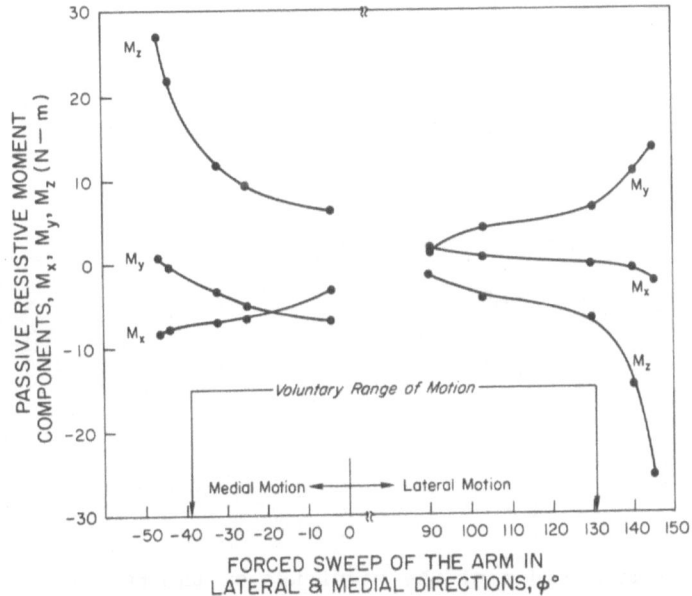

Fig. 14. Components of the passive resistive moment vector at the
shoulder joint during forced sweep of the arm.

184

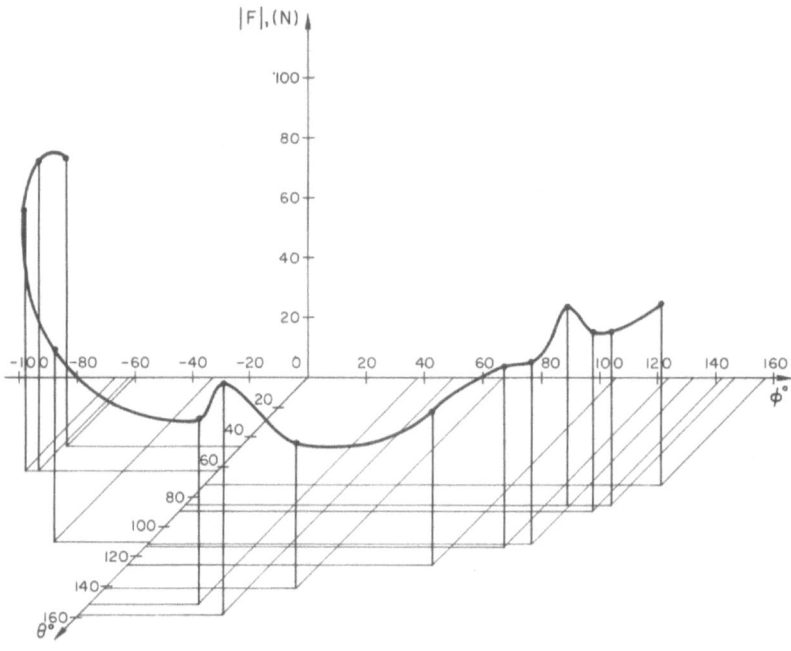

Fig. 15. Maximum values of the magnitude of the passive resistive force at the shoulder joint for various forced sweeps of the arm.

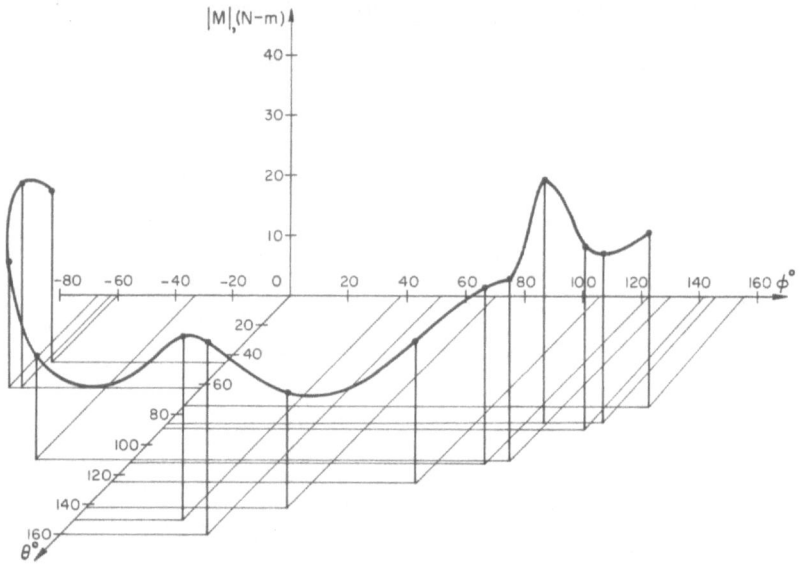

Fig. 16. Maximum values of the magnitude of the passive resistive moment at the shoulder joint for various forced sweeps of the arm.

the forced sweep tests, one can obtain a more complete picture on
the behavior of the passive resistive force and moment vectors at
the joint. Figs. 15 and 16 display in essence a summary of numerous tests. In these figures only the maximum values of the
magnitudes of the passive resistive force and moment vectors are
plotted. In this section we presented some representative
numerical results on the shoulder joint of a subject. More extensive results on all major joints of the human body can be found in
reference [60].

5.3 Concluding remarks

The immediate application of the research work discussed in the
previous section is the development of more realistic joint models
for the articulated total body models of the human body. One of
the primary tasks of the joint modeling is the distribution of the
passive resistive moments as forces on the bony structure and
various ligaments of the joint. One can expect that the total
number of unknowns, i.e., contact and ligaments forces, will
exceed the number of equations that can be written for each joint;
thus, the problem becomes indeterminate. In the case of the
shoulder joint, the humerus, scapula and clavicle can provide up
to 18 equations of equilibrium (or motion). Each contact force
constitutes six unknowns; three for the force components and three
for the coordinates of its application on a particular body
component. To deal with this indeterminate situation, one can
invoke the simplex technique of linear programming, [61], by
establishing an optimization criterion. The optimization
criterion may consist of minimizing contact and/or ligament forces
or some weighted combinations of these two sets of quantities.
Depending upon the orientation of the masses of humerus and torso,
i.e., depending on the variables θ, ϕ, and ψ, the contact force
and the ligament force quantities which enter the optimization
process should vary. Anatomical and kinesiological insight can
assist one in the selection process.
      One can also consider the possibility of applying a simpler
method based on the combination principle to deal with the
indeterminate problem. Defining n as the degree of indeterminancy
and m as the total number of unknowns based on a systematic
combination, any n number of the m quantities can be assumed to
have zero value, thus making the remaining m-n quantities
determinate. Of course, here one must consider all possible
combinations of unknowns and solve for them using the determinate
system. Most of these solutions would be inadmissible and the
conditions of inadmissibility can be as follows: 1. Any of the
ligaments included in the system has a compressive force. 2. Any
of the contact forces becomes tensile. 3. Any of the ligament
or contact forces reach an unreasonably large magnitudes in
comparison with externally applied force and moment values.

186

Utilizing these conditions and possibly some others one can get a unique solution of the indeterminate system of equations.

A final, but by no means the least significant, remark, is that although one can base the development of the joint models on data which are collected on human subjects by means of quasi-static testing of the joints, these joint models must somehow reflect dynamic and viscoelastic effects since their final appli-cation is on the articulated total body model of the human body. It is a well established fact that biological materials display strain rate sensitivity of varying magnitudes. Thus, the force response of a ligament at a given strain level will be different at different rates of loading; in general, the higher the rate of loading, the higher the magnitude of force. There are only a very few studies reported in the literature which deal with strain rate effects on ligaments. One must investigate their applicabil-ity on the modeling task or at least get some indications about the type of modifications one can make on the static data so that they can be more suitably applied for dynamic situations.

REFERENCES

1. E. J. Marey, J. de l'Anat. et de la Physiol. (9), 1873, 42.
2. B. Bresler and J. P. Frankel, Trans. Am. Soc. Mech. Engrs. (72), 1950, 27.
3. W. G. Hyzer, Engineering and Scientific High Speed Photography, New York: MacMillan, 1963.
4. J. V. Mascelli and A. Miller, American Cinematographer Manual, Hollywood, Cal. Amer. Soc. of Cinematographers Holding Corp., 1966.
5. A. Steindler, Kinesiology of the Human Body, Thomas, Springfield, 1964, 62.
6. M. A. Mac Conaill, Physiotherapy (50), 1964, 359.
7. W. W. Murphy, D. H. Garcia and R. G. Bird, ASME Paper No. 66-WA/BHF-2, 1966.
8. M. J. Adrian, Kinesiology Review, 1968, 12.
9. L. B. Ringer and M. J. Adrian, The Research Quarterly (40), 1969, 353.
10. M. P. Murray, S. B. Sepic and E. J. Barnard, Physical Therapy (47), 1967, 272.
11. S. J. Clayson, et al., Archives of Physical Medicine (47), 1966, 255.
12. T. E. Shoup, Proceedings of the Third Canadian Congress of Applied Mechanics, Calgary, Alberta, 1971.
13. J. B. Saunders, V. T. Inman and H. D. Eberhart, The Journal of Bone and Joint Surgery (35-A), 1953, 543.
14. J. R. Leighton, Archives of Physical Medicine and Rehabilita-tion (36:5), 1955, 71.
15. H. Young, The Journal of Bone and Joint Surgery (45-A), 1963, 1627.

16. F. R. Finley and P. V. Karpovich, The Research Quarterly (35), 1964, 379.

17. R. Contini, H. Gage and R. Drillis, Biomechanics and Related Bioengineering Topics, R. M. Kenedi, ed. Pergamon Press, New York, 1965, 413.

18. W. T. Liberson, Archives of Physical Medicine and Rehabilitation (46), 1965, 37.

19. V. Klissouras and P. V. Karpovich, The Research Quarterly (38), 1967, 41.

20. R. Beckett and K. Chang, Journal of Biomechanics (1), 1968, 147.

21. P. D. Gollnick and P. V. Karpovich, The Research Quarterly (35), 1964, 357.

22. L. Freedman and R. H. Munro, The Journal of Bone and Joint Surgery (48-A), 1966, 1503.

23. C. L. Taylor and A. C. Blaschke, Annals New York Academy of Sciences (51), 1951, 1251.

24. T. J. Engen and W. A. Spencer, Archives of Physical Medicine and Rehabilitation (49), 1968, 9.

25. J. A. Roebuck, Jr., Kinesiology Review, 1968, 5.

26. J. P. Paul, Proceedings of the Institution of Mechanical Engineers (181), 1967, 8.

27. H. Eberhart and V. Inman, Annals New York Academy of Sciences (51), 1951, 1213.

28. L. G. Hallen and O. Lindahl, Acta Orthopaedica Scandinavica (36), 1965, 400.

29. J. B. Morrison, Biomedical Engineering (4), 1969, 573.

30. S. T. Dempster, Annals New York Academy of Sciences (63), 1955, 559.

31. L. W. Lamoreux, ASME Paper No. 72-MECH-80, 1972.

32. G. K. McKee, Proceedings of the Institution of Mechanical Engineers (181), 1967, 85.

33. R. C. Johnston and G. L. Smidt, The Journal of Bone and Joint Surgery (51-A), 1969, 1083.

34. E. Y. S. Chao, et al., Journal of Biomechanics (3), 1970, 459.

35. G. L. Smidt, Physical Therapy (51), 1971, 9.

36. G. L. Smidt, Journal of Biomechanics (6), 1973, 79.

37. E. Bahniuk and M. J. Wijnschenk, ASME Paper No. 63-WA-282, 1963.

38. D. Bousso, Bio-medical Engineering (4), 1969, 313.

39. F. C. Risteen and L. E. Torfason, ASME Paper No. 70-MECH-55, 1970.

40. C. H. Barnett, Journal of Anatomy (87), 1953, 91.

41. C. W. Radcliffe, Transactions of the Sixth Conference on Mechanisms, Purdue University, 1960, 143.

42. A. Burstein and V. H. Frankel, ASME Paper No. 67-DE-38, 1967.

43. C. C. D. Shute, Proceedings of the Institution of Mechanical Engineers (181), 1967, 9.

188

44. F. Freudenstein and L. S. Woo, Bulletin of Mathematical Biophysics (31), 1969, 215.
45. V. H. Frankel, A. H. Burstein and D. B. Brooks, The Journal of Bone and Joint Surgery (53-A), 1971, 945.
46. D. T. Reilly and M. Martin, Acta Orthopaedica Scandinavica (43), 1972, 126.
47. F. G. Evans, Proceedings of the C.P.C. Symposium on Biomechanics, J. M. Cooper, ed., Indiana University, 1970, 3.
48. G. J. Sammarco, A. H. Burstein and V. H. Frankel, Orthopedic Clinics of North America (4), 1973, 75.
49. H. O. Beck and W. E. Morrison, The Journal of Prosthetic Dentistry (12), 1962, 873.
50. D. C. Cannon, Instrumentation for the Investigation of Mandibular Movements, M.S. Thesis, Case Institute of Technology, 1965.
51. T. Messerman, The Journal of Prosthetic Dentistry (17), 1967, 36.
52. F. J. Knap, B. L. Richardson and J. Bogstad, Journal of Dental Research (49), 1970, 289.
53. C. T. Thompson, A System for Determining the Spatial Motions of Arbitrary Mechanisms - Demonstrated on a Human Knee, Ph.D. Thesis, Stanford University, 1972.
54. G. L. Kinzel, B. M. Hillberry, A. S. Hall, D. C. Van Sickle, and W. M. Harvey, Journal of Biomechanics (5), 1972, 283.
55. M. Chasles, Bull. Sci. Math. (14), 1830, 321.
56. M. Skreiner, Journal of Mechanisms (1), 1966, 115.
57. F. Klein, Geometry translated by E. R. Hednick and C. A. Noble, No. S151, Dover Publications, Inc., New York, N.Y., 1939.
58. M. Bocher, Introduction to Higher Algebra No. S1238, Dover Publications, Inc., New York, N.Y., 1964.
59. H. Goldstein, Classical Mechanics, Addison-Wesley, Cambridge, Mass., 1959.
60. A. E. Engin, "Measurement of Resistive Torques in Major Human Joints," The Ohio State University Research Foundation Final Report to U.S. Air Force, Air Force Systems Command, Aeronautical Systems Division, 1978.
61. G. B. Dantzig, Linear Programming, McGraw-Hill, New York, N.Y., 1968.

JOINT REPLACEMENTS *

J.P. Paul

Bioengineering Unit, University of Strathclyde
Wolfson Centre, 106 Rottenrow, Glasgow G4 0NW
Scotland

ABSTRACT. Some of the mechanical factors affecting the design and success of joint replacements in the human are considered. Particular attention is paid to the selection of the relevant loading system and its analysis. Loads on the joints of a normal subject can only be analysed by virtue of assumptions simplifying the multiple indeterminacy in these structures. Particular attention is paid to the loading of the hip and knee joint relative to the walking activity and the loads transmitted by joint replacements. Fixation requirements are considered. Similarly, the appropriate loading to be considered for the upper extremity is reviewed - data is presented on the loading at levels in the finger, wrist, elbow and shoulder and joint forces are presented for many of the articulations. The implications of the studies relative to the present families of joint replacement are discussed.

1. CRITERIA FOR ORTHOPAEDIC IMPLANTS

Implants are used in modern surgery in a wide range of different conditions, each with its appropriate philosophy. Some implants have a structural function, e.g. orthopaedic implants for fractures, or vascular replacements for attenuated areas of blood vessels. Many implants have a specific function after implant, such as joints, which require to permit

*Part of the work reported here was supported by the Arthritis and Rheumatism Council

190

angular movement, hydrocephalous tubes which make a path for fluid transport, cardiac pacemakers to improve the heart's regularity of cycling, cardiac and other valves to restore hydraulic efficiency. Stimulators may be implanted, either to assist continence or to allow functional stimulation frequently of the extremities. Many implants have a cosmetic aim and are used mainly as space fillers or restorers of a more aesthetic form to a deficient structure. Occasionally the implant may be diagnostic, as in the case of the 'radio pill'. It may be for therapeutic purposes as in the use of indwelling electrodes which may allow the acquisition of an electroencephologram, or it may be used for tissue destruction. Many materials are inserted to assist surgery and, mainly, they are adhesives or sutures. In the future one might see artificial organs of some kind implanted, although it would appear that the problem of the energy source will prevent the artificial heart from being available for many years. Studies are underway to have implants to relay to the brain structure signals corresponding to vision or to hearing, but the implementation of this concept is for the distant future.

1.1 Criteria for implants

1. They should be non poisonous (as implanted and also as they may be after use when subjected to the effect of leaching or exposed in fine articulate form as wear debris.) Plastics components frequently include chemicals to give resistance to ultra violet radiation, to preserve plasticity and to increase the volume of the product. If any of these are leached out the mechanical properties of the remaining material will be considerably altered. Some materials which have been found to satisfy long term testing for implantability in the compact form as components may transpire to be unsuitable when the very large areas associated with wear debris are exposed to body fluids.

2. The material should give no obvious signs of carcinogenicity. The physical form of the material is thought to have some relationship to this as well as its chemical composition.

3. The device should allow sufficient function at the site where implanted and it should be able to maintain this function years after implantation.

4. The intrinsic strength of the implant should be adequate and the connection transmitting load between the implant and the

skeletal structure should be designed to avoid over-stressing of bone material.

5. The implant should be dimensionally compatible with the existing anatomy of the individual.

6. It should be reasonably possible to insert a **device** using normal surgical techniques without excessive **destruction** of adjacent tissues.

7. There should ideally be a possibility of removal of the implant and adoption of an alternative strategy for the patient's rehabilitation in the event of failure. In this context failure may mean fracture or loosening of the device, or the occurrence of pain or infection.

2.   REASONS FOR JOINT REPLACEMENT

Joint replacement is a procedure being increasingly used in current surgical practice for the relief of pain and restoration of function to joints. The patients treated include those with rheumatoid arthritis, osteoarthritis and abnormalities of the joint structure due to trauma or congenital factors. In most cases relief of pain is immediate and function is significantly improved over the original. Unfortunately, early success in pain relief and functional restoration may not last for more than two years and the patient is then faced with the prospect of additional major surgery, which may present difficulties due to the materials remaining from the first attempt.

In current practice the materials used or considered for use include metals and alloys, plastics, ceramics and vitreous carbon. Polymethyl-methacrylate plastic in the form of a 'cold' setting resin is used to match the profiles of the implants to the corresponding bone surfaces. Metals used include cobalt chrome molybolenum stainless steel, cobalt chrome alloy, pure titanium and titanium alloys. International standard specifications for the chemical composition, metallurgical condition and preparation of materials for implants are now available in draft form and work is proceeding on corresponding documents for plastics. It is interesting that many of these metals and alloys were developed for other commercial purposes and found to have suitable characteristics for, first, dental use and, subsequently, for general implantation. It is an interesting economic fact that the amount of these metals required by the manufacturers each year is scarcely enough to justify the special 'melts' that are necessary to have the purity and chemical composition assured for these materials.

3. REQUIRED FUNCTION OF THE IMPLANTED JOINT

Generally the joints in the human body allow at least one major movement
together with other accessory movements.   For instance, at the hip the
major angulation is in flexion and extension but, equally important to
normal function, is the ability to abduct and rotate the limb about its own
axis.   Similarly, although the basic action provided by the knee joint is
flexion, this is associated with relative rotation about the axis of the
tibia and translation in the anterior/posterior direction of the femur
relative to the tibia.   It is an open question whether the implanted
device should attempt to provide these accessory movements in full or
in partial form or restrain them altogether.   At the hip joint the available
replacements allow three fundamental rotations to take place.   At the
knee joint, the interphalangeal joint and the elbow joint, the major
movement is flexion; and there exist designs of joint replacements which
are in the form of pure hinges.   In the normal joint, moments about the
long axis of a body segment and moments tending to adduct or abduct
at these joints are carried by development of tension in the appropriate
ligamentous structure.   Because of the stiffness of the mechanical
construction of the hinges this is unlikely to happen and the suggestion
has been made on many occasions that the tendency of hinge type joint
replacements to loosen in their fixture to the bone can be ascribed to the
transmission of these moments completely by the implant.   It would
appear that in many cases the implant has not been specifically designed
to interface and transmit such a loading in an adequate way to the host
bone material and it may be that the hinge joint should remain a possible
candidate provided care and attention is given to the nature and magnitude
of all the load actions to which it will be subjected in service.   There is
certainly a place for the fully constrained type of joint where the progress
of the joint disability has been such as to lead to large deformation of the
bone structure.   Similarly, if the relative movements in the normal
joint are significantly different from rotation about a single axis and
if the axis of the implanted device is displaced from the mean
instantaneous centre then flexion of the joint will automatically
produce tension in the ligamentous structure and probably result in
pain or reduced functional movement.   If a hinge is being inserted
then all those structures which constrain the movements of the one
relative to the other should be made non functional.

Conversely, where a joint replacement is fitted which is purely of the
'resurfacing' type it is essential that there be sufficient ligamentous
restraint to retain the integrity of the joint to transmit all of the

accessory loadings which occur and again, the path of relative movement produced by the new surfaces whould correspond as closely as possible to the original locus of instantaneous centres.

4   LOADING

During function the compressive force transmitted at the surface of a joint corresponds to the effect of gravity and acceleration on the body mass, the effect of external loads on the body structures and the tensions which are developed in muscles and ligaments.   In the design of joint replacements it would appear logical to consider the most pessimistic and adverse conditions only if they can be shown to occur frequently.   More generally one would look to the repetitive loading actions or activities which the normal patient regularly undertakes to provide the cycles of load to which a joint replacement should be tested.   This raises a very general question as to what are the regularly occuring and major functions of the legs and arms.   Obviously these are quite different and the leg may be defined as having the function of structurally supporting the body either with the assistance of the contralateral limb or on its own and allowing relative movement between the body and its environment. Many studies relating to leg loading have analysed the artificial situation of standing stationary on one leg - saying that walking is in fact a series of incidents of this type.   This is in fact untrue, because, during walking on a level surface, there exists a mediolateral component of force between ground and foot which is absent during stationary standing and this corresponds to the fact that in a stationary position the centre of mass must be over the foot, whereas, in walking, the centre of mass is generally not over the area covered by the foot.   The other important point is that in stationary standing there is very little activity of the muscles which flex or extend the articulations of the leg. In walking however these muscles are used and obviously the loading they produce on the joint has to be taken into consideration in the full specification of the loading system.   (See Figs. 1 and 2)

Obviously there are activities more stressful to the joints than level surface walking at moderate speed and studies have been undertaken which show that in negotiation of stairs and inclines the values of joint forces can approach nine or ten times body weight.   Similarly there will presumably be high values of load developed by the muscular reflexes during unbalanced situations such as tripping or falling.   Nevertheless it appears not illogical to cover the main service specification of joint replacements for the lower limb by reference to tests in level walking, recognising that the other occasion- ally occuring events would be dealt with in the design under the heading of 'safety factor'. (See table 1)

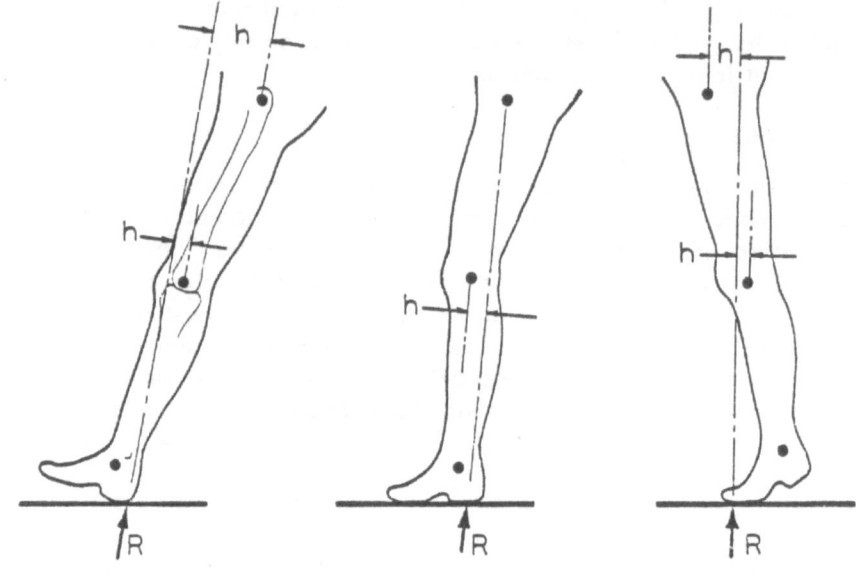

Fig. 1

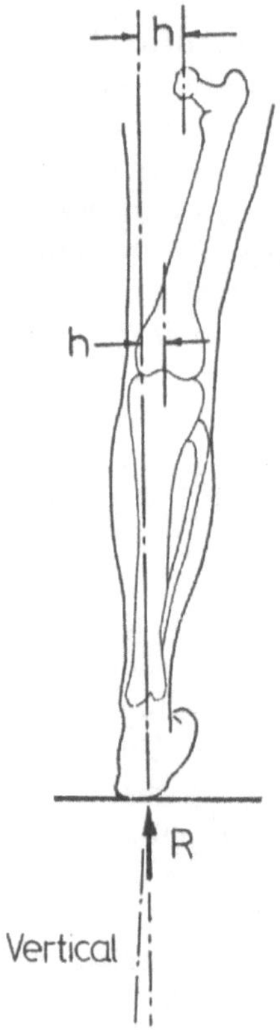

Fig. 1 and Fig. 2 show leg positions
during level walking with resultant
ground/foot force.
For values see Fig. 3

Fig. 2

Vertical

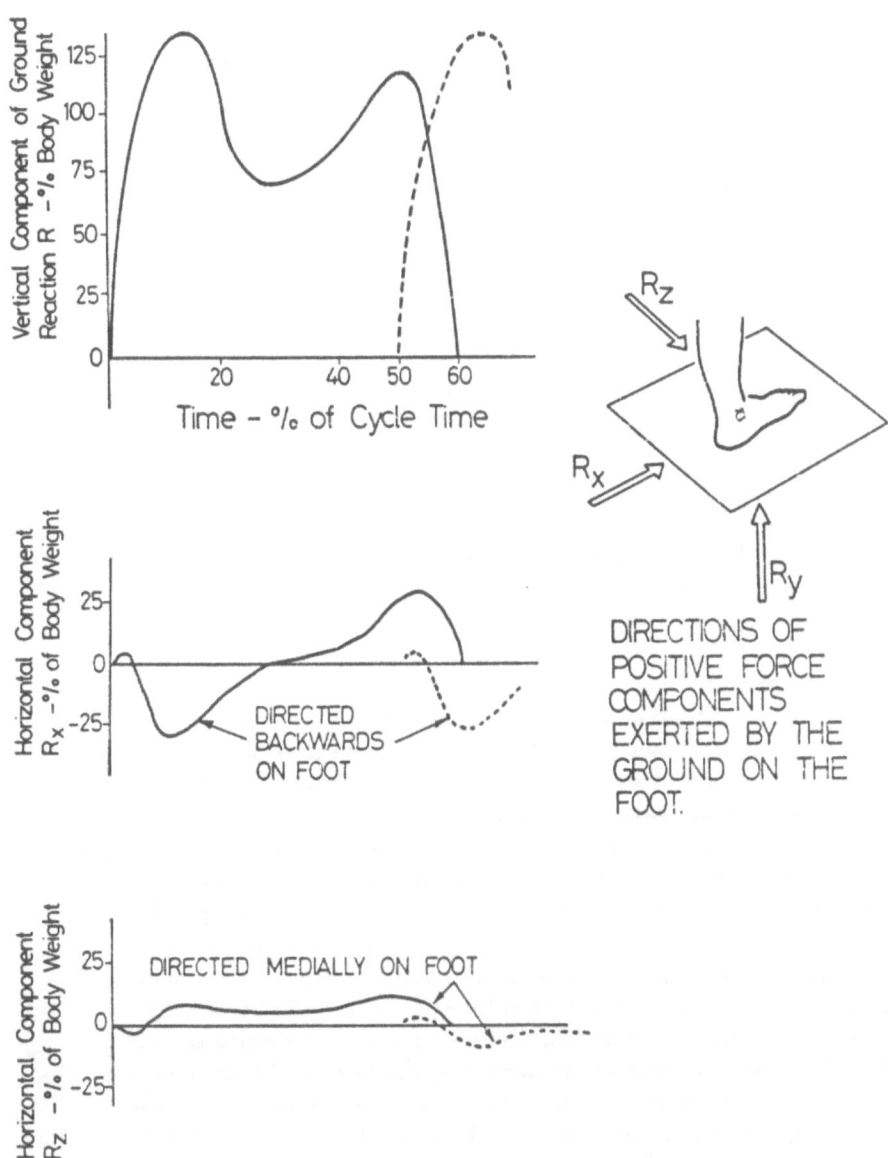

Fig. 3 Variation with time of the components of force transmitted
between ground and foot for a walking test subject.

196

Activity	Number of Tests	Tibio-Femoral Joint	Patella/Femoral Joint	Torque About Tibial Axis Nm
Level Walking	22	2.8	0.6	18
Fast Level Walking	6	4.3	1.5	-
Stair Ascent	7	4.4	1.8	33
Stair Descent	6	4.9	2.9	21
Ramp Ascent	8	3.7	1.6	30
Ramp Descent	8	4.4	2.6	22

Table 1   Knee joint force expressed as a multiple of body weight.

4.1 Load Measurement

There is only one set of experiments reported in the literature in which a transducer has been incorporated to measure the forces transmitted at one of the joints of the leg, although it is understood that other tests are either underway or about to be reported. The work of Rydell in 1965 is extremely valuable as being the only data of its kind. This refers to actual measurements of the force transmitted by femoral head replacement devices during a range of activities of the test subject. There were two test subjects who required the treatment because of traumatic injury to the femoral head. The tests were conducted for one week each before the wiring to the internal electrical strain gauges was finally severed. The way normally adopted of measuring the loading between body segments is to measure the force exerted at the extremity, in this case at the ground on the foot, in all its components and also its position relative to the articulations of the leg. If successive measurements are taken of the limb configuration its path in space can be determined and, by various techniques, the components of acceleration can be evaluated for use in conjunction with information relating to the mass properties of the body segments. The determination of acceleration from displacement measurement and the determination of the mass properties of body segments are both inaccurate procedures but, fortunately, the contribution of the mass related terms to the loadings at the articulations is not large during the stance phase, which is when the major loading occurs. The moments transmitted between the body segments at the ankle, the knee and the hip can now be determined. (See Figs. 4, 5 and 6)

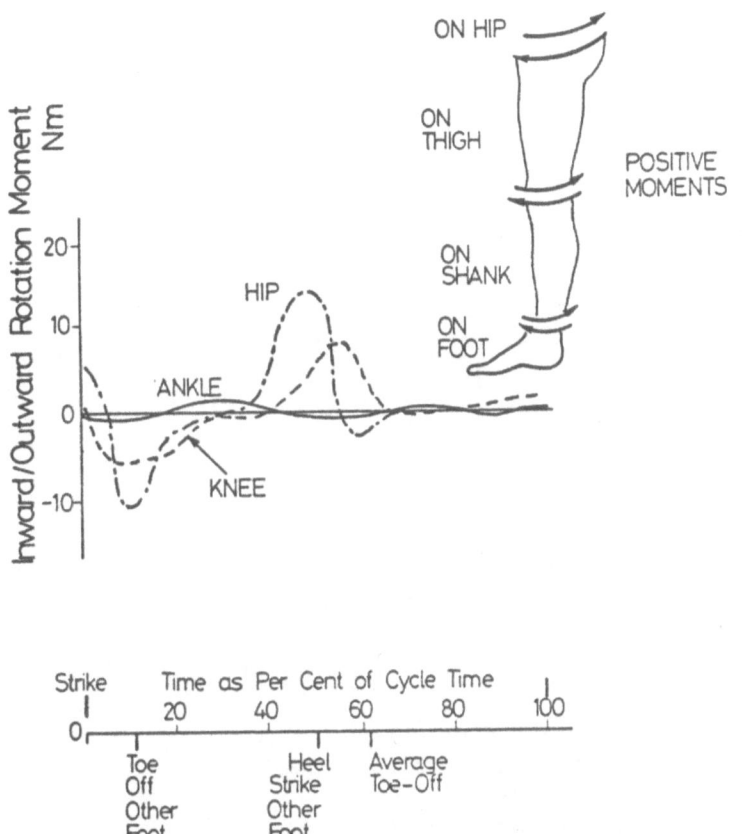

Fig. 4   Inward/Outward rotation moments at intersegment junctions of the leg during normal level walking.

198

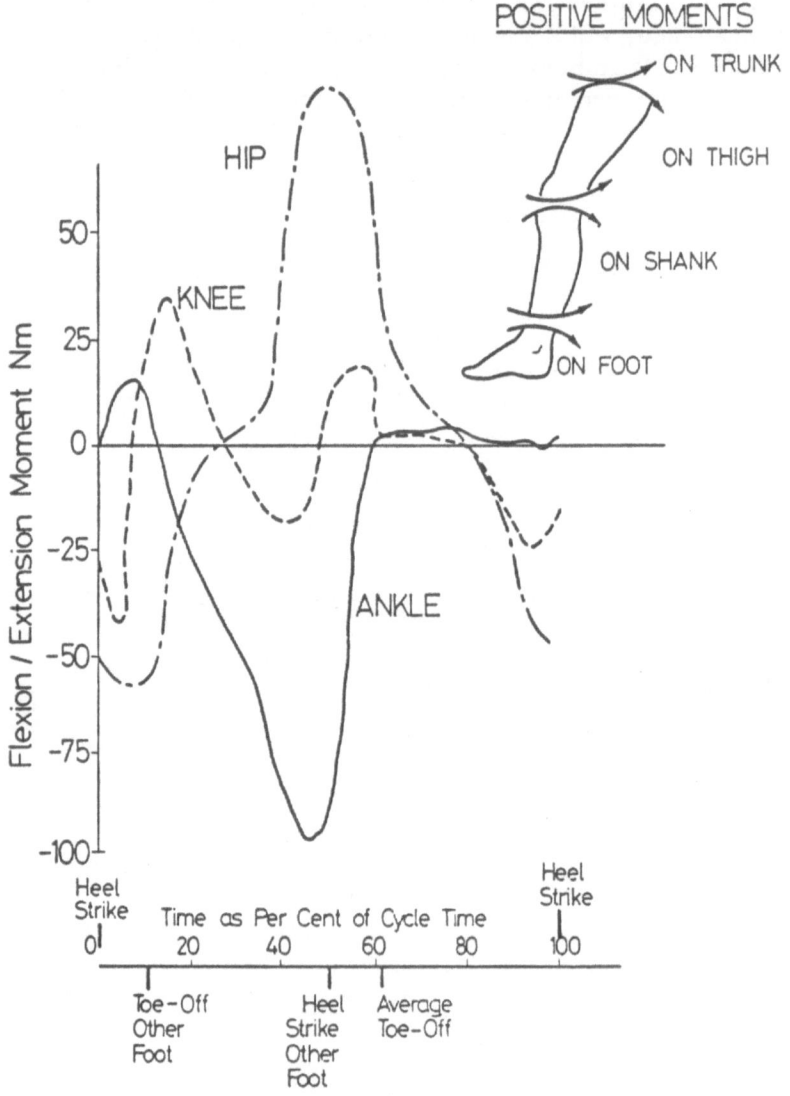

Fig. 5 Flexion/Extension moments at intersegment junctions of the leg during normal level walking.

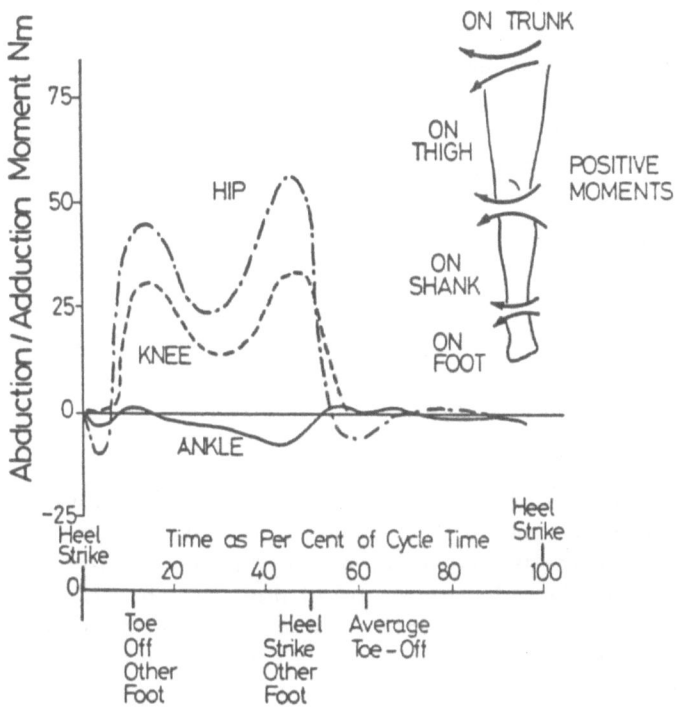

Fig. 6   Abduction/adduction moments at intersegment
junctions of the leg during normal level walking.

It is important to realise however that the resultant forces and the
resultant moments transmitted at the articulations need further
analysis before the values of the forces in the connective tissues
and in the joint surfaces can be determined.   Their anatomical
structure is first investigated in postmortem dissection analyses
and the dimensions defining the positions of the major load bearing
structures relative to the external landmarks of the articulations
are related to measurements which may be taken from outside
relating to the scale of the structures for a particular patient
relative to those which have been acquired and averaged in the
in the dissecting room.   Generally, next, the forces in the
extensor or flexor muscles are calculated from a knowledge of
the externally applied load.   In making this calculation it has to

be appreciated that simplification of the detailed anatomical structure is being undertaken in that, generally more than one muscle participates in each activity and, for this type of analysis, it is usual to group the muscles according to their function, phasic activity and anatomical position. Knowing the value of the force in the appropriate group of muscles the adduction/abduction loading is next investigated. As far as the hip joint and similar joints are concerned this moment will be balanced by appropriate tension in the relevant muscles.

At the knee a moment in this direction can be resisted either by taking a greater share of the compressive joint load in one compartment than in the other, or by considering one compartment of the joint to be completely unloaded and there to exist a tension in the lateral ligamentous structure adjacent to it. The tension in this ligament together with the compression in the joint compartment, comprises the means of transmitting the moment in question together with the resultant force. The ligamentous structure is generally assumed to resist any shear forces and also any rotational actions taking place about the long axis of the members. In this way the values are obtained for all the structures carrying tensile load and the vector sum of these is obviously the compressive load on the joint, when due account is taken for the external load actions. It will be noted that the final allocation of load to the anatomical structures is by equilibrium equations but, in this case, it is important to realise that the equilibrium considered is the dynamic equilibrium corresponding to the inclusion of the instantaneous value of ground to foot force and also the appropriate inertial force actions on the body segments situated between the ground and the articulation of interest. The curves of variation of hip and knee joint force averaged from thirtylsix tests are shown in Figs. 7 and 8. The abscissa in each case is time normalised to percentage of cycle time commencing at heel strike and the ordinate is the joint force in multiples of body weight. The three curves coerespond to slow, medium and fast walking which were in the ranges up to 1.1, 1.1 to 1.5 and 1.5 to 2.0 metres per second. It is obvious that greater stride length, which corresponds to walking at higher speed, is responsible for the increased loading both at the hip and the knee.

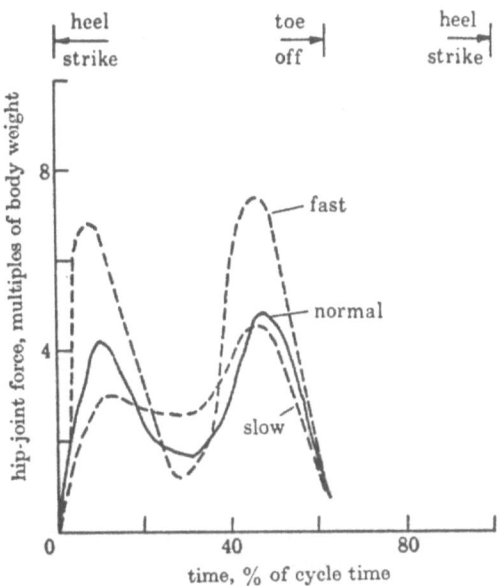

Fig. 7   Force transmitted by the hip joint expressed as a multiple of
body weight during level walking.

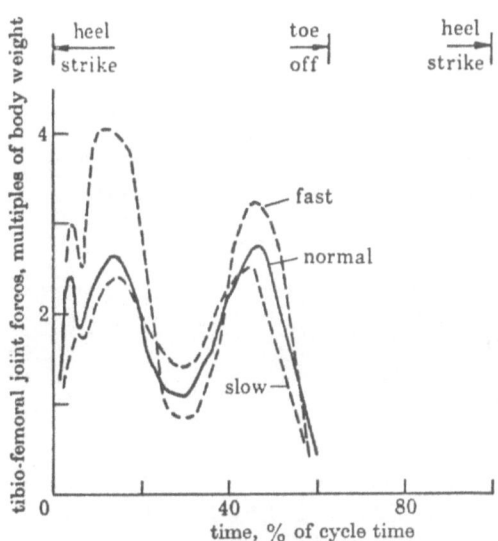

Fig. 8   Force transmitted by the tibio-femoral part of the knee joint
during level walking

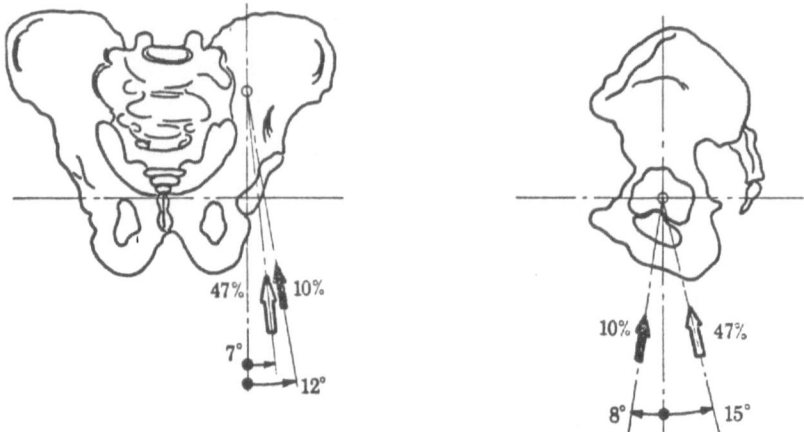

Fig 9.   Direction relative to the pelvis of resultant hip joint force, identified as maximal by reference to Fig. 7.

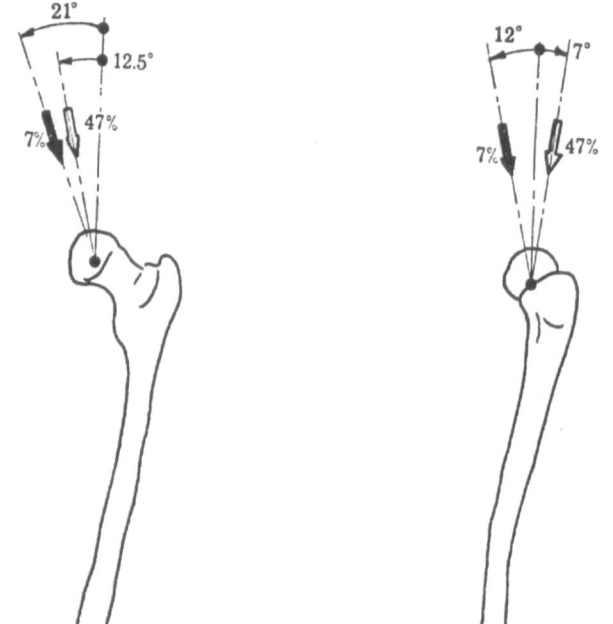

Fig. 10.   Direction relative to the femur of resultant hip joint force identified as maximal by reference to Fig. 7.

It is equally important to be aware of the directions in which
the forces are acting relative to the anatomical structures.
Fig. 9 shows two views of the pelvis and the directions of the
resultant hip joint force have been transferred to the diagram
for the two instants corresponding to the maxima of the curves
of Figs. 7 and 8.   These directions are averaged from all of
the test results.   Corresponding results are shown in Fig. 10
for the hip joint force relative to the head of femur at the
corresponding two curves in the cycle.

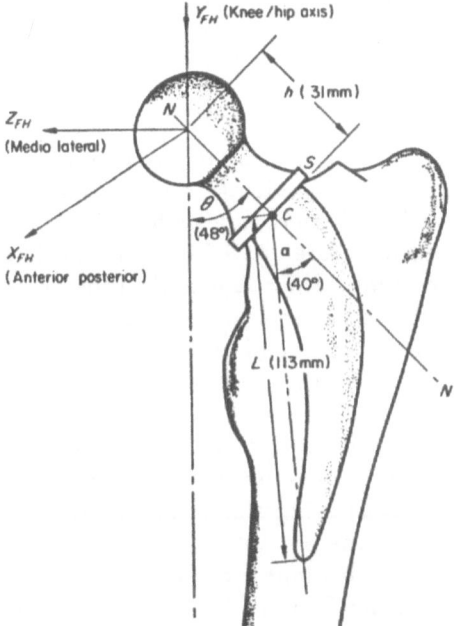

Fig 11.   Idealised view of femoral head prosthesis

If a typical form of femoral component of a total joint replacement
is taken as shown in Fig. 11 the forces to which it is subjected in
the frontal view are basically along the line from head of femur to
the femoral condyles and from medial to lateral.   Early in the
cycle the force acts in the posterior direction and later acts on the
head in the anterior direction.   If the components are combined
the resultant force is certainly not along the axis of the femoral
neck, thus the physiological loads tend to tilt the prosthesis relative
to the femur with the proximal part of the prosthesis impinging on
the medial border on the femur and the distal part on the lateral.

204

The effect of the anterior/posterior component force is also to tilt
the prosthesis, making contact with the femur cyclically at the
proximal end and distal end on both aspects.   The anterior/posterior
component does however tend to rotate the prosthesis about the
axis of its stem but, because of the substantial cross section of the
stems of most upper femoral prosthetic replacements, the tendency
for the prosthesis to turn in the bone is not great.   This is in contrast
to knee prostheses, particularly of the hinged type. Having a
comparatively slender stem the twisting moments transmitted at the
joint to the femur and to the tibia are transmitted as shear forces at
the radius of the circle including the tips of the stem.   It is felt
that this type of loading may be the cause of some of the reported
problems in loosening of this type of prosthesis.

Although every attempt is made, for instance, by the use of profiled
rasps, to cut the femoral cavity to a shape approximating as closely
as possible to that of the implant, obviously the close fit necessary
for gradual transmission of load from prosthesis to bone cannot be
achieved.   Many surgeons therefore use a 'filler' in the form of
polymethylmethacrylate cement, which is mixed in the operating
theatre and is fluid as installed but sets hard in a short time.   There
has been a little work on the mechanical characteristics of this
cement material but much work still remains to be done, particularly
in relation to the strength of the interface between the cement and
the implant and between the cement and the bone.   It has been
suggested from time to time that there would be advantages in the use
of prostheses made of materials having elastic constants of the same
order of magnitude as bone.   The present author can see no great
justification for this, since the implant is of necessity of basically
different geometrical dimensions from the host area.   The major form
of deformation of the prosthesis relative to the bone and vice versa
is in bending and the relevant parameter is the second moment of
area, which can obviously not be made equal in both cases. It is
interesting to note also that at the neck of the implant, it is the
implant which carries the full amount of load, i.e., compression
and bending, with some torsion, whereas the cut surface of the bone
is by definition unstressed.   In the transition from there to the tip
of the prosthesis the stresses in the implant must diminish to zero and
those in the bone increase to the values relevant to the loading of the
shaft.   Obviously there is no way in which the bone can be fully
stressed along its length and there will always be an incompatibility
between the curvatures of the implant $(EI/M)_1$ and that for the bone,
$(EI/M)_2$

Failures have been reported of Charnley type prostheses at a distance approximately one third of stem length away from the tip, where it appears that the medial aspect of the femur has not been able to support the upper portion of the prosthesis sufficiently. With the lower end fixed firmly in cement the device has been loaded more or less as a cantilever from that level and fatigue fractures have been reported. Apparently this occurs more frequently in patients who are active and overweight but it is one of the ways in which the replacement can be seen to be running very close to the design strength limits. Similarly, although I believe no prosthesis has been required to be removed because of excessive wear, there are recorded cases of substantial penetration by the spherical head of the femoral component into the high density polyethylene of the acetabular part.

The optimal design of the interface between the prosthesis and the shaft of the femur is difficult. The bone material is distributed in an uneven way, is anisotropic and strain rate dependent. The mechanical properties of the polymethylmethacrylate cement are not completely known in respect of the behaviour under complex stress systems and there is no reliable information on the coefficient of friction developed between it and natural and inserted components. Some studies have been carried out on anatomical specimens bearing networks of strain gauges into which prepared endo-prostheses have been fitted before testing under specific loading conditions. Stress analysis has been undertaken using finite element stress analysis techniques. At one stage there was much work done by loading appropriate birefringent models to obtain the characteristic photo-elastic stress analysis patterns. It is not possible however to reproduce with these models the internal anatomical construction of the bone, nor the effect of variation in elastic constants for bone. In all cases these stress analyses are dependent on a knowledge of the magnitude and direction of the loads in the structures and, regrettably, account is rarely taken of the true directions of the resultant loads. Similarly, I know of no such analysis where the effect on the bone of the loads distributed to it by muscular and ligamentous structures is taken into account.

5   UPPER LIMB LOADING

On the philosophy that the investigations into the loadings on joints should be related to the problems of the disabled and the possible design of joint replacements, the upper limb presents certain difficulties in respect of awareness of the activities causing the greatest stress at the articulations. From discussions with therapists and with patients it

206

transpired that, for the fingers, difficulty was experienced in turning
stiff taps or unscrewing tight bottle caps and, in some cases, simply in
gripping, as in pinching.   Investigations were therefore instituted in
which measurements were made of the loading on individual fingers
during the tap turning and pinching activities.   This was accomplished
by making a contact surface of the appropriate shape which would be
in touch with one finger at a time only.   This was connected through
a force transducer to the remainder of the tap or pinching cylinder to
make a rigid assembly.   Thus, when the test was being performed, the
hand was in the natural position for the activity and yet the force of a
single finger was being measured and described in terms of 3 component
forces and   3 moments about appropriate axes.   (See Fig. 12)

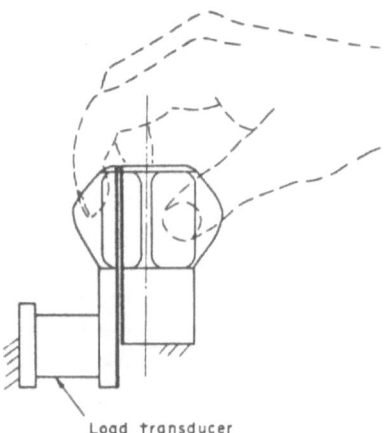

Load transducer

Fig 12   Instrumented fixture for finger force
measurement during tap turning. One
sector of the tap is detached and assembled
to a rigid six quantity force transducer.

6.   DATA OBTAINED

A patient with problems at the joints of the elbow and shoulder
frequently finds difficulty in grooming and dressing.   These are
activities involving large ranges of movement but of generally
comparatively small forces.

The activities which were conceived to be stressful to these joints
and also relevant to the activities of the candidate patient were

prescribed bearing in mind that the patient with generalised joint
disease will frequently be disabled in the leg at the time when any
arm disablement occurs.   It is likely that he may use his arms therefore to assist his repositioning in bed or standing from a seated position.
An alternative considered related to bringing chair and table closer
together.   The tests devised to represent some of the problems of daily
living were in two categories.   In one, the subject held in his hand
a mass of one kilogram while he undertook movements representing
reaching and eating activities.   The force transducer was mounted
to act as the arm of a chair and the test subject rose from the chair
with his heels on the ground and legs straight as far as he could.
The final test was accomplished with the test subject seated and he
then reached forward and pulled a loaded table towards him.   The
force which he exerted was measured by a six quantity force transducer
connected to the device and gripped by the test subject during the
activities which were measured by cine cameras, salient points on the
surface anatomy being marked for recognition and measurement.
As with the leg, anatomical dissection studies were undertaken to
determine the position and lines of effective force transmission of the
relevant structures acting at each joint.   From a knowledge of the
loading and the appropriate structures calculations were made of the
forces transmitted and data is shown for the interphalangeal and
metacarpophalangeal joint of the index finger in Table II

Activity	Subject	PIP Joint Longitudinal Force Radial cpt	Ulnar cpt	MP Joint Longitudinal Force
Tap Turning	1		53	151
	2		56	173
	3		43	184
	4		54	171
Pinching	1	37	42	83
	2	35	75	153
	3	36	50	98
	4	38	49	75

Table II

Forces developed at the MP joint and in the
radial and ulnar compartments of the IP joint
of the index finger in two activities. Force values in Newtons.

Maximum loading was found for the elbow to occur in the table pulling exercise where forces were calculated at 2.4 kN maximum. Data is not yet available on the load conditions at the shoulder joint, although the moments to be transmitted suggest that the forces are likely to be slightly in excess of those of the elbow. If the pressure at the joints is taken to be uniformly distributed over the appropriate compartments the intensity of pressures at the hip, elbow and index finger may be compared for the activities of walking, chair rising and tap turning respectively. These are 1.9, 3.0, (4.3 and 2.9)MN/m^2. The bracketed figures refer respectively to the IP and MP joints of the index finger. Thus, not surprisingly, the stresses seen to be acting at these different joints in different activities are nominally close in magnitude. This is not surprising, since one would expect the same basic biological material to be used for the functional parts of the joint. It is an indication also that if joint replacement is practiced and the dimensions of the replacement part correspond approximately to the joint being excised, then materials which have been demonstrated to be satisfactory for joint replacement at one level may well be satisfactory at other levels provided the design can be arranged to transmit the loading developed by function to the supporting bone material without prejudicing its viability.

REFERENCES

Bresler, B and Frankel, J.P., The forces and Moments in the Leg during Level Walking, Trans. Am. Soc. Mech Eng. 72, 27 - 36 (Paper No. 48 - A - 62) 1950

Barbenel, J.C., and Paul, J.P., Biomechanics in Medical Engineering, Ray C.D. Ed. Year Book Medical Publishers Chicago, 1971

Berme, N., Paul, J.P. and Purves, W.K., A Biomechanical Analysis of the Metacarpophalangeal Joint, J. Biomechanics Vol. 10 pp. 409 - 412 Pergamon Press, 1977

Dvir, Z., Biomechanics of the Shoulder Joint, PhD Thesis University of Strathclyde, 1978

Eberhart, H.D., Inman, V.T. and Saunders, J.B. de C., Fundamental Studies of Human Locomotion and other information relating to design of Artificial Limbs , University of California, Berkeley, Eberhart, H.D. Editor, 1947

Frankel, V.H., Burstein, A.H., Orthopaedic Biomechanics, Lea and Febiger, Philadelphia, 1971

Harrington, I.J., The effect of congenital and pathological conditions on the load actions transmitted at the knee joint, in Total Knee Replacement, Proc. Conf. Inst. Mech. Eng., London, 1974

Inman, V.T. Functional aspects of the Abductor Muscles of the Hip, Jnl. Bone Jt. Surg. 39, 3, 607, 1947

Morrison, J.B., Bioengineering Analysis of Force Actions transmitted by the Knee Joint, Biomed. Engng 3, 164 – 170, 1968

Nicol, A.C., Paul, J.P. The Forces and Moments transmitted at the Articulations of the Upper Extremity of the Human during Certain Normal Activities Proc Sixth International Symp. on External Control of Human Extremities, Dubrovnik, Vol 2., 1978

Paul, J.P., Forces transmitted by Joints in the Human Body Proc. Inst. Mech. Eng. 181 3J 8 – 15, 1967

Paul, J.P., Comparison of EMG signals from leg muscles with corresponding force actions calculated from walkpath measurements Proc. Conf. Human Locomotor Engineering, Inst. Mech. Eng. London pp 16 – 26., 1971

Paul, J.P. and Poulson, J. The analysis of forces transmitted by joints in the human body Proc. of Fifth International Conference on Experimental Stress Analysis, Udine, Italy, CISM, Udine 1974

Paul, J.P. Forces Transmitted by Joints in the Human Body Proc. Symposium Lubrication and Wear in Living and Artificial Human Joints, Proc. Inst. Mech Eng V181 3J, 8 – 15

Barbenel, J.C. and Paul, J.P. Biomechanics in Medical Engineering Ray C.D. Ed. Year Book Medical Publishers, Chicago

Paul, J.P. Force Actions transmitted by Joints in the Human Body Proc. Roy. Soc. London B 192 163-172, 1975

Paul, J.P. Loading on Normal Hip and Knee Joints and on Joint Replacements , Engineering in Medicine, Ed. Schaldach M., Springer Verlag. Berlin, 1975.

Paul, J.P. Biomechanics of the Upper Limb in Arthritic Patients, Proc. Conf. IRMA III Basle, 1978

Rydell, N. Forces acting on the femoral head prosthesis, Acta Orthop. Scand. Suppl. 88, 1966

Swanson, S.A.V., and Freeman, M.A.R., The Scientific Basis of Joint Replacement, Pitman Medical Publishing Co. Tunbridge Wells, 1977

Schaldach, M. Editor, Engineering in Medicine, Springer Verlag, Berlin, 1975

Walker, P.S., Human Joints and their Artificial Replacements, C.C. Thomas, Springfield, Illinois, 1977

RELATIONS BETWEEN THE MICROSCOPIC STRUCTURE AND FRACTURES
OF HUMAN COMPACT BONE*

F. Gaynor Evans, Ph.D.

Department of Anatomy, The University of Michigan,
Ann Arbor, Michigan, U.S.A.°

ABSTRACT. Statistically significant correlation coefficients
suggest the following relations between some mechanical properties
of adult human compact bone and its histological components in the
break area:(1) The percentage of secondary osteons in the break
area increases torsional shear stress, shear modulus, energy
absorbed to failure, compressive strength, fatigue life, and
Rockwell superficial hardness but decreases ultimate tensile
strength. (2) The average area/secondary osteon decreases ultimate
tensile strength, single (punching) shear strength, and modulus
of elasticity. Percentage of interstitial lamellae increases
ultimate tensile strength but decreases fatigue life. (3)
Percentage of spaces in break area decreases all mechanical
properties. Collagen fiber orientation also influences mechanical
properties. Classifying osteons as light, intermediate, and dark
on the basis of their appearance in polarized light, suggests that
the percentage of dark osteons increases tensile stress, strain
and single shear strength. The percentage of light osteons decreases
single shear strength, and tensile stress and strain. Intermediate
osteons increases torsion shear strength, shear modulus, and tensile
strain, but decreases single shear strength and modulus. The
percentage of intermediately and markedly radiolucent osteons
decreases tensile stress and strain.

* This research was supported in part by Research Grant AM03865
from the National Institutes of Health, U.S. Public Health Service,
Department of Health, Education and Welfare.
° Present address.

INTRODUCTION

Bone or osseous tissue is a visco-elastic, anisotropic, composite material (Welch, 1971; Piekarski, 1973) found only in the skeleton (internal and/or external) of vertebrate animals. Bone is one of the major tissue components of the human body constituting, according to Wilmer (1940), 22% of the total body components at 6 lunar months and 18% in the newborn and the adult. The only more abundant components are (1) muscle which forms 25% at 6 lunar months and 45% in the newborn and the adult, and (2) skin and fat which form 25% in the newborn and the adult.

Whether or not any object, including a bone, fails or fractures as the result of the application of a force is a function of the kind and amount of material composing the object, the way in which that material is distributed, and the chemical and mechanical properties of the material. In the case of a bone the material involved is osseous tissue.

During the daily activities of life the bones of the human body, individually and collectively, are subjected to a variety of force systems as a result of gravity, muscular activity, pressure of adjacent structures, and atmospheric pressure. Whether or not a bone fractures as a result of any one or more of these factors depends on many biological and non-biological variables.

Among the biological variables to be considered are the age, the sex, the race and the state of health of the individual. The last variable involves vitamins, hormones, nutrition, and general physiology of the individual, which, in turn, may affect the amount, the type, the distribution and the degree of calcification and of ossification of the bone as well as its biochemical and mechanical properties.

Non-biological variables influencing whether or not failure of a bone occurs from application of a force are the type, the magnitude, the point and rate of application, and the direction of the force applied to it. Other non-biological variables affecting the biomechanical behavior of bone under a load are whether or not the bone is fresh, embalmed, frozen or preserved in some other way, and whether it is wet or dry. Other variables are temperature and humidity conditions during the preparation and testing of a bone. If standardized test specimens are used the orientation of the specimens within the intact bone also influences the results of a test.

The biological and non-biological variables mentioned above are applicable to the biomechanical behavior under load of an intact bone or a standardized test specimen of bone. In studying

213

the mechanical properties of bone or osseous tissue, which are important in the fracture mechanism, the use of standardized test specimens is the method of choice.

There is a voluminous literature on the gross and microscopic anatomy, the embryology, the biochemistry, the physiology, the pathology, and the fracture of human bone. However, there is considerably less literature on the mechanical properties of bone which are related to the fracture mechanisms, see reviews by Ascenzi and Bell (1972), Carter and Spengler (1978), Currey (1970), Hayes (in press), Herrmann and Liebowitz (1972), Knese (1970), Kraus (1968), Reilly and Burstein (1974), and Swanson (1971), and books by Evans, (1957, 1973) and by Yamada (1970).

Literature on the relations of the microscopic structure of bone, generally compact or cortical bone, to its fracture mechanisms, especially for human bone, is less abundant than that on mechanical properties. Although much of the data on the mechanical properties of compact bone and their relation to the microstructure and fracture of bone was obtained from non-human bone the following discussion, for the purpose of my assignment in this study institute, is restricted to human compact (cortical) bone.

GROSS ANATOMY OF BONES

In an adult human being osseous tissue normally forms 206 named bones of the skeleton in addition to sesamoid bones in the tendons of some muscles.

On the basis of their shape bones are classified as (1) flat bones - the scapula (shoulder blade) and some of the skull bones, (2) long bones - the major bones of the upper and the lower limb, and (3) short or irregular bones - the bones of the wrist, the ankle, and the vertebral (spinal) column. From their embryonic development bones are categorized as membrane (dermal) bones and as cartilage (replacing) bones. Cartilage bones are first preformed in cartilage and later become ossified into bone while membrane bones ossify directly from membrane without passing through a cartilaginous stage. Except for the clavicle (collar) bone, which is the most commonly fractured bone in the body, dermal bones are confined to the skull. The rest of the bones of the skeleton, including some of the skull, are cartilage bones.

Bone is also classified as compact (cortical) and spongy (cancellous). Compact bone is the dense hard bone on the surface of a bone while spongy bone is the soft trabecular bone inside a bone. In a typical long bone, e.g. the femur (thigh) bone, the compact bone forms an external shell surrounding the bone except for the articular cartilage covering the joint surfaces.

214

The compact bone is quite thick in the middle third of the length
of a long bone but gradually thins out towards the ends of the bone.
The spongy or trabecular bone is found within the head, neck, and
greater trochanter of the proximal part of the bone and the condyles
of the distal part of the bone.

MICROSCOPIC ANATOMY OF COMPACT BONE

Hancox (1972) considers bone to be the most complex material
in the body whose diversity of function is reflected in its unique
physical and chemical characteristics. The elementary constituents
of bone, according to Pritchard (1972) are (1) collagen fibers,
which form nearly one-third of the dry weight of bone, (2) crystals,
generally considered to be hydroxyapatite, about 30-50 A wide and
up to 600 Å long, (3) the cement or amorphous ground substance
which is a continuous phase with discrete fibrils and crystals
embedded in it and (4) the osteocytes or bone cells. The crystals
or inorganic component of bone constitute nearly two-thirds of the
dry weight of bone matrix. The collagen fibers embedded in the
organic matrix contribute greatly to its strength and toughness
while its hardness and rigidity are due to its inorganic components.

On the basis of its microscopic structure bone is classified
often as bundle bone, woven or fibrous bone, and fine-fibered
lamellar (Haversian) bone. Bundle bone has a matrix dominated
by regularly arranged coarse fiber collagenous bundles with
osteocytes that follow the pattern of the fibers. When the fibers
are parallel the osteocytes are found as columns between the
fiber bundles. Woven bone has coarse, loosely packed fiber bundles
of varying size up to 30μ in diameter. The fibers form an irregular
interlacing course through the matrix. Woven fiber bone is also
characterised by an abundance of large randomly packed osteocytes
and the fact that the matrix stains bluish or purplish with
hematoxylin, presumably because of its high basophil content. In
microradiographs woven bone is conspicuous because it is more
highly calcified than other bone that is present.

Fine fibered bone is often called lamellar bone because it
consists of lamellae which are 3-7μ thick. However, some fine-
fibered bone is not lamellar in nature. In ordinary histological
preparations fine-fibered bone has a clear eosinophil matrix with
small, ovoid osteocytes spaced at regular, rather wide, intervals.
Under polarized light one can easily determine if lamellation is
present. The adult human skeleton is almost entirely fine-fibered
or lamellated bone.

A mature human long bone is essentially tubular in the middle
third of its length. The wall of the tube is composed of lamellar
bone with various orientations within the wall of the shaft. On
the outer surface of the shaft just beneath the periosteum,

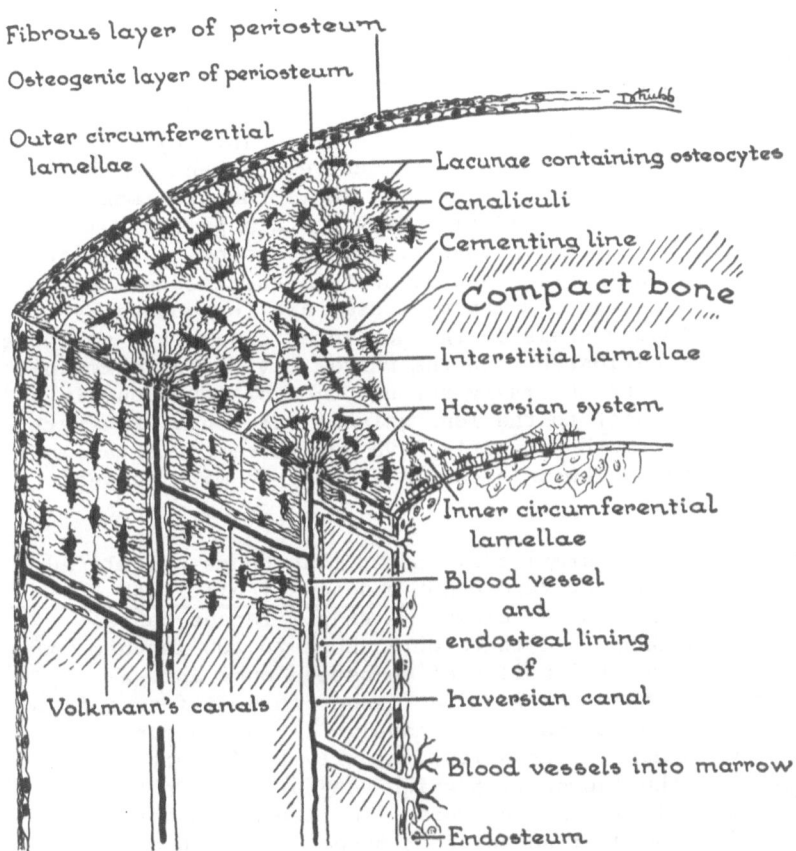

Fibrous layer of periosteum

Osteogenic layer of periosteum

Outer circumferential lamellae

Lacunae containing osteocytes

Canaliculi

Cementing line

Compact bone

Interstitial lamellae

Haversian system

Inner circumferential lamellae

Blood vessel and endosteal lining of haversian canal

Volkmann's canals

Blood vessels into marrow

Endosteum

Diagram of the histological structure of a human long bone. From Arthur W. Ham, HISTOLOGY, 6th ed. Lippincott, Philadelphia, 1969.

a layer of specialized connective tissue investing the bone except for the joint surfaces, are the outer circumferential lamellae. In each of these regions there may be several layers of circumferentially oriented lamellae. Between the outer and the inner circumferential lamellae there is a mosaic of lamellae in the form of complete osteons (Haversian systems), incomplete osteons, and interstitial lamellae. (Figure 1).

A Haversian system or osteon consists of 4-20 lamellae encircling a central Haversian canal (22-110μ in diameter) containing one or more blood vessels. Rather uniformly distributed throughout an osteon are lenticular cavities, varying from 20 x 10 x 5 μm to 27 x 13 x 7 μm in size (Boyde, 1972) that are usually filled with an osteocyte (bone cell). The volumes of such lacunae would be 525 and 130 μm^3, respectively. Lacunae are connected with one another by extremely small tunnels (mean diameter 0.2 μm) called canaliculi which contain protoplasmic processes of the osteocytes. Boyde reported around 32 canaliculi radiating from one-half of a lacuna. Within the lacunae and canaliculi the osteocyte and its processes are surrounded by tissue fluid. Blood vessels in the Haversian canals are connected with those in the periosteum and the marrow cavity by Volkmann's canals which course transversely through the cortical bone in a direction perpendicular to the long axis of the bone. However, the osteocytes and the bone matrix have no systematic organization with respect to the Volkmann's canals as they do with respect to the Haversian canals.

Frost (1960) for normal adult human long bones calculated that osteocyte lacunae average 0.80% and canaliculi 1.45% of vascular-free cortical bone volume. A single lacuna has an average volume of $310\mu^3$ and there were about 26,100 lacunae/mm^3. Canaliculi of innermost lamellae of an osteon open into a Haversian canal so they can receive tissue fluid diffusing from the blood vessels in the Haversian canal. In the outermost lamellae of an osteon the canaliculi usually form short loops reaching back to the lacuna from which they arise. On rare occasions canaliculi in the outermost lamellae of an osteon communicate with those of an adjacent osteon (Weimann and Sicher, (1947)). Complete and incomplete osteons surrounded by cement lines separating them from adjacent bone material are called Secondary Osteons in contrast to Primary Osteons which are not surrounded by cement lines or Haversian lamellae. Secondary osteons do not appear during the first 2 or 3 years of life.

In most textbooks osteons, in cross section, are illustrated by being nice and round. However, they are more often elliptical. Furthermore, they are not simple cylinders of osseous tissue but frequently are branched (Filogamo, 1946a; Koltze, 1951; Cohen and Harris, 1958).

The collagen fibers of bone lie in the lamellae and vary in their orientation from one lamellae to another within a single osteon as well as from one osteon to another. The orientation of the collagen fibers can be seen by polarized light or by scanning electron microscopy.

Collagen fibrils are characterized by a periodic banding whose repeat distance along the fibril is roughly 640 Å. The tropocollagen molecule is about 2800 Å long, 13.6 Å in diameter and has a molecular weight of about 290000. Normally the collagen fibrils seen by electronmicroscopy are formed by lateral aggregations of tropocollagen molecules which overlap longitudinally by specific amounts (Hancox, loc. cit.).

Hydroxyapatite crystals are found within the collagen fibers. Usually the long axis of the crystal is parallel to that of the collagen fiber with which it is associated. Various opinions have been expressed regarding the nature of the cement lines (Sokoloff, 1973). By microradiography one can visualize the degree of mineralization in bone.

For more information on the structure and composition of bone see Bloom and Fawcett (1975), Bourne (1972), Eanes and Posner (1970), Glimcher (1976), Ham (1969), Miller and Martin (1968), Robinson (1975), and Vaughan (1975).

TENSILE, COMPRESSIVE AND SHEARING PROPERTIES:

MODULUS OF ELASTICITY

Apparently the first to comment on the effects of the microstructure of bone on its biomechanical behavior was Rauber (1876) who noted that "the cell containing bone substance is given an arrangement of particular importance for the strength of bone by the usual development into lamellae." Rauber points out that the Haversian canals are oriented predominantly parallel with the long axis of a long bone. According to him the outer and the inner circumferential lamellae are "particularly suited and needed to absorb bending stresses and to counteract a displacement and dislocation of haversian systems." However, no data were presented to support these opinions.

Maj (1938) investigated the relation between porosity and the bending strength of standardized test specimens of compact bone from the anterior and posterior aspects of the femur of a 79-year-old man.

Test specimens were obtained at 2 cm. intervals from strips of bone cut the length of the femur. Porosity was determined by computing the volume occupied by the cavities of the specimens.

A similar analysis was made of the metatarsal bones of an ox.

Data obtained showed that the breaking load decreased and the porosity increased from the approximate middle of the femur toward its extremities. This was especially true of specimens from the posterior aspect of the femoral shaft. However, the increase in the porosity of the specimens was not proportional to the decrease in the breaking load.

Maj concluded from his studies that the degree of porosity was not responsible for the variations in breaking load except in the distal part of ox metacarpal bones where the porosity was approximately 50%. According to Maj, differences in the strength of compact bone of different areas of a single skeletal segment are probably a function of intrinsic properties of the bone and variations in the density and orientation of the collagen fibers. He also showed that porosity of compact bone was greater than commonly believed.

Later Maj (1942) studied regional variation in the bending strength of standardized specimens from rings of bone, about 2 cm thick, from the middle of the diaphysis of the humerus, ulna, femur and tibia of 40 individuals from 5 to 90 years of age. All the specimens were oriented in the major axis of the diaphysis. Six humeral, 3 ulnar, 9 femoral, and 6 tibial specimens were tested.

Variations in bending strength were more evident in human bones than in lower animals and were greater and more marked in the femoral and humeral specimens than in those of tibial and ulnar ones. Average maximum values for bending strength of specimens from specific zones of the diaphysis were distributed with certain regularity and had a somewhat constant relationship. Minimum values were very inconsistently distributed, and for the femoral, the humeral, and to a lesser extent for the tibial specimens it was difficult to determine which sections of the bone were the stronger.

With respect to the age of the individual from whom the specimens were obtained, Maj's study showed that (1) the highest fracture loads were found in the greatest statistical percentage in the middle of the third decade and in the fifth decade of life; (2) the lowest fracture loads were most often found in individuals in the 8th and 9th decades of life; (3) in human bone lower fracture loads were more frequently obtained in the period of minimal resistance, and (4) the average value for fracture strength from the 25th to the 35th years of life corresponds to that from the 50th to the 70th years of life. Thus the bending strength of bone between the 25th and 35th year of life is approximately inter-mediate to that between the sixth and seventh decades of life.

Maj had no satisfactory explanation for the rather low fracture strength of bone from individuals from 25 to 35 years of age. He did not think changes occurring in fracture strength of bone with advancing age could be explained by differences in density, size, and structure of Haversian systems nor the prevalent direction of collagen fibers. He believed that the causes of individual variability in fracture strength were primarily biological, some acquired and others congenital, and thought that the variability is an explanation of chemical-physical diversity within the fundamental elements of bony tissue, that is, the collagen fibers, the osteomucoid substance, and the mineral salts.

Yokoo (1952) studied the effect of Haversian lamellae orientation on the compressive strength of diaphyseal compact bone from the long bones of 43 human subjects from 27 to 80 years of age. He found that the compressive strength of compact femoral bone in a direction perpendicular to the Haversian lamellae was only 3/5 as strong as that in a direction parallel to Haversian lamellae. However, the maximum contraction perpendicular to the Haversian lamellae was 1.2 times greater than that parallel to the lamellae.

Okamoto (1955), who studied wet compact bone from the femur of a 32-year-old man and also bone from a cow, reported that the collagen fibers were not significant in compression but had considerable significance in tension. Cement substance was very important in both tension and compression, especially in the latter.

Aoji (1959) determined the relation of the size of Haversian systems and canals, the distribution ratio of Haversian canals, and the area percentages of the Haversian systems, canals, and interstitial lamellae to the tensile and compressive strength of the middle portion of the shaft of fresh long bones from the extremities of 28 subjects ranging from 24 to 83 years of age.

In tension Aoji reported that ruptures occurred in the boundary of Haversian systems and interstitial lamellae. In compression failure of the lamellae occurred at the interstitial portion. Although the Haversian systems "resisted hard" against both tension and compression the interstitial lamellae "resist hard only against tension but not against compression. Compression strength is inversely proportional to the area percentage of the interstitial lamellae, while tensile strength is inversely proportional to the area percentage of the Haversian canals."

The relation between the chemical components and strength of compact bone was investigated by Uehira (1960) in specimens from the middle of the femoral diaphysis of individuals from new-born to 80 years of age. Similar investigations were made on bones from 12 cows, 14 dogs, 5 cats, 10 rabbits, 5 guinea pigs, and 6 rats.

Although no age changes, after puberty, were found in the quantitative relation of the chemical components of the bone the compressive strength of the bone decreases with advancing age because of the decrease in the strength of the organic cement substance. Decrease in tensile strength with age is due to an increase in the ratio of the cross sectional area of the Haversian canals.

My own studies on the relations of the tensile, compressive, shearing, fatigue, and torsion properties of human compact bone to its histological structure are an outgrowth of previous investigations on the skull, the femur, and the pelvis by means of electric strain gauges and a strain sensitive lacquer called "Stresscoat." Electric strain gauges, applied directly to the bone, and the cathode ray oscilloscope were first used by Gurdjian and Lissner (1944) to study the mechanism of skull fracture in dogs. Later Stresscoat was used to study the mechanism of skull fracture in dogs and monkeys, living and dead, as well as in man by Gurdjian and Lissner (1945, 1946, 1947), by Gurdjian, Lissner and Webster (1947), and by Gurdjian, Webster, and Lissner (1949). Evans and Lissner also used Stresscoat to study femoral and pelvic deformations and fractures (Evans, 1957).

Data obtained in these investigations showed that linear fractures of the skull in the dog, the monkey and man, as well as similar fractures of the human femur and pelvis all arose from failure of the bone from the tensile stresses and strains produced within it by bending of the bone as a result of the force applied to it. In compression fracture or those produced by high velocity missiles, e.g. bullets, the fracture mechanism is somewhat different.

The importance of tensile stresses and strains in the fracture mechanisms of the skull, the pelvis and the femur, as demonstrated by the above-mentioned Stresscoat studies, prompted Evans and Lebow (1951) to determine the tensile stress and strain, shearing stress, and hardness of compact bone from various regions of the femoral shaft. They were particularly interested to learn if specimens from the regions of the shaft where the first Stresscoat cracks appeared, indicating sites of highest tensile strain where failure would occur with sufficient load, also had the highest ultimate tensile strength. Some correlations between the sites of the Stresscoat patterns and tensile properties of the bone were found. Later Evans and Lebow (1952) compared the ultimate tensile stress and strain of standardized test specimens of compact bone from various thirds of the human femoral, tibial, and fibular shaft.

Data obtained in these studies motivated Evans to initiate a series of investigations on the relations between various mechanical properties of human compact bone and its microscopic structure.

Information resulting from these investigations was used to account for differences in the tensile stress and other mechanical properties of human compact bone.

In his first study, Evans (1958) examined cross sections of embalmed femoral and fibular specimens in ordinary light and in polarized light.

From data obtained by ordinary light studies, Evans explained the greater tensile strength of the fibular specimens on the basis that they had fewer but larger secondary osteons than did the femoral specimens. This suggests that many small osteons and their fragments tend to reduce the tensile strength of human compact bone. The reduction in tensile strength is not due to the osteons per se but to the fact that they and their remnants are surrounded by cement lines which are areas of weakness as indicated by a definite tendency for fractures to follow the cement lines. Consequently, the more osteons and their remnants there are per unit area of bone the more cement lines or substances there are where failure or fracture can occur.

The polarized light data revealed that the fibular specimens had a marked tendency to be darker than the femoral ones indicating that their collagen fiber bundles were more nearly parallel with the long axis of the osteon than in the femoral specimens. Thus, the collagen fibers in the fibular specimens were better oriented for resisting tension than were those in the femoral specimens.

Evans and Bang (1966) determined the ultimate tensile strength, single shearing strength, tensile strain, modulus of elasticity and Rockwell superficial hardness of 45 wet tested standardized femoral and 32 fibular specimens. Tensile stress, strain and modulus were determined parallel with and shearing stress and hardness perpendicular to the long axis of the specimen. An analysis of variance revealed that the mean tensile stress and modulus in the fibular specimens were significantly greater (1%) than in the femoral specimens. However, femoral specimens had a significantly greater (1%) number of osteons/mm^2 and percentage of osteons and of spaces in the break area than did the fibular specimens. The percentage of interstitial lamellae in the break area was significantly greater (1%) in the fibular specimens.

Among the femoral specimens a significant negative correlation (1%) was found between percentage of spaces in the break area and tensile stress, modulus, and hardness as well as a positive correlation (2%) between tensile strain and the percentage of osteons in the break area. Fibular specimens had a positive correlation (1%) between tensile strain and percentage of osteons in the break area and the number of osteons/mm^2; a negative correlation (1%) between tensile strain and percentage of interstitial lamellae in the break area and between single shearing strength and average area/osteon; and a negative correlation (2%) between tensile strain and percentage of spaces in the break area.

The femoral specimens had many small osteons and their remnants but relatively little interstitial lamellae while fibular specimens had the opposite composition. Consequently, the femoral specimens had more cementing substance per unit area of bone than did the fibular specimens. These differences may explain, in part, the significantly lower tensile stress and modulus of the femoral specimens compared with the fibular ones.

In their second study Evans and Bang (1967) compared the mechanical properties and histological components of cross sections taken as close as possible to the fracture site, of femoral, tibial, and fibular specimens of adult human compact bone. They found that the corrected break area, i.e. the cross section area minus the major spaces, of 56 femoral specimens had 47% secondary osteons, 11% remnants of osteons, and 42% interstitial lamellae. Seventy-six tibial specimens had 37% osteons, 9% remnants, and 54% interstitial lamellae while 37 fibular specimens had 35% osteons, 13% remnants, and 50% interstitial lamellae. These were significant (1%) differences.

Analysis of variance revealed the following histological differences at the 1% significance level: (1) femoral specimens had larger osteons and osteon remnants which formed a greater percentage of the break area than tibial sections; (2) the percentage of the corrected break area formed by interstitial lamellae was greater in the tibial than in the femoral sections; (3) femoral sections had more osteons/mm^2 and a greater percentage of the break area formed by osteons than did fibular sections; (4) fibular specimens had a larger percentage of the corrected break area formed by interstitial lamellae than the femoral sections; (5) the number of osteons/mm^2 and the percentage of the break area formed by osteons was greater in the tibial than in the fibular sections; and (6) fibular sections had larger osteons and osteon remnants than did tibial sections.

An analysis of variance between the means showed that the tibial specimens had a significantly higher ultimate tensile and shearing strength, tensile strain, modulus of elasticity, and density than the femoral specimens. Tibial specimens were also more dense than fibular specimens. Fibular specimens had a greater tensile and shearing strength and modulus of elasticity than the femoral specimens. All differences were at the 1% significance level.

Correlation coefficients between the mechanical properties and the histological structure of the three types of specimens revealed a strong positive correlation between ultimate tensile strength (0.02 level) and the percentage of interstitial lamellae in the corrected break area. Hardness had a positive correlation (0.01 level) with the number of osteons/mm^2 and the percentage of the break area formed by osteons. Strong negative correlations (0.01 level) were found between ultimate tensile strength and the percentage of the break area formed by osteons; between the single shearing strength and the average area/osteon remnant (0.02 level); and between hardness and the percentage of spaces in the original break area (0.001 level). A negative correlation was found between the modulus of elasticity and the average area/osteon (0.05 level) and between modulus of elasticity and the percentage of the original break area formed by the spaces (0.01 level). A negative correlation was also found between single shearing strength and the average area/osteon (0.05 level).

From the correlations between the tensile properties of human compact bone and its microscopic structure, Evans and Bang concluded that secondary osteons and their fragments tend to decrease the tensile strength and modulus of elasticity of bone while interstitial lamellae tend to increase them. Secondary osteons and their fragments do not per se tend to reduce the tensile properties of human bone but the cement substance, which surrounds the histological components and separates them from adjacent components appears to be the weakest material present and the site of microfractures. Fractures of cross sections of bone due to tensile stress and strain created by tension applied to opposite sides of the section or by drying have a marked tendency to follow the cement lines. Thus, the more secondary osteons and their remnants there are in a given area of bone the more cement lines it has where microfractures can occur.

Factors affecting the elasticity of bone were investigated by Smith and Walmsley (1959) in bone from the human tibia, the horse radius, the metacarpus of an ox and a sheep, and the dog femur. Their specimens were tested under axial tension and compression and by bending. Effects of stress duration, water content, temperature and vascularity on bone deformation and elasticity were also studied. An additional variable investigated was the effect of partial lamination.

Data obtained in their studies indicated that bone deformation under stress varies with stress duration and fluid content and temperature of the specimens. The relation between modulus of elasticity in tension to that in bending is partially dependent on the vascular pattern of the bone.

Dempster and Coleman (1960) determined the tensile strength of standardized specimens of human compact bone along and across the "grain." On the basis of photomicrographs taken of wet- and dry-

tested undecalcified specimens they concluded that "the weaker
structural elements are the cement lines surrounding osteons and
the planes between the lamellae of the Haversian system." Maj and
Toajari (1937) had noted the tendency of fractures to follow
cement lines between osteons. However, they believed it was more
frequent in calcified than in undecalcified bone. McElhaney (1966)
reported that fractures produced at a high strain rate of loading
seemed to follow the cement lines surrounding the osteons. Similar
effects of secondary osteons and their cement lines on the strength
characteristics and microfractures of compact bone have also been
noted by Aoji (1959), Bird et al., (1968), Carter and Hayes (1977),
Currey (1959, 1962), Heřt et al. (1965), Okamoto (1955),
Piekarski (1970), Pope and Outwater (1974), Simkin and Robin (1974),
Sweeney et al. (1965), and Uehira (1960).

A classic series of studies on mechanical properties of
portions of single osteons was made by Ascenzi, Bonucci and their
associates. In their initial study, Ascenzi and Bonucci (1964)
determined the tensile strength of longitudinal sections of single
osteons isolated from longitudinal sections 20 to 50 micra thick,
of femoral shafts. The longitudinal sections of single osteons
were dissected out under a polarizing light microscope at a
magnification of 80 to 100 times. Bone was removed from all sides
of a longitudinally sectioned osteon in the middle region of the
original bone sample. The ends of the sample which were larger
were put into square lugs to provide good fixation in the tensile
testing apparatus. Ultimate tensile strength was calculated from
the cross sectional area of the isolated middle part of the osteon.
Specimens were tested in both the wet and the dry condition to
determine the effect of moisture. Cross sectional areas were
measured in each state.

On the basis of collagen fiber bundle arrangement in
successive lamellae 2 types of osteons were chosen for study.
In the first type of osteon the collagen fibers have a marked
longitudinal spiral course which changes so slightly that the
fibers of one lamella have about a 0° angle with those of the
next lamella. In polarized light osteons of the first type are
uniformly bright in longitudinal section. In the second type of
osteon the collagen fibers in one lamella make about a 90° angle
with the fibers of the next lamella. Osteons of the second type,
when seen in polarized light, have an alternation of light and
dark lamellae in longitudinal section.

Ascenzi and Bonucci found that dry osteons, both at the
initial and final stages of calcification, had a significantly
higher ultimate tensile strength than wet osteons. Osteons with
a marked longitudinal arrangement of collagen fiber bundles in
successive lamellae had a higher ultimate tensile strength than
osteons with fiber bundles running alternately so that their

direction in successive lamellae changes through an angle of about 90°. The degree of calcification does not significantly change the tensile strength of osteons with the same orientation of their collagen fibers.

Ultimate tensile strength is the same magnitude in both calcified and decalcified osteons which indicates that the collagen fibers are essential in determining some of the mechanical properties of bone. Human and ox osteons have the same ultimate tensile strength.

In the second publication (Ascenzi, Bonucci and Checcucci, 1966), tensile properties of single osteons were determined with a microwave extensometer specifically developed for the purpose. The technique for dissection of a sample of a single osteon was the same as that used previously (Ascenzi and Bonucci, 1964). It was found that drying increased the tensile strength and modulus of elasticity of individual osteons but reduced their tensile strain. Wet tested specimens had a greater tensile strain than did the dry ones as evident from the stress-strain curve which was almost a straight line to failure for the dry specimens and a curve for the wet specimens. In wet osteon samples the degree of calcification produced a significant variation in the stress-strain curve which indicated an increase in the modulus of elasticity with increasing amounts of calcium salts. The tensile modulus of elasticity of the organic matrix of decalcified osteons corresponds to that of collagen. Osteons with a marked longitudinal arrangement of the collagen fiber bundles in successive lamellae appeared to have a greater ultimate tensile strength and modulus of elasticity but lower tensile strain than in osteons whose fiber bundles run alternately in such a way that their direction in successive lamellae changed at an angle of about 90°. Individual age appears to have little effect on tensile properties of osteons. Comparisons of tensile properties of single osteons and of macroscopic specimens suggest that the osteon is the mechanical unit of compact bone. Tensile behavior is the same in human and ox osteons.

Compression properties of segments of single osteons were also investigated by Ascenzi and Bonucci (1968). Segments of single osteons were dissected out, from 500 micra thick cross sections of human and ox femoral shafts. A thickness of 500 micra is a critical limit because if the cross sections were thicker they would not be transparent enough for examination under polarized light, which was used in their study. During the dissection of the osteons care was taken not to overheat them. The length and cross sectional area of the dissected osteons were accurately measured and calculated with an eyepiece micrometer. Samples were measured wet as that was the condition in which they were tested. Length to cross section ratio was between 2.5:1 and 3:1. Tested osteons varied in degree of calcification and orientation of their collagen bundles. The Haversian canal was in the long axis of the test osteon and its diameter was kept as constant as possible.

On the basis of the cross section appearance of the osteons in polarized light they were classified into 3 types. In Type I osteons the collagen fibers had a marked transverse spiral course in successive lamellae and the osteons are uniformly bright in polarized light. In Type II osteons the collagen fibers in one lamella had a marked longitudinal spiral course while in the next lamella the fibers had an almost transverse course so that fibers in successive lamellae made an angle of nearly 90°. In polarized light Type II osteons have an alternation of light and dark lamellae. In Type III osteons the collagen fibers had a marked longitudinal spiral course with the pitch to the spiral changing so little that the angle of the fibers was practically the same in successive lamellae. Type III osteons are uniformly dark in polarized light although they are often bordered by a bright lamella which was always removed during dissection of the osteon.

Ascenzi and Bonucci found that: (1) ultimate compressive strength was greatest in osteons with transversely oriented collagen fiber bundles (Type I osteons), lowest in osteons with longitudinally oriented fiber bundles (Type III osteons), and intermediate in osteons with fiber bundles that changed through an angle of about 90° in successive lamellae (Type II osteons); (2) modulus of elasticity was greatest in Type I osteons; (3) in all 3 types of osteons the stress-strain curves for fully calcified osteons were markedly different from those of osteons with a low calcium content which had a much lower modulus of elasticity; (4) there was no measurable age effect on the compressive properties of the osteons; (5) comparison of the compressive properties of segments of single osteons with that in macroscopic bone samples supports the view that the osteon is the mechanical unit of compact bone; (6) fractures in osteon samples start with microscopic fissures induced by shearing stress; (7) in every case these fissures form an angle of 30°-35° with the osteon axis and do not vary with the microscopic structure of the osteon; and (8) electron microscopy reveals bone crystal distortion and breaking of collagen fibrils at the edges of the fissures.

Data obtained by Ascenzi and Bonucci shows that osteons with transversely oriented collagen fiber bundles (Type I osteons) have the greatest compressive strength while those with longitudinally oriented collagen fibers (Type III osteons) have the lowest and supports conclusions of Gebhardt (1905) from a study of metallic models. Gebhardt assumed that when fiber bundles and crystallites are loaded almost parallel with their long axis, as in Type III osteons, they easily bend and fracture. However, transversely oriented fibers and crystallites, as in Type I osteons, form a ring that prevents bending. Consequently, they have the greatest compressive strength.

Evans and Vincentelli (1969) investigated the relation of collagen fiber orientation, as revealed by polarized light, to the tensile properties and single shearing strength of 16 femoral, 28 tibial and 9 fibular specimens of adult embalmed human compact bone in an attempt to determine whether or not the results reported by Ascenzi and his associates for single osteons also applies to larger specimens.

In an attempt to reduce the number of variables a histological analysis was made of cross sections, taken as close as possible to the fracture site, of bones from two cadavers. Osteons, from their appearance in polarized light, were classified as light (bright), intermediate, and dark.

Histological analysis of the cross section revealed that femoral sections had the highest and tibial sections the lowest percentage of light osteons. The percentage of dark osteons was considerably greater in the tibial than in either the femoral or fibular sections in which the percentage of dark osteons was approximately equal. Fibular sections had the highest and femoral sections the lowest percentage of intermediate osteons although the differences among the 3 bones were not as great as for the light and dark osteons.

The highest percentage of light osteons plus fragments were in the femoral and the lowest in tibial sections respectively. Tibial sections had the greatest percentage of dark osteons plus fragments and femoral sections had the least. Fibular sections had the highest percentage of intermediate osteons and fragments while the tibial section had the lowest.

The percentage of the break area formed by dark osteons plus their fragments was significantly greater (0.001 level) in the tibial than in either the femoral or fibular sections. Femoral sections had a significantly greater (0.001 level) percentage of light osteons plus fragments than did the tibial sections. The percentage of light osteons plus their fragments was significantly greater (0.01 level) in the fibular sections than in tibial sections.

A very high positive correlation (0.001 level) was found between single shearing strength and the percentage of dark osteons in the break area. There was also a high positive correlation (0.01 level) between single shearing strength and the percentage of intermediate osteons in the break area. Modulus of elasticity and tensile strain had a positive correlation at the 0.02 level and the 0.05 level, respectively, with the percentage of inter- mediate osteons in the break area. Negative correlations

(0.001 level) were found between shearing strength and percentage of light osteons and at the 0.05 level between modulus of elasticity and light osteons.

Evans and Vincentelli thought that perhaps the lack of a positive correlation between tensile strength and modulus of elasticity and the percentage of dark osteons in their specimens which they had expected from Ascenzi and Bonucci's study (1967), was due to the fact that the dark osteons alone formed too small a proportion (20%) of the break area to have any significant effect. Dark osteons and their fragments combined constituted only about 30% of the break area.

Ultimate tensile strength, tensile strain and modulus of elasticity were determined from tests in which the load was applied to the specimen parallel with its long axis while shearing strength was determined by applying the load perpendicular to the long axis of the specimen. Consequently, the predominant direction of the collagen fibers of the dark osteons was perpendicular or normal to the direction of the shearing force while in the light osteons and fragments the predominant direction of the fibers would be more nearly parallel to the shearing force. Thus, the light osteons would not resist shearing as well as the dark ones because shearing occurs more easily parallel to the direction of the collagen fibers than transverse to them.

Although Evans and Vincentelli classified osteons as dark, light and intermediate, as did Ascenzi and Bonucci (1968), their interpretation of the collagen fiber orientations was similar to that of Smith (1960) who recognized three different types or patterns of collagen fiber orientation. According to Smith, osteons differed from one another in the relative numbers of longitudinal and circumferential fibers they contained and in the degree of lamination they exhibited. Smith correlates the instance of the three fiber patterns with relative ages and regions of the bone in which they occur.

Filogamo (1946b) by studying serial cross sections of osteons in polarized light found that variations in collagen fiber orientation occurred along the axis of the osteon. If the specimens were from old individuals 20% of the samples showed marked variation, while only minor variations were found when the specimens were taken from younger individuals.

Vincentelli and Evans (1971) also investigated the relations of tensile properties, collagen fiber orientation and calcification in unembalmed tibias from above-knee amputations of 4 white men from 23 to 74 years of age. Unembalmed material was used, instead of embalmed as in their previous study, because calcification, one of the variables, was probably influenced by embalming.

Osteons, from their appearance in polarized light, were classified as light, intermediate, and dark, or, on the basis of microradiographs, as slightly radiolucent, intermediately radiolucent, and markedly radiolucent.

Ultimate tensile strength has a significant (0.01 level) positive correlation with dark osteons and an equally significant negative correlation with light osteons. Modulus of elasticity had no significant correlation with any of the three types of osteons. Tensile strain had a very highly significant (0.001 level) negative correlation with light osteons and an equally high positive correlation with dark osteons. None of the mechanical properties had any significant correlation with the intermediate osteons.

When the light osteons were combined with their remnants ultimate tensile strength had a highly significant (0.001 level) negative correlation with the light group and a slightly significant (0.05 level) negative correlation with the intermediate group. The negative correlation of tensile strain with the light group was the same as previously but the positive correlation with the dark group was reduced to the 0.05 significance level. Modulus of elasticity had no significant correlations with any group.

In their previous study, Evans and Vincentelli (1969) with specimens from embalmed femurs, tibias, and fibulas combined no significant correlations were found between ultimate tensile strength and light, intermediate, or dark osteons. A possible explanation for this lack of correlation in the embalmed bones is that in all 3 bones the light osteons formed less than 25% and the dark osteons less than 20% of the break area. The intermediate osteons were more abundant, forming approximately 25-30% of the break area.

An analysis of the microradiographic data revealed that the only significant correlation was a negative one between intermediate radiolucent osteons and ultimate tensile strength, and between markedly radiolucent osteons and ultimate tensile strain. However, the correlations were only at the 0.05 significance level.

Vincentelli and Evans determined the effect of various degrees of calcification on correlations between collagen fiber orientation and mechanical properties by partialing out the intermediate radiolucent group of osteons, that is, the group having the highest correlation with mechanical properties. Interstitial lamellae, which also formed a part of the break area, were likewise partialed out. Partial correlation coefficients showed that the correlations between histological components and mechanical properties still persisted although in some cases the significance level of some of the correlations was lower.

In order to estimate how accurately bone mechanical properties can be predicted from collagen fiber orientation and degree of mineralization, multiple correlations using the tensile properties as the dependent variables, and all the histological and micro-radiographic components as the independent variables were also computed. It was found that ultimate tensile strength and strain each had a positive correlation, at the 0.01 significance level, with the percentage of the break area formed by the various independent variables. However, the magnitude of the correlation between tensile strength and the histological and microradiographic variables was greater with the original than with the corrected break area (i.e. the original break area minus all the spaces, represented by the Haversian canals, Volkmann's canals, resorption areas, etc.)

The fact that Vincentelli and Evans found more significant correlations between the tensile properties of their specimens and osteons with different orientations of collagen fibers than they did with osteons of varying degree of calcification suggests that collagen fibers have a greater influence on the tensile properties of adult human compact bone than degree of calcification does.

Shearing strength of single human osteons, with respect to degree of calcification and collagen fiber orientation in successive lamellae, was investigated by Ascenzi and Bonucci (1972). From the data obtained they concluded that (1) osteons whose collagen fiber bundles had a markedly longitudinal spiral course in successive lamellae were the weakest in resisting shearing stress. This suggested that in other types of osteons the compactness of bone was strengthened by lamellae with collagen fibers having a marked transverse spiral course. (2) Ultimate shearing strength and modulus of elasticity increase as calcification progresses. (3) Shearing strength of single osteons is markedly lower than the tensile and compressive strength of the same type of osteons. (4) Osteons loaded in their long axis have a range of elastic deformation barely more than 1% the length of the specimen. (5) With the technique used in their study the shearing of osteons appears to be preferentially related to lamellar structure. In osteons eccentrically loaded the parts that slip out are rather triangular in shape and often one or two fractures occur. (6) The cementing substance surrounding osteons may have a greater resistance to shearing than the osteon itself.

The conclusion by Ascenzi and Bonucci that osteons with collagen fibers having a markedly longitudinal spiral course in successive lamellae were the weakest in resisting shearing is the opposite from the data of Evans and Vincentelli (1969) who found

231

a very highly significant (0.001 level) positive correlation
between shearing strength and the percentage of dark osteons
(i.e. osteons whose fibers have a predominantly longitudinally
spiral course) and an equally high negative correlation between
shearing strength and the percentage of light osteons in the break
area. The differences between the results of the two studies,
although both used punching shear tests, is due to the fact that
Ascenzi and Bonucci applied the shearing force parallel to the
long axis of the osteon while Evans and Vincentelli applied it
perpendicular to the long axis of the osteon. Thus, in Ascenzi
and Bonucci's study shearing occurred parallel with the
longitudinally oriented fibers while in Evans and Vincentelli's
study shearing occurred perpendicular to the longitudinally
oriented fibers.

Relations of the compressive properties of human compact bone
to collagen fiber orientation and degree of calcification were
also investigated by Evans and Vincentelli (1974) in 65 standardized
specimens of wet, unembalmed bone from tibias of 6 adult men.
Osteons were classified as light, intermediate, and dark from
their appearance in polarized light and as slightly radiolucent,
intermediately radiolucent, and markedly radiolucent from their
appearance in microradiographs. Ultimate compressive strength
had a significant positive correlation (0.01 level) with the
percentage of intermediate and of slightly radiolucent osteons and
a significant negative correlation (0.001 level) with the percentage of spaces in the cross section. Compressive strain had a
highly significant (0.001 level) positive correlation with the
percent of light osteons in the break area. There were no other
significant linear correlations between the compressive properties
and histological variables.

Multiple correlation coefficients between compressive strength
or strain and the histologic and microradiographic variables were
higher and more significant than those found with modulus of
elasticity as the dependent variable. The significant positive
correlation between compressive strength and percentage of osteons
in the cross section, regardless of their collagen fiber orientation,
suggests that osteons tend to increase the compressive strength of
human compact tibial bone.

In order to compare their results with those of Ascenzi and
Bonucci for individual osteons, Evans and Vincentelli excluded 14
of their specimens with a large percentage of interstitial
lamellae and then calculated the correlation coefficients between
the compressive properties and histological variables of the
remaining 51 specimens with more than 75% Haversian bone. The
correlation of compressive strength with intermediate osteons was
considerably higher than with the entire samples of 65 specimens.
However, the correlation between compressive strain and light

osteons was slightly reduced, although still significant. No
new significant correlations were found.

The results of Evans and Vincentelli's investigation are not
directly comparable with those of Ascenzi and Bonucci (1968) for
several reasons: (1) Type I osteons of Ascenzi and Bonucci were
never found in Evans and Vincentelli's specimens and their light
osteons resembled the illustrations of Ascenzi and Bonucci's
Type II osteons. Also Evans and Vincentelli's sections were only
70μ thick compared to 500μ for Ascenzi and Bonucci's sections.
Furthermore, Evans and Vincentelli investigated tibial specimens
while Ascenzi and Bonucci studied femoral specimens; (2) Evans
and Vincentelli's dark osteons were similar to Ascenzi and
Bonucci's Type III osteons and usually had a light lamella around
the circumference of the osteon. This light lamella was removed
by Ascenzi and Bonucci before testing the osteon. An inner light
lamella bounding the Haversian canal was frequently present in
Evans and Vincentelli's material. According to Gebhardt's
theory (1905), the presence of these light lamellae should markedly
change the compressive properties of the dark osteons; (3) Ascenzi
and Bonucci did not test osteons corresponding to Evans and
Vincentelli's intermediate type which formed 17.9 percent of the
cross sectional area of their specimens. These osteons had
several light lamellae alternating with dark areas of variable
width. However, the light and dark areas were approximately equal.

Fracture formation and its relation to different collagen
fiber patterns and the microscopic structure for ox compact bone
have been investigated by Simkin and Robin (1974).

In addition to their studies on individual osteons Ascenzi,
Bonucci and Simkin (1973) also investigated the role of collagen
fiber bundle orientation in the mechanical properties of single
osteonic lamellae. In these studies cylindrical osteon samples
were subjected to diametrial compression perpendicular to their
long axis. When necessary the direction of loading could be
continually changed.

The data obtained showed that (1) in type I osteons in which
the collagen fiber bundles in successive lamellae changed through
an angle of about 90°, circular type fractures occurred in
lamellae whose collagen fiber bundles had a markedly longitudinal
spiral course while lamellae with fiber bundles having an almost
transversely oriented spiral course were unaffected; (2) in
osteons whose fiber bundles have a marked longitudinal spiral
course in successive lamellae (Type II) fracture extended radially
from the Haversian canal toward the periphery of the osteon until
all the lamellae were affected; (3) these findings were independent
of the degree of calcification of the osteon which supports the
view that the compactness of osteonic bone is strengthened by the

presence of lamellae with an almost transversally oriented spiral course; (4) the first fractures appeared between collagen fibrils, indicating that the interfibrillar substance is considerably weaker than the fibrils, and (5) in Type I osteons the fractures in lamellae whose fibers have a markedly longitudinal spiral course are circular thus making it possible to isolate lamellae with fiber bundles having an almost transverse spiral course. The sections were studied under polarized light.

Ascenzi and Bonucci (1976) investigated the mechanical similarities between alternate osteons and cross-ply laminates. Their study was based on fully calcified osteons with an alternation of dark and bright lamellae, when seen in polarized light, obtained from longitudinal sections of adult human femoral shafts. The specimens were tested in pure tension in a direction parallel with their long axis. Tensile strain occurring in a specimen during a test was measured with a microwave extensometer especially designed for the purpose. The specimens were tested wet at a temperature of about 20°C. A knee or change in slope of the stress-strain curve occurred at low stresses. A model for understanding these phenomena is provided by the mechanical behavior of a fiber-reinforced cross-ply laminate plastic. Data from their tests as well as those from an electron microscope examination of loaded osteons suggests that the change in slope (knee) of the stress-strain curve of the osteons at low stress is due to the failure of the interfibrillar cementing substance in lamellae whose fiber bundles are oriented perpendicular to the loading direction plus yielding of canaliculi previously filled with osteocyte processes.

Ascenzi and Bonucci (1977) have some evidence of a state of initial stress in osteonic lamellae from human femoral shafts. In this study lamellar samples whose collagen fibers had a transverse spiral course were prepared from osteons with alternating lamellae. When the diameter of the lamellae is large with respect to their height the samples lose the cylindrical shape they normally have in whole osteons and undergo spontaneous deformations. This suggests that the lamellae have a state of initial stress. The deformations are more complex than those expected by Volterra's theory of dislocation.

Cutting each lamellar sample along a line parallel with its axis eliminates the stress. The shape of the lamella was then analyzed. From their data Ascenzi and Bonucci concluded (1) the capacity of lamellae whose fibers have a transverse spiral course to support a tensile load oriented parallel to the osteon axis is essentially dependent upon the state of initial stress and (2) calcification has no basic part in producing the initial stress.

Scanning electron microscopy has been used by Frasca, Harper, and Katz (1977) to study collagen fiber orientation in secondary human osteons. In this investigation decalcified osteons were used to determine correlations in collagen fiber orientation with their appearance in polarized light. It was found that osteons that appeared "dark" in polarized light contained fiber orientation with little or no transverse component while "bright" osteons had fiber orientation with transverse and longitudinal components. "Intermediate" osteons had fiber orientations which were richer in longitudinal than in transverse components.

In all the investigations thus far discussed, the strength tests of the bone specimens were conducted under slowly applied loads. However, the mechanical property values obtained when the load is slowly applied differ from those when the load is rapidly applied because bone is a rate sensitive material. This was first demonstrated by McElhaney and Byars (1965) for the compressive properties of standardized compact bone specimens from ox and human femurs. Bird et al. (1968) found a similar phenomenon for the compressive properties of beef femoral bone. Human skull bone was also found to be rate sensitive, as far as its tensile properties are concerned by Roberts and Melvin (1969), Melvin et al. (1969) and Wood (1971). However, none of these investigators correlated their mechanical property data with the histological structure of their specimens.

Apparently the only investigation of the relations between the impact properties of human compact bone and its microscopic structure is that of Saha and Hayes (1976) who determined the correlation between the tensile impact strength and energy absorbing capacity of longitudinal test specimens from both femurs of an embalmed adult human subject and the right femur of a 38-year-old male autopsy specimen with no history of bone disease.

Saha and Hayes determined the impact tensile strength of their specimens with a pendulum type tensile impact tester at a strain rate of 133 sec^{-1}. Recorded load time histories of their specimens revealed marked nonlinearities in the stress-strain behavior of some specimens including plastic deformation and strain hardening effects. The latter result emphasized that fracture energy alone did not completely represent the tensile impact behavior of bone. Mean tensile impact strengths and impact energies found for 49 fresh human specimens were 126.3±33.1 MN/m^2 and 18790 ± 7355 J/m^2, respectively. Quasi-static tensile strength for 13 fresh human specimens were 34% less than the impact tensile strength.

Statistically significant correlations were found between (1) ultimate strain and impact energy absorbing capacity; (2) modulus of elasticity and both tensile impact stress and yield stress, and (3) maximum stress and impact energy absorbing capacity.

Statistically significant negative correlations were also found between the percentage of secondary osteons in the fresh human specimens and both the maximum stress in tensile impact and the impact energy absorbing capacity. The correlation between elastic and strength properties were independent of their dependence on the microscopic structure of the specimens.

TORSION PROPERTIES OF HUMAN COMPACT BONE

Although torsion properties of human compact bone have been determined by Rauber (1876), Hazama (1956), Knets et al. (1973) and Pfafrod et al. (1972, 1975), Evans (1978) appears to be the only one who has correlated the torsion properties with the various histological components of the bone.

Evans' data was obtained from torsion tests of 123 standardized tubular specimens of compact bone from femurs of 14 adult embalmed human cadavers. In the study torsion shear stress, shear modulus, and energy absorbed to failure were correlated with the percentage of various histological components in cross sections of the specimens taken as close as possible to the fracture site.

Positive correlations, at the 0.01 significance level, were found between (1) torsion shear stress and the number of complete secondary osteons, (2) shear modulus and the number of complete osteons, and (3) energy absorbed to failure and the percentage of complete osteons. Negative correlations, at the 0.01 significance level, were found between (1) torsion shear stress and percentage of spaces, (2) shear modulus and the percentage of spaces, and (3) energy absorbed to failure and the percentage of spaces.

Positive correlations, at the 0.05 significance level, were found between (1) torsion shear stress and the percentage of complete osteons, (2) shear modulus and the percentage of interstitial lamellae, and (3) energy absorbed to failure and number of complete osteons. Negative correlations, at the 0.05 significance level, were found between (1) torsion shear stress and percentage of osteon remnants, and (2) shear modulus and percentage of osteon remnants.

Implications from the above correlations are (1) all torsion properties tend to be reduced by the percentage of spaces in the break area, and (2) torsion shear stress and modulus also tend to be reduced by the percentage of osteon remnants in the break area. All torsion properties tend to be increased by the number of complete osteons in the break area and (2) modulus tends to be increased, to a lesser extent, by the percentage of interstitial lamellae in the break area.

236

FATIGUE LIFE OF HUMAN COMPACT BONE

Fatigue life of compact bone was first determined by Evans and Lebow (1957) who recorded the number of cycles to failure, at a constant stress of 3.52 kgf/mm^2 and a rate of 1800 repetitions per minute, of standardized specimens of unembalmed femoral, tibial, and fibular bone from above-knee amputations of 5 adult men. In a second study Lease and Evans (1959) made a study of the fatigue of intact metatarsal bone II through V from the embalmed bodies of 8 men and 3 women. In a third investigation King and Evans (1967) analyzed the fatigue life of 248 uniform specimens, tested at 12 different stress levels, of compact femoral bone from 17 embalmed adult human cadavers by assuming the Weibell probability distribution.

Seireg and Kempke (1969) reported on the fatigue life of tibias of living male rats. The fatigue properties of unembalmed compact femoral bone from 22 subjects 35 to 98 years of age were determined by Swanson et al. (1971). A total of 68 specimens from 14 men and of 39 specimens from 7 women were tested. The specimens were obtained from femurs removed at autopsy. The amplitude of bending as well as effects of surface finishing were also investigated.

Evans and Riolo (1970) seem to be the only ones who have determined the correlations between the fatigue life of human compact bone and its microscopic structure. Their investigation was based on 47 standardized specimens of unembalmed tibial compact bone obtained from above-knee amputations of 7 Caucasian men from 23 to 56 years of age. None of the amputations had been performed for primary bone lesions and all the men had been active up to a relatively short time before surgery.

Fatigue life (cycles to failure) of the specimens was determined in a Model SF-2 Sonntag flexure fatigue machine. Water dripped on the specimens during a test to prevent drying. All tests were made at a constant stress of 344.7 x 10^6 dynes/cm^2. Cross sections of the specimens, taken as close as possible to the fracture sites, were analyzed with respect to the number and the percentage of the various histological components in the break area.

Positive correlations, at the 0.01 significance level, were found between the fatigue life of the specimens and the percentage of secondary osteons and of osteons plus their remnants in the break area. An equally significant negative correlation existed between fatigue life of the specimens and the percentage of interstitial lamellae in the break area.

These correlations suggest that osteons tend to increase and interstitial lamellae tend to decrease the fatigue life of human

compact tibial bone. This is just the opposite effect that osteons
and interstitial lamellae have on the tensile strength of human
compact bone.

Elastic after-effect, plasticity, and fatigue in compact bone
from the radius of a horse and the metacarpus of an ox have been
investigated by Smith and Walmsley (1957).

A study of the correlations between fatigue life, microscopic
structure and density of bovine compact bone has been made by
Carter, Hayes, and Schurman (1976).

EFFECTS OF AGE ON MECHANICAL PROPERTIES AND
HISTOLOGY OF NORMAL COMPACT BONE

Evans (1976) determined the tensile properties (breaking load,
strength, strain), modulus of elasticity, and density, plus the
histological structure of cross sections at the fracture site for
207 standardized specimens of compact bone from the embalmed
femur, tibia, and fibula of 17 men from 35 to 75 years of age.
The men were divided into a younger (41.5 years old average) and
an older (71 years old average) group.

The average tensile properties, modulus of elasticity, and
density of specimens from the younger men were greater than those
of specimens from older men. However, specimens from older men
had a greater percentage of spaces and more osteons/mm^2 and osteon
remnants/mm^2 in the cross sections than did specimens from younger
men. Specimens from the latter group had a slightly larger percentage of osteons, osteon remnants, and interstitial lamellae
than specimens from older men. Evans believed that the differences
in the tensile properties, resulting in a greater incidence of
fracture in older men, can be explained by the quantitative and
qualitative differences found in the histological composition of
the bone in the younger and the older men.

In another study Evans (1977) reported that, with advancing
age, tensile strength declined the most, modulus of elasticity was
second, and tensile strain was third. Changes were also found in
the percentage of various histological components of cross sections
of the specimens at the fracture site. With advancing age increases
occurred in (1) the percentage of spaces in the original break area
and of interstitial lamellae in the corrected break area, i.e. the
original break area minus the major spaces; (2) the percentage of
osteon remnants as well as the number of osteons/mm^2 and the number
of osteon remnants/mm^2. Decreases with advancing age were found in
(1) the percentage of osteons in the corrected break area, (2) the
size (area in mm^2) of the osteons, and (3) the size (area in mm^2)
of osteon remnants; in all cases the osteons were of the secondary

238

type. The material used in the study consisted of 70 femoral,
101 tibial, and 36 fibular specimens from embalmed bodies of
17 men from 36 to 75 years of age.

From the data obtained in this study Evans concluded that
(1) cement lines are areas of weakness at which microfractures or
cracks occur, and (2) the decrease in the tensile properties of
human compact bone with advancing age appear to be primarily the
result of (a) a quantitative decrease in the amount of bone as a
result of increased porosity and (b) qualitative changes in the
microstructure of the bone. The latter is due to an increase in
the number of osteons/mm^2 as a consequence of which there is an
increase in the amount of cement lines, where cracks can occur,
as well as an increase in the number of Haversian canals, lacunae,
and canaliculi which increase the porosity of the bone. Haversian
canals, lacunae, and canaliculi are also discontinuities in bone
which can act as areas of higher stress concentration where cracks
can be initiated. However, a crack initiated at one such area,
e.g. a lacuna, might be stopped when it had been propagated to
the next lacuna.

SUMMARY

Statistically significant correlation coefficients between
some of the mechanical properties of standardized test specimens
of adult human compact bone and the percentage of the cross
sectional area at the fracture site formed by (1) spaces, (2) by
secondary osteons, (3) by remnants or fragments of secondary
osteons, and (4) by interstitial lamellae suggest the following:
1 - Ultimate tensile strength tends to be increased by the percentage of interstitial lamellae but decreased by the percentage
of secondary osteons in the break area.
2 - Modulus of elasticity tends to be decreased by the percentage
of spaces in the cross sectional area and by the average area/
secondary osteons.
3 - Single (punching) shearing strength, perpendicular to the long
axis of the specimens, tends to be decreased by the average area/
osteon and per osteon remnant in the cross sectional area.
4 - Rockwell superficial hardness tends to be increased by the
percentage of secondary osteons in the cross sectional area and by
the number of osteons/mm^2, but decreased by the percentage of spaces
in the cross sectional area. Hardness was determined in a direction
perpendicular to the long axis of the specimens.
5 - Fatigue life, determined with a Sonntag flexure fatigue
machine, tends to be increased by the percentage of secondary
osteons and of osteons plus their remnants but decreased by the
percentage of interstitial lamellae in the cross sectional area.
6 - Torsional shear stress, shear modulus, and energy absorbed to
failure tend to be increased by the percentage of and the number of
secondary osteons, but are reduced by the percentage of spaces in

the break area.

7 - Cement lines surrounding secondary osteons and the substance
between individual lamellae of secondary osteons are areas of
weakness where microfractures can and do occur. Therefore, the
more secondary osteons and their remnants in a given area of bone
the more cement lines there are for fracture to occur.

Statistically significant correlation coefficients between
the tensile, shearing, and compression properties of standardized
specimens of adult human compact bone and the percentage of the
cross sectional area at the fracture formed by light, intermediate,
and dark osteons, classified on the basis of their appearance in
polarized light, suggest the following:

1 - Single (punching) shear strength tends to be increased by the
percentage of dark secondary osteons alone or when combined with
their remnants in the cross sectional area.

2 - Torsion shear strength, modulus of elasticity, and tensile
strain tend to be increased by the percentage of intermediate
secondary osteons in the cross sectional area.

3 - Single (punching) shear strength (perpendicular to the long
axis of the specimens) and modulus of elasticity tend to be
decreased by the percentage of light secondary osteons alone or
combined with their remnants in the cross sectional area.

4 - Tensile stress and strain tend to be increased by the percentage of dark osteons in the cross sectional area.

5 - Tensile stress and strain tend to be decreased by the percentage of light osteons and their remnants and by the percentage
of interstitial lamellae in the cross sectional area.

6 - Tensile stress and strain tend to be decreased by the percentage of intermediately radiolucent and markedly radiolucent
osteons, respectively, in the cross sectional area.

7 - Mechanical properties and histological composition of bone
vary from one bone to another and from one region to another in
a single bone.

REFERENCES

1. Aoji, O. Metrical studies on the lamellar structure of human long bones. J. Kyoto Pref. Med. Univ. 65: 941-965, 1959.
2. Ascenzi, A. and G.H.Bell. Bone as a mechanical engineering problem. In THE BIOCHEMISTRY AND PHYSIOLOGY OF BONE, G.H. Bourne, ed., Ch. 9, pp. 311-352. Academic Press, N.Y., 1972.
3. Ascenzi, A. and A. Benvenuti. Evidence of a state of initial stress in osteonic lamellae. J. Biomechanics 10: 447-453, 1977.
4. Ascenzi, A. and E. Bonucci. The ultimate tensile strength of single osteons. Acta Anat. 58: 160-183, 1964.
5. _____. The tensile properties of single osteons. Anat. Rec. 158: 375-386, 1967.
6. _____. The compressive properties of single osteons. Anat. Rec. 161: 377-392, 1968.
7. _____. The shearing properties of single osteons. Anat. Rec. 172: 499-510, 1972.
8. _____. Mechanical similarities between alternate osteons and cross-ply laminates. J. Biomechanics 9: 65-72, 1976.
9. Ascenzi, A., Bonucci, E. and A. Checcucci. The tensile properties of single osteons studied using a microwave extensimeter. In STUDIES ON THE ANATOMY AND FUNCTION OF BONE AND JOINTS, F. G. Evans, ed., pp. 121-141. Springer, Berlin,1966.
10. Ascenzi, A., Bonucci, E. and A. Simkin. An approach to the mechanical properties of single osteonic lamellae. J. Biomechanics 6: 227-236, 1973.
11. Bird, F., Becker, H., Healer, J. and M. Messer. Experimental determinations of the mechanical properties of bone. Aerosp. Med. 39: 33-48, 1968.
12. Bloom, W. and D.W.Fawcett. A TEXTBOOK OF HISTOLOGY, 10th ed., p. 858. Saunders, Philadelphia, 1975.
13. Bourne, G.H., ed. THE BIOCHEMISTRY AND PHYSIOLOGY OF BONE, 2nd ed., 3 vols. Academic Press, N.Y., 1971-1972.
14. Boyde, A. Scanning electron microscope studies of bone. In THE BIOCHEMISTRY AND PHYSIOLOGY OF BONE, G.H. Bourne, ed., Vol. 1, Ch. 8, pp. 259-310. Academic Press, N.Y., 1972.
15. Carter, D.R. and W.C.Hayes. Compact bone fatigue damage: a microscopic examination. Clin. Orthop. 127: 265-274, 1977.
16. Carter, D.R., Hayes, W.C. and D.J.Schurman. Fatigue life of compact bone--II. Effects of microstructure and density. J. Biomechanics 9: 211-218, 1976.
17. Carter, D.R. and D.M.Spengler. Mechanical properties and composition of cortical bone. Clin. Orthop. (in press).
18. Cohen, J. and W.H.Harris. The three-dimensional anatomy of Haversian systems. J. Bone Jt. Surg. 40-A: 419-434, 1958.
19. Currey, J.D. Differences in the tensile strength of bone of different histological types. J. Anat. 93: 87-95, 1959.
20. _____. Strength of bone. Nature 195: 513-514, 1962.
21. _____. The mechanical properties of bone. Clin. Orthop. 73: 210-231, 1970.

22. Dempster, W.T. and R. F. Coleman. Tensile strength of bone along and across the grain. J. Appl. Physiol. 16: 355-360, 1960.

23. Eanes, E.D. and A.S.Posner. Structure and chemistry of bone mineral. In BIOLOGICAL CALCIFICATION, H. Schraer, ed., pp. 1-26. Elsevier-North-Holland, Amsterdam, 1970.

24. Evans, F. Gaynor. STRESS AND STRAIN IN BONES, p. 245. Thomas, Springfield, IL, 1957.

25. _____. Relations between the microscopic structure and tensile strength of human bone. Acta Anat. 35: 385-301, 1958.

26. _____. MECHANICAL PROPERTIES OF BONE, p. 322. Thomas, Springfield, IL, 1973.

27. _____. Mechanical properties and histology of cortical bone from younger and older men. Anat. Rec. 185: 1-11, 1976.

28. _____. Age changes in mechanical properties and histology of human compact bone. Yearbook of Physical Anthropology 20: 57-72, 1977.

29. _____. Relations between torsion properties and histology of adult human compact bone. J. Biomechanics (in press).

30. Evans, F. Gaynor and S. Bang. Physical and histological differences between human fibular and femoral compact bone. In STUDIES ON THE ANATOMY AND FUNCTION OF BONE AND JOINTS, F. Gaynor Evans, ed., pp. 142-155. Springer, Berlin, 1966.

31. _____. Differences and relationships between the physical properties and the microscopic structure of human femoral, tibial, and fibular cortical bone. Am. J. Anat. 120: 78-88, 1967.

32. Evans, F. Gaynor and M. Lebow. Regional differences in some of the physical properties of the human femur. J. Appl. Physiol. 3: 563-572, 1951.

33. _____. The strength of human compact bone as revealed by engineering technics. Am. J. Surg. 83: 326-331, 1952.

34. _____. Strength of human compact bone under repetitive loading. J. Appl. Physiol. 10: 127-130, 1957.

35. Evans, F. Gaynor and M. L. Riolo. Relations between the fatigue life and histology of adult human cortical bone. J. Bone Jt. Surg. 52A: 1579-1586, 1970.

36. Evans, F. Gaynor and R. Vincentelli. Relation of collagen fiber orientation to some mechanical properties of human cortical bone. J. Biomechanics 2: 63-71, 1969.

37. _____. Relations of the compressive properties of human cortical bone to its histological structure and calcification. J. Biomechanics 7: 1-10, 1974.

38. Filogamo, G. Le forme et la taille des osteones chez quelques mammifères. Arch. Biol., Paris 57: 137-143, 1946a.

242

39. Filogamo, G.   Precizazioni sulla disposizione e sull'orientamentc
    dell fibre collagne degli osteoni nell'uomo.   Ric. Morfologia
    22: 1-5, 1946b.
40. Frasca, P., Harper, R.A. and J. L. Katz.   Collagen fiber
    orientation in human secondary osteons.   Acta Anat. 98:
    1-13, 1977.
41. Frost, H.M.   Measurement of osteocytes per unit volume and
    volume components of osteocytes and canaliculi in man.
    Henry Ford Hosp. Med. Bull. 8: 208-211, 1960.
42. Gebhardt, W.   Über funktionell wichtige Anordnungsweisen der
    feinen und grösseren Bauelemente des Wirbeltierknochen.
    II Spezieller Teil.   Arch. Entw. Mech. 20: 187-322, 1905.
43. Glimcher, M.J.   Composition, structure and organization of
    bone and other mineralized tissues and mechanism of
    calcification.   In HANDBOOK OF PHYSIOLOGY, Sect. 7,
    Endocrinology, vol. 7, pp. 25-116.   G.D.Aurbach, ed.
    American Physiological Society, Washington, D.C., 1976.
44. Gurdjian, E.S. and H.R. Lissner.   Mechanism of head injury as
    studied by the cathode ray oscilloscope.   Preliminary Report.
    J. Neurosurg. I: 393-399, 1944.
45. _____   Deformation of the skull in
    head injury.   A study with the "stresscoat" technique.   Surg.,
    Gynec. and Obst. 81: 679-689, 1945.
46. _____   Deformation of the skull in
    head injury studied by the "stresscoat" technique, quantitative
    determinations.   Surg., Gynec. and Obst. 83: 219-233, 1946.
47. _____   Deformations of the skull
    in head injury as studied by the "stresscoat" technic.
    Am. J. Surg. 73: 269-281, 1947.
48. Gurdjian, E.S., Lissner, H.R. and J.E.Webster.   The mechanism
    of production of linear skull fracture.   Further studies on
    deformation of the skull by the "stresscoat" technique.
    Surg., Gynec. and Obst. 85: 195-210, 1947.
49. Gurdjian, E.S., Webster, J.R. and H.R. Lissner.   Studies on
    skull fracture with particular reference to engineering
    factors.   Am. J. Surg. 78: 735-742, 1949.
50. Ham, A.W.   HISTOLOGY, 6th ed.   Lippincott, Philadelphia, 1969.
51. Hancox, N.M.   BIOLOGY OF BONE, p. 198.   Cambridge University
    Press, Cambridge, 1972.
52. Hayes, W.C.   Biomechanical measurements of bone.   In CRC
    HANDBOOK OF ENGINEERING IN MEDICINE AND BIOLOGY.   Chemical
    Rubber Co., Cleveland, Ohio (in press).
53. Hazama, H.   Study on the torsion strength of the compact
    substance of human beings.   J. Kyoto Pref. Med. Univ. 60:
    167-184, 1956.   (Japanese text, English summary).
54. Herrmann, G. and H. Liebowitz.   Mechanics of bone fracture.
    Ch. 10 in FRACTURE, vol. VII, Fracture of Nonmetals and
    Composites, H. Liebowitz, ed.   Academic Press, New York, 1972.

55. Heřt, J.P., Kučera, P., Vávra, M. and V. Volenik. Comparison of the mechanical properties of both the primary and Haversian bone tissue. Acta Anat. 61: 412-423, 1965.

56. King, A.I. and F. G. Evans. Analysis of fatigue strength of human compact bone by the Weibull method, in DIGEST OF THE SEVENTH INTERNATIONAL CONFERENCE ON MEDICAL AND BIOLOGICAL ENGINEERING, B. Jacobson, ed., p. 514. Stockholm, 1976.

57. Knese, K.-H. Mechanik und Festigkeit des Knochengewebes. In HANDBUCH DER MEDIZINISCHEN RADIOLOGIE. Bd. IV/1 L. Diethelm ed., pp. 417-439. Springer, Berlin, 1970.

58. Knets, I.V., Pfafrod, G.O., Saulgozis, Yu.-Zh., Laizan, Ya B. and Kh. A. Yanson. Degree of deformation and strength of the compact bone tissue during torsion. Polymer Mech. 5: 911-918, 1973. (In Russian).

59. Koltze, H. Studie zur äusseren Form des Osteone. Z. Anat. EntwGesch. 115: 584-596, 1951.

60. Kraus, H. On the mechanical properties and behavior of human compact bone. In ADVANCES IN BIOMEDICAL ENGINEERING AND MEDICAL PHYSICS, S. Levine, ed. Interscience, New York, 1968.

61. Lease, G. O'D. and F. G. Evans. Strength of human metatarsal bones under repetitive loading. J. Appl. Physiol. 14: 49-51, 1959.

62. Maj, G. Osservazione sulle differenze topografiche della resistenza meccanica del tessuto osseo di uno stesso segmento scheletrico. Monit. Zool. Ital. 49: 139-149, 1938.

63. _____. Studio sulle variazioni individuali e topografiche della resistenza meccanica del tessuto osseo diafisario umano in diverse età. Arch. Ital. Anat. Embriol. 67: 612-633, 1942.

64. Maj, G. and E. Toajari. Osservazioni sperimentali sul meccanismo di resistenza del tessuto osseo lamellare compatto alle azioni meccaniche. Chir. org. movimento 22: 541-557, 1937.

65. McElhaney, J.H. Dynamic response of bone and muscle tissue. J. Appl. Physiol. 21: 1231-1236, 1966.

66. McElhaney, J.H. and E.F.Byars. Dynamic response of biological materials. ASME Publ. 65-WA/HUF-9, 1-8, 1965.

67. Melvin, J.W., Robbins, D.H. and V.L.Roberts. The mechanical behavior of the diploë layer of the human skull. Proc. Eleventh Midwestern Mechanics Conf. 5: 811-816, 1969.

68. Miller, E.J. and G.R.Martin. The collagen of bone. Clin. Orthop. 59: 195-232, 1968.

69. Okamoto, T. Mechanical significance of components of bone tissue. J. Kyoto Pref. Med. Univ. 58: 1004-1006, 1955 (Japanese text, English summary).

70. Pfafrod, G.O., Knets, I.V., Saulgozis, Yu. Zh., Kregers, A.F. and Kh. A. Yanson. Age-related changes in the strength of compact bone tissue under torsion. Polymer Mech. 3: 493-503, 1975 (In Russian).

71. Pfafrod, G.O., Saulgozis, Yu. Zh., Knets, I.V., and Kh. A. Yanson. Experimental determination of the shear modulus of compact bone tissue. Polymer Mech. 4: 697-705, 1972 (in Russian).

72. Piekarski, K. Fracture of bone. J. Appl. Physics 41: 215-223, 1970.

73. _____. Analysis of bone as a composite material. Internat. J. Eng. Sci. 11: 557-565, 1973.

74. Pope, M.H. and J.O.Outwater. Mechanical properties of bone as a function of position and orientation. J. Biomechanics 7: 61-66, 1974.

75. Pritchard, J.J. General histology of bone. In THE BIOCHEMISTRY AND PHYSIOLOGY OF BONE, 2nd ed., vol. 1., G.H.Bourne, ed., Ch. 1. Academic Press, N.Y. 1972.

76. Rauber, A.A. ELASTICITÄT UND FESTIGKEIT DER KNOCHEN. Engelmann, Leipzig, 1876.

77. Reilly, D.T. and A.H.Burstein. The mechanical properties of cortical bone. J. Bone Jt. Surg. 56A: 1001-1022, 1974.

78. Roberts, V.L. and J.W. Melvin. The measurement of dynamic mechanical properties of human skull bone. Applied Polymer Symposium 12: 235-247, 1969.

79. Robinson, R.A. Physiochemical structure of bone. Clin. Orthop. 112: 263-314, 1975.

80. Saha, S. and W.C.Hayes. Tensile impact properties of human compact bone. J. Biomechanics 9: 243-252, 1976.

81. Seireg, A. and W. Kempke. Behavior of in vivo bone under cyclic loading. J. Biomechanics 2: 455-461, 1969.

82. Simkin, A. and G. Robin. Fracture formation in differing collagen fiber pattern of compact bone. J. Biomechanics 7: 183-188, 1974.

83. Smith, J.W. The arrangement of collagen fibers in human secondary osteons. J. Bone Jt. Surg. 42B:588-605, 1960.

84. Smith, J.W. and R. Walmsley. Elastic after-effect, plasticity and fatigue in bone. J. Anat. 91: 603-604, 1957.

85. _____. Factors affecting the elasticity of bone. J. Anat. 93: 503-523, 1959.

86. Sokoloff, L. A note on the histology of cement lines. In PERSPECTIVES IN BIOMEDICAL ENGINEERING, R. M. Kenedi, ed., pp. 135-138. University Park Press, Baltimore, 1973.

87. Swanson, S.A.V. Biomechanical characteristics of bone. In ADVANCES IN BIOMEDICAL ENGINEERING, R.M. Kenedi, ed., vol. 1, pp. 137-187. Academic Press, N.Y., 1971.

88. Sweeney, A.W., Byers, R.K. and R.P. Kroon. Mechanical characteristics of bone and its constituents. ASME Pub. #65-WA/HUF-7:1-17, 1965.

89. Uehira, T. On the relation between the chemical components and the strength of the compact bone. J. Kyoto Pref. Med. Univ. 68: 923-940, 1960 (Japanese text, English summary).

90. Vaughan, J.M. THE PHYSIOLOGY OF BONE. Clarendon Press, Oxford, 1975.

91. Vincentelli, R. and F. G. Evans. Relations among mechanical properties, collagen fibers and calcification in adult human cortical bone. J. Biomechanics 4: 193-201, 1971.

92. Weimann, J.P. and H. Sicher. BONE AND BONES, p. 464. Mosby, St. Louis, 1947.

93. Welch, D.O. The composite structure of bone and its response to mechanical stress. In RECENT ADVANCES IN ENGINEERING SCIENCE, vol. 5. A.C.Eringen, ed. Gordon and Breach, N.Y., 1971.

94. Wilmer, H.A. Changes in structural components of human body from six lunar months to maturity. Proc. Soc. Exper. Biol. Med. 43: 545-547, 1940.

95. Wood, J.L. Dynamic response of human cranial bone. J. Biomechanics 4: 1-12, 1971.

96. Yamada, H. STRENGTH OF BIOLOGICAL MATERIALS, p. 297. Williams and Wilkins, Baltimore, 1970.

97. Yokoo, S. The compressive test upon the diaphysis and the compact substance of the long bones of the human extremities J. Kyoto Pref. Med. Univ. 51: 291-313, 1952 (Japanese text, English summary).

DETERMINATION OF DYNAMIC ELASTIC PROPERTIES OF SPONGY BONE*

M. Anliker and J. Goodbread

Institute for Biomedical Engineering, University of Zurich and ETH Zurich, Switzerland

ABSTRACT. New interferometric techniques have been developed to quantify surface displacements associated with flexural, axial and torsional waves in bars. These techniques have been utilized in an experimental analysis of the propagation of small stress waves in samples of spongy bone excised from the knee condyles of macerated human femurs. The values for Young's modulus E and the shear modulus G deduced from wave speed and density measurements indicate a pronounced anisotropy of spongy bone. They also exhibit a moderate correlation between the density and the two elastic parameters E and G, which suggests that E and G are roughly proportional to the square of the density. A noninvasive method of quantifying spongy bone density and other mineralization parameters on the basis of a computer tomograph especially designed for this purpose is presented and some initial results obtained on humans and rats are described.

* This work has been supported in part by the Swiss National Science Foundation, Grants No. 4.0600.72, 6.140-0.74 and 3.121.-0.77.

1. INTRODUCTION

The primary purpose of this exposition is to present some results of recent investigations of the mechanical properties of human bone. Special emphasis is thereby given to work in which one or both of the authors have to some extent been personally involved. Besides this, an attempt is made to demonstrate the need for a multidisciplinary approach in studying properties of bone.

From a physiological point of view bone serves two important functions. In its various forms it provides the rigid supporting and load bearing system for the entire body. Just as importantly, it serves as a reservoir for the calcium stores of the body. These two functions are intimately related. There is strong evidence that the quantity and distribution of bone material change in response to mechanical loading (1). Similarly, disturbances in calcium metabolism may lead to drastic changes in distribution of bone.

Pathological changes in bone tissue lead, in general, to changes both in strength and in quantity or quality of bone material. Osteomalacia, for example, alters the ratio of components in the bone. It is associated with a loss of the calcium hydroxyapatite mineral fraction and consequently with a lowering of the ratio of mineral to organic matrix. Osteoporosis, on the other hand, appears to decrease the total amount of material, while having little effect on the mineral-to-matrix ratio (2).

A comprehensive clinical evaluation of bone status should include an assessment of the mechanical integrity of bones. The latter is defined by the bone mineral mass, its geometric distribution and the elastic properties of the bone material. Whereas noninvasive clinical methods of determining the mineral mass of certain bones and its geometric distribution have become available through computed tomography (3,4), there exists still no corresponding validated technique of measuring the elastic properties of the bone material. Information on elastic properties is insofar desirable as they may not only depend on the amount of bone mineral present but also on the bonding between the constituents and the lamellar structure of bone.

To arrive at a method of determining noninvasively
these properties, two pathways can readily be identified. The first is to investigate a possible correlation
between elastic properties of excised samples with some
other properties, such as the density. The second possibility is to obtain data on the elastic moduli of excised samples in such a manner that the results may serve
as a guideline toward development of a direct noninvasive measurement for example on the basis of sound
transmission. Mechanical properties of materials with
respect to small time varying deformations may be
inferred from the natural frequencies of samples of
simple geometry or from the propagation characteristics
of transient stress waves in such samples. For example,
the speed and attenuation of axial or flexural stress
waves in beam-shaped samples are directly related to
the dynamic mechanical behavior of the beam material.

Following the first approach, Bundy (5) studied
the elastic moduli of samples of compact bone from the
shaft of the human femur with regard to spatial variation
and anisotropy. He found:
1) There is significant variation of both Young's
   and shear moduli as a function of location
   within the bone.
2) Compact bone is anisotropic with respect to
   its elastic moduli.
3) Young's modulus correlates well with density,
   while the shear modulus correlates poorly with
   density.

Similarly, Pugh, Rose and Radin (6) have examined
the relationship between Young's modulus of spongy bone
samples from human knee codules and the density. Samples were taken from a single location, and the direction
of measurement was the same in all cases. They concluded that:
1) Young's modulus correlated poorly with density.
2) For certain samples with uniform distribution
   of trabecular thickness, better correlation was
   obtained when trabecular contiguity, a measure
   of the degree of cross bracing of the structure,
   was used as an independent variable.

The second approach has been pursued by several investigators for the case of compact bone. Thompson (7)
studied the flexural vibrations of excised dog radii

and observed that variations in geometry along the radius shaft had a significant influence on the resonant
frequencies. Viano et al. (8) measured the resonance
frequencies and mode shapes of excised human femur
shafts for lateral, axial, and torsional vibrations. With
geometrical and density information provided by tomographic scanning, they were able to determine average
values of Young's and shear moduli for the bones.

These studies bear directly on the work of Jurist
et al. (9) which has been directed at developing an
in vivo audio frequency resonance measurement for the
clinical evaluation of the elastic status of the human
ulna. Some success has been reported in differentiating
osteoporotic from normal bones on the basis of resonant
frequency and bone geometry. However, according to the
results of Viano et al. (8), the method applied does
not permit a separation of various causes for changes
of the resonance frequencies, such as variations of the
cross section along the bone, changes of the boundary
conditions at the two ends of the ulna and alterations
of the elastic properties of the bone material. In
addition, compact bone density ρ and Young's modulus
E both decline with increasing age. This implies that
resonance frequencies of flexural or axial waves are
not especially sensitive indicators of osteoporosis because they are directly proportional to E/ρ. As an
alternative, even shear waves do not seem to offer a
noninvasive approach eventhough the shear modulus G
decreases more strongly with age than does Young's modulus, because the transmission shear waves through the
soft tissue surrounding the bones is accompanied by
high losses.

In the following a review is given of recent experimental investigations of mechanical properties of spongy
bone samples excised from the knee condyles of human
femurs (10,11). This work constitutes essentially an
extension of efforts made by Bundy (5) and by Pugh,
Rose and Radin (6). To illustrate the complexities and
multidisciplinary aspects which may characterize projects of biomechanics, some of the interesting features
of the measuring procedures, instrumentation, electronic
signal processing techniques and computed tomography developed in conjunction with the osteoporosis research
carried out in Zurich (12) are described. First, a no-
vel interferometric approach to study the propagation

of small amplitude stress waves in bar-like test specimens is presented, together with a dispersion curve
obtained for bending waves in a spongy bone sample.
Then, the determination of elastic properties with
the aid of the axial and torsional buffer bar techniques is discussed and a new method of quantifying extremely small angles of rotation is introduced. Subsequently the relationship between the density of the
spongy bone specimens and the elastic parameters derived from measurements of the transmission times of
small stress pulses is examined. Finally, the noninv-
vasive determination of mineralization parameters by
means of computed tomography is briefly described in
the light of future research on bone diseases and their
treatment (12).

2. EXPERIMENTAL ANALYSIS OF STRESS WAVES IN BEAM-LIKE BONE SAMPLES WITH PHASE STABILIZED INTERFEROMETERS

The transmission properties of transient stress waves
propagating in a beam are readily evaluated from recordings of the corresponding surface displacements at
different points along the length of the beam. To allow
for examination of small samples and the study of the
material properties at high frequencies, it is convenient to utilize an interferometric technique for the
measurement of the surface displacements. One of the
principal advantages of optical techniques is that no
contact is required with the moving structure. Moreover,
with interferometric methods, it is possible to resolve
surface displacments as small as 0.01 nm at frequencies
ranging up to the order of 1 MHz. Displacements of such
small magnitude ascertain a linear behavior of the
mechanical structure and repeatability of the stress
wave measurements. For mildly dispersive systems, the
need for Fourier analysis of the transient stress
signals to determine the phase velocity and attenuation
as a function of frequency may be avoided by inducing
perturbations in the form of finite trains of sine
waves. This was demonstrated for example in studies of
wave transmission in blood vessels (13,14).

252

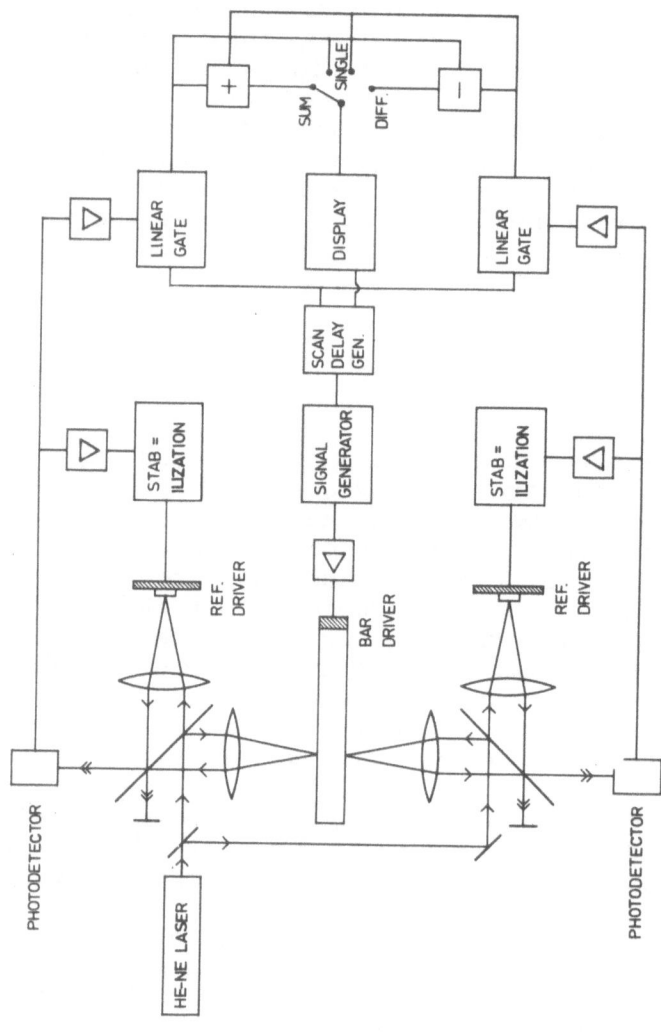

Fig. 1. Schematic Illustration of Measuring System for Small Bending and Axial Waves in Bars

2.1 Overview of experimental arrangement

The system used in examining the mechanical properties
of bone samples in the form of beams is based on the
optical homodyne techniques described by Sizgoric and
Gundjian (15). It is schematically shown in Figure 1
and consists of a He-Ne laser, a pair of stabilized
Michelson interferometers, a wave generator, a pair of
photodiodes and of electronic signal processing equipment. Included in the latter are box-car integrators
(linear gates), as well as a set of recording and
display instruments. The beam and the optical components
are mounted on an aluminum slab resting on a table which
is isolated against vibrations. For the purpose of
measuring bending- and axial waves the interferometers
are positioned on opposite sides of the beam in such a
way that they detect lateral displacements at corresponding coordinates. A servo loop which controls the position of a reference mirror provides stabilization
of each of the interferometers against drift and low
frequency vibrations up to 50 Hz. The reference mirrors
are cemented to piezoelectric bending plates so that
their position can be altered electrically with minimal effort.

Fig. 1. Schematic Illustration of Measuring System for
Small Bending and Axial Waves in Bars

The piezoelectric transducer fixed to one end of the
bar induces transient stress waves in the form of
finite trains of sine waves. The corresponding lateral
displacements are measured with the aid of two Michelson interferometers positioned on opposite sides of
the bar. Repetitive generation of the stress waves and
the use of box-car integraters permit the measurement
of surface displacements with amplitudes as small as
0.01 nanometers (nm). Axial- and bending components of
the stress perturbations induced by the piezoelectric
element can be separated by adding and subtracting the
response of the two inferometers.

Stress waves in the form of finite trains of sine waves are induced by means of a piezoelectric transducer (Philips PXE5) cemented to one end of the beam. The corresponding excitation voltage is derived from a Wavetek Mod. 144 function generator with a counting-gating circuit which permits the number of sine waves in the train to be selected in the range from 1 to 19. To produce waves of sufficient strength, the excitation signal can be amplified up to peak-to-peak values of about 160 Volts. The amplifier used for this purpose consists of a chain of three cascade differential amplifiers with an emitter follower current amplifier as the final stage. With a capacitive load of 500 pF the bandwidth is 1.2 MHz and the maximum differential output voltage 160 Volts.

In practice it is not possible to induce stress waves of only one kind. Because of imperfections in the transducer and in its attachment to the bar the waves generated are in general of a composite nature. By mounting the transducer laterally or axially at the end of the beam one usually induces bending as well as axial waves of sufficient amplitude to be observable in the recordings. However, these two types of waves can easily be separated by employing two interferometers as illustrated in Figure 1 and by making use of the fact that axial waves produce contractions and expansions of the cross section while bending waves displace it laterally. Hence by adding and subtracting the electronically processed signals from the two interferometers one obtains the axial and the bending components of the stress waves.

2.2 Analysis of interferometer response

To analyze the interferometer response to the ω_0 bar motion the reference beam and the beam reflected from the bar are expressed as

$$u_r = A_r \sin(\omega_0 t) \text{ and } u_b = A_b \sin(\omega_0 t + \emptyset)$$

respectively where ω_0 is the circular frequency of the laser light. With K representing a proportionality factor the detector voltage is given by

$$V = \frac{K}{\tau} \int_0^\tau (u_r + u_b)^2 \, dt$$

If f_m denotes the largest frequency component in the bar motion to be measured and if

$$\frac{2\pi}{\omega_o} \ll \tau \ll \frac{1}{f_m}$$

the detector voltage can also be written as

$$V = K\left[\frac{A_r^2 + A_b^2}{2} + \frac{A_r A_b}{\tau} \int_0^\tau \{\cos\Phi - \cos(2\omega_o t + \Phi)\} dt\right]$$

By utilizing a silicon PIN photodiode (Monsanto MD1) as a light detector, the bandwidth is greater than 10^8 Hz with a load resistance of 50 Ω. Therefore the condition for τ is easily met when stress waves with frequencies on the order of 1 MHz are to be detected. When Φ changes negligibly during the time interval τ, the detector voltage can be simplified to

$$V = K\left(\frac{A_r^2 + A_b^2}{2} + A_r A_b \cos\Phi\right) \tag{1}$$

Decomposing the phase difference Φ into a stationary part Φ_o and a time dependent part $\Phi(t)$ which varies with the lateral surface motion of the bar, $x(t)$, one obtains:

$$\Phi = \Phi_o + \Phi(t) \quad \text{and} \quad \Phi(t) = \frac{4\pi}{\lambda_o} x(t)$$

where λ_o is the wave length of the laser light.

With $x(t) \ll \frac{\lambda_o}{4\pi}$; V reduces to

$$V = K \frac{A_r^2 + A_b^2}{2} + A_r A_b \left(\cos\Phi_o - \frac{4\pi}{\lambda_o} x(t) \sin\Phi_o\right) \tag{2}$$

The sensitivity of the detector voltage with respect to lateral displacements of the bar is:

$$\frac{dV}{dx} = -\frac{4\pi}{\lambda_o} K A_r A_b \sin\Phi_o \qquad (3)$$

Accordingly maximal sensitivity is achieved when

$$\sin\Phi_o = -1, \text{ or when } \Phi_o = \frac{3\pi}{2} \pm 2n\pi, \; n = 1,2,\ldots$$

For small deviations from such phase values up to $\pm 0.045 \; \pi$, i.e. for bar displacements in the range $x \leqslant 6$ nm, the sensitivity is constant within 1 %. The servo loop was designed to maintain maximal sensitivity within this range. Consequently the operating point of the interferometer system is defined by the detector voltage corresponding to maximal sensitivity:

$$V_{op} = K \frac{A_r^2 + A_b^2}{2} \qquad (4)$$

In view of the fact that V_{op} depends on A_r and A_b, one has to redetermine V_{op} whenever the motion of a new surface point on the bar is to be examined, because any rearrangement of the optical system components can be expected to cause a change in the optical conditions and thus in the intensity of the beams from the reference mirror and the bar surface. Similarly the maximal sensitivity

$$\frac{dV}{dx}_{max} = \frac{4\pi}{\lambda_o} K A_r A_b \qquad (5)$$

will be altered by such rearrangements. Quantification V_{op} and $\frac{dV}{dx}_{max}$ is achieved by measuring the extrema V_{max} and V_{min} of the detector voltage when the reference mirror is displaced by a distance in excess of one wave length λ_o through an appropriate variation of the driver voltage. From equation (1) it follows that V_{op} and $k \; A_r A_b$ may be expressed in terms of the maximum and minimum voltage:

$$V_{op} = \frac{V_{max} + V_{min}}{2} \tag{6}$$

$$\text{and} \quad K \, A_r A_b = \frac{V_{max} - V_{min}}{2} = \frac{1}{2} \, V_{pp} \tag{7}$$

where V_{pp} is the peak-to-peak voltage.

Thus, knowing the wave length λ_0 of the laser light, both V_{op} and $\frac{dV}{dx}\,_{max}$ are defined by the values for V_{max} and V_{min}.

2.3 Signal processing and stabilization

For convenience the preamplified detector signal is electronically divided by expression (7) and thereby automatically normalized with respect to the sensitivity. To allow for corrections of drift and low frequency disturbances of magnitudes up to $\pm 10 \, \lambda_0$ the optical system must be sufficiently well adjusted to provide constant sensitivity and constant V_{op} for reference mirror displacement of such an extent. This implies a constant amplitude of the beam from the reference mirror for this displacement range. Likewise the amplitude of the beam from the bar surface must also remain constant throughout the measurement range of ± 6 nm. The lenses in the two legs of the interferometer were inserted to minimize effects of rotation of the mirror and bar surfaces on the beam amplitudes. They offer the additional advantage of easy separation of the incident from the reflected beam to prevent light from returning into the laser. To avoid amplitude variations due to phase aberrations, the mirror and bar surface are placed slightly in front of the focal point. Adequate intensity of the reflected light was assured by attaching an aluminized polyester self-adhesive film (MMM Corp. polyester film No. 850) to the beam.

The signals from the photodetector are used as parallel inputs to two different amplifiers. One of these constitutes a low frequency channel which is flat from DC to 100 kHz and serves as input to the

258

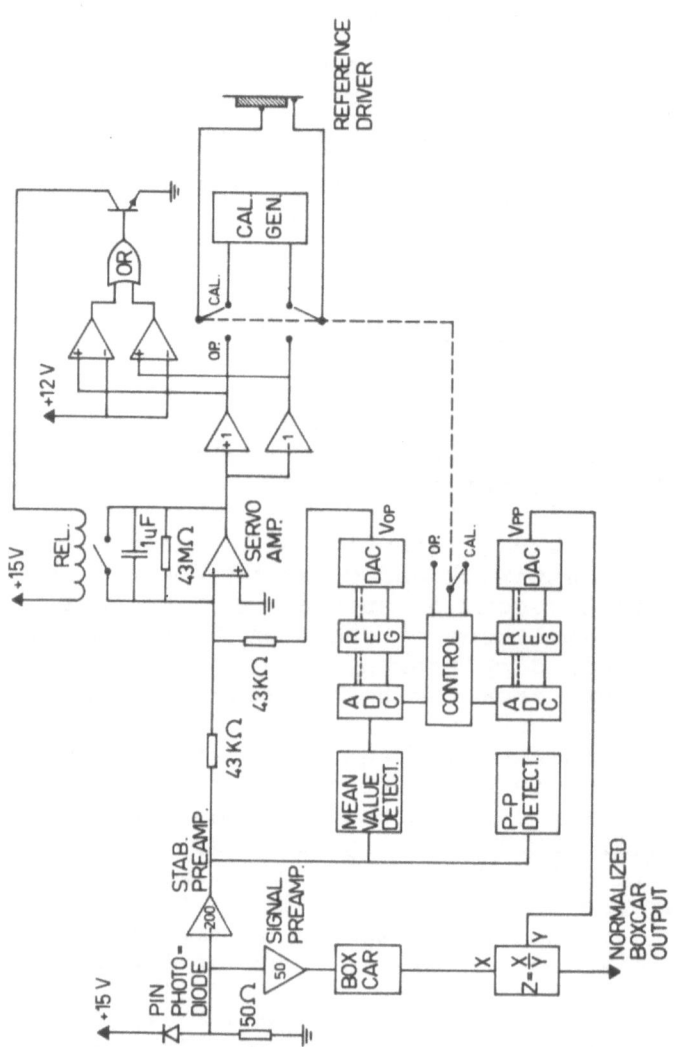

Fig. 2. Stabilization and Normalization Circuit

stabilization and normalization circuit as shown in
Figure 2. The other is a video amplifier with a gain
of 50 and a bandwidth of 90 MHz. This channel is the
input to the signal processing electronics.

The box-car integrator forms the heart of the
signal processing system. Its principal components are
a linear gate and a scan delay generator (Brookdeal
Electronics, Models 415 and 425 A). The latter is
triggered by a pulse coincident with the start of the
excitation signal. After a delay interval it generates
a pulse which opens the linear gate for a sampling of
the amplified photodetector signal. At each repetition
of the trigger, a progressively greater delay is introduced. The successive samples are then low-pass filtered. The output of the linear gate is therefore a time-
stretched reproduction of the input with an attendant
noise reduction. A voltage proportional to the delay
time is produced by the scan delay generator and provides a time base for an x - y recorder or similar
display device.

Fig. 2. Stabilization and Normalization Circuit

In the calibration mode (CAL) a signal generator
(CAL GEN) is used to activate the reference driver in
a controlled manner such that it moves through a distance of 20 wave-lengths of the laser light. The corresponding voltage V_{op} from the mean signal detector is
digitized and stored in the register (REG). At the same
time the average peak-to-peak voltage V_{pp} induced by the
reference driver is also digitized and stored as a
measure of the sensitivity of the signal detection
system. In the operating mode (OP) the voltage V_{op} is
the reference signal for the servo amplifier in the
feedback loop for stabilization against low frequency
distrubances and drift. Moreover, the peak-to-peak voltage V_{pp} is now employed as normalization factor.

The stabilization circuit allows for two modes of operation designated "calibrate" and "operate" (see Fig. 2). In the calibration mode a triangular wave form of 50 Hz is applied to the reference mirror driver. At a peak-to-peak amplitude of 30 Volts the total displacement of the reference mirror amounts to $\pm$ 10 λ_0. The associated amplified photodiode response is averaged by a mean value detector, then digitized to an accuracy of 8 bits and held in a storage register as V_{op}. For measurements of the beam displacement the "operate" mode is employed and V_{op} in the storage register is converted back into analog form and compared at the inverting input terminal of the servo operational amplifier with the amplified photodiode output as evident from Fig. 2. A feedback resistor of 43 M Ω gives the servo amplifier a DC-gain of 1'000. The amplified error voltage is applied to the reference driver which changes the path length difference in such a way that the error signal is minimized. The minimum feedback capacitance for unconditional dynamic stability of the servo system was found to be 1 μF. If the path compensation exceeds $\pm$ 10 λ_0 a reset circuit is triggered which sets the driver voltage to zero and thus allows the system to restabilize itself. Normalization of the sensitivity is effected by electronically dividing the output of the box-car integrator by V_{pp}. This voltage is obtained from the calibration signal by means of a peak-to-peak detector. It is digitized and stored in the same manner as V_{op}.

2.4 Evaluation of measuring system and results

For the purpose of testing the measuring system, series of elementary wave propagation experiments were performed in a Plexiglas bar and a beam-like sample of compact bone from a human femur. Perturbations were generated by a laterally mounted transducer in the frequency range from 5 kHz to 130 kHz and by an axially attached one for frequencies between 90 kHz and 200 kHz. The excitation signal was obtained by passing a train of sine waves through cascaded active low and high-pass filters (Multimetrics, Model AF 120) with the cutoff points set to the central frequency of the wave train. Filtering proved necessary to suppress the sidelobes of the spectrum of a train of sine waves, since in dispersive systems like bars

these sidelobes give rise to stress wave components
which travel with velocities different from that
corresponding to the central frequency.

Theory predicts axial stress waves to be propagated at higher speed than bending stress waves.
Accordingly we expect a finite train of sinusoidal
perturbations to exhibit a growing separation of the
corresponding trains of axial- and bending waves with
increasing distance from the transducer. This is
evident from Fig. 3 which depicts the surface displacements recorded with one of the interferometers.
The phase velocity of the signal was evaluated from
the slope of the lines connecting corresponding zero-
crossings. Only zero-crossings of the central part
of the wave trains were used for this purpose in
order to avoid effects of fore- and after-runners.
Consistency of the evaluations can be deduced from
the variations in the steepness of the slopes which
correspond to an error on the order of 2 %.

The resulting phase velocities for flexural waves
propagating in the Plexiglas bar are illustrated in
Fig. 4 together with the theoretical dispersion curve
predicted on the basis of the Timoshenko beam theory.
For the theoretical prediction of the dispersion, the
Poisson ratio was taken to be 0.33 (16) and the geometric parameter k' for shearing stiffness was chosen
as 0.83 (17). The velocity of longitudinal waves of
infinite wavelength in a bar, c_o, was determined by
fitting the curve corresponding to the generalized form
of Rayleigh's equation (18) for the phase of axial
waves with long wave lengths to the experimentally determined phase velocities of the longitudinal stress
waves. The value obtained for the Plexiglas bar was
2171 m/sec. The method described was also applied to
a 3 mm thick beam of compact bone machined out of the
diaphysis of a human femur. A plot of the phase velocity of bending waves in this bone sample is given in
Fig. 5.

The experimental results given here agree within
an error interval of about 2 % with the theoretical
predicitons on the basis of Timoshenko beam theory.
In view of this agreement the use of the instrumentation
and the methodology for the evaluation of the mechanical properties of bone and other materials from the

262

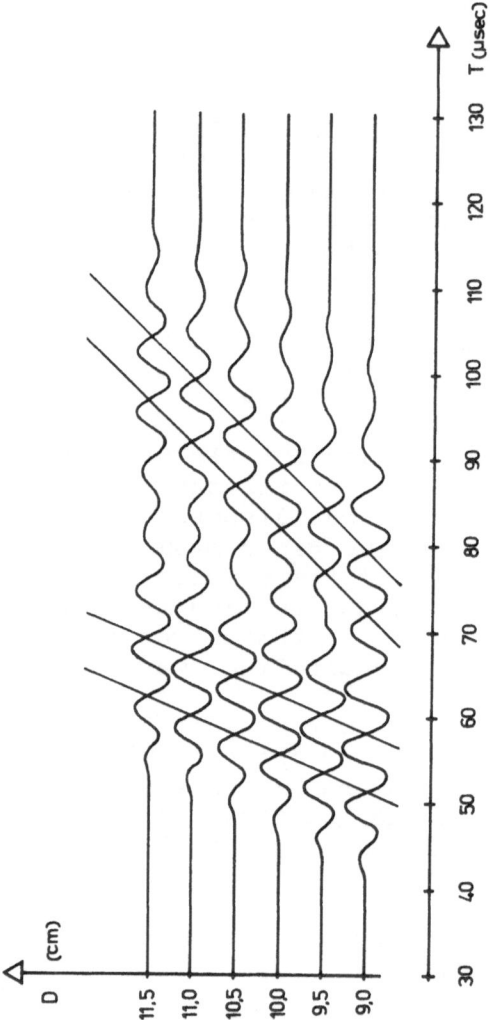

Fig. 3. Sample Recordings of a Train of 3 Filtered Sine Waves with a Frequency of 140 kHz Propagating Along a Plexiglas Bar.

Axial and flexural waves are clearly separated from each other because the recording was made at points sufficiently far from the bar end at which the stress perturbations were generated. D denotes the distance from the transducer and T the time elapsed since the beginning of excitation.

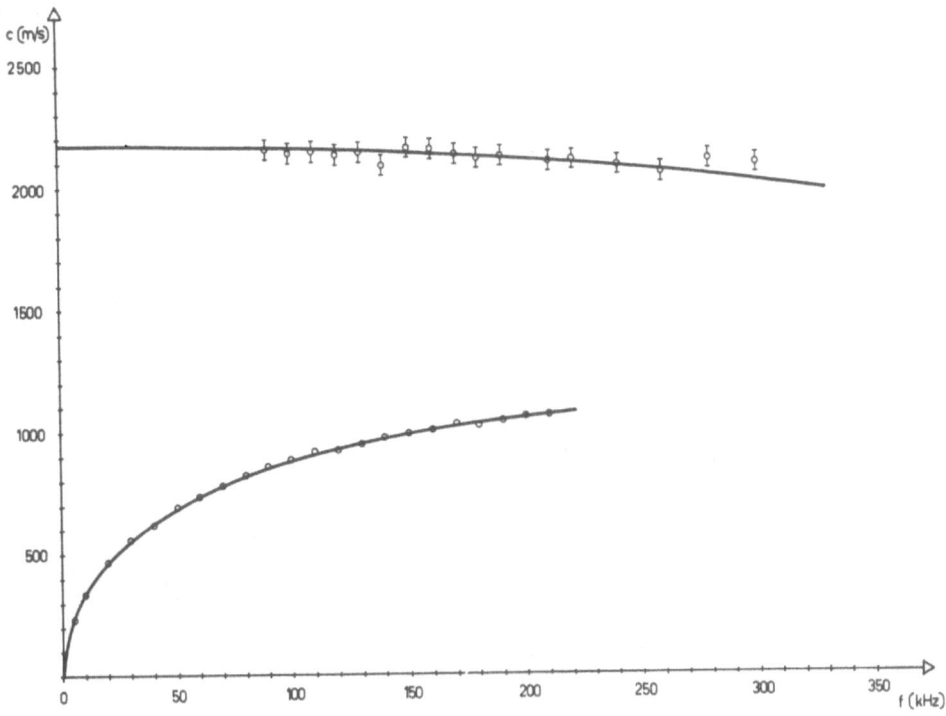

Fig. 4. Dispersion Data for Flexural and Axial Waves in a Plexiglas Bar

The solid lines represent the theoretical dispersion curves based on Rayleigh's equation (axial waves, upper curve) and Timoshenko beam theory (flexural waves, lower curve). The experimental results are given by circles. In the case of flexural waves the error is less than 2 %.

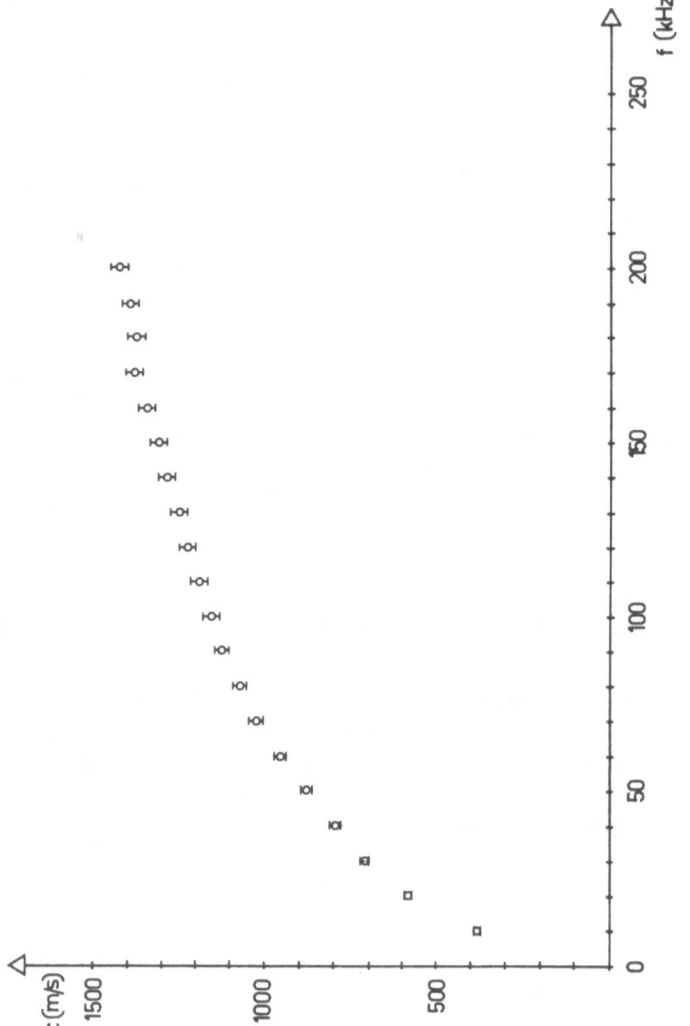

Fig. 5. Dispersion Data for Flexural Waves in a Bone Sample

The phase velocities shown were obtained from a 3 mm thick beam cut out from a human femur.

stress wave transmission data of beam-like samples seems to be justified. However, it is often exceedingly difficult to excise spongy bone samples which are both, sufficiently slender and sufficiently homogeneous to meet the prerequisites of beam theory. For a general experimental analysis of the dynamic elastic properties of spongy bone specimens it therefore proved necessary to make use of alternate techniques.

3. BUFFER BAR TECHNIQUES APPLIED TO BONE SAMPLES

A method frequently employed in practice in determining dynamic elastic moduli of solids is the measurement of the transmission time of stress pulses with the aid of the buffer bar technique (19,20). This technique seems to lend itself also to the quantification of elastic parameters of spongy bone samples. Yet, in view of the trabecular structure of spongy bone, a basic restriction must be imposed on the wave length spectrum of the stress pulses, if the desired data on the elastic properties should pertain to the macroscopic mechanical behavior. As the average intertrabecular distance is of the order 1 mm, the major wave length components of the stress pulses should not be less than ~10 mm. For a wave speed of 600 m/s this would for example imply that the dominant frequencies contained in the stress pulses should be below 60 kHz. For measurement purposes it is assumed that the cylindrical spongy bone samples behave like linearly elastic solids and that the speeds of axial and torsion waves in these samples together with their average densities provide information on the effective or average Young's modulus for the direction of the axis of the cylinder and on the corresponding effective shear modulus. By excising samples whose axes have different orientations with respect to the femur axis and determining their values for E and G, the degree of anisotropy in the macroscopic elastic behavior of spongy bone in the knee condyles can be assessed.

3.1 The axial buffer bar technique

A schematic diagram of the design of an axial buffer bar system is given in Fig. 6. The displacements of the end mirror caused by the transient stress signal

266

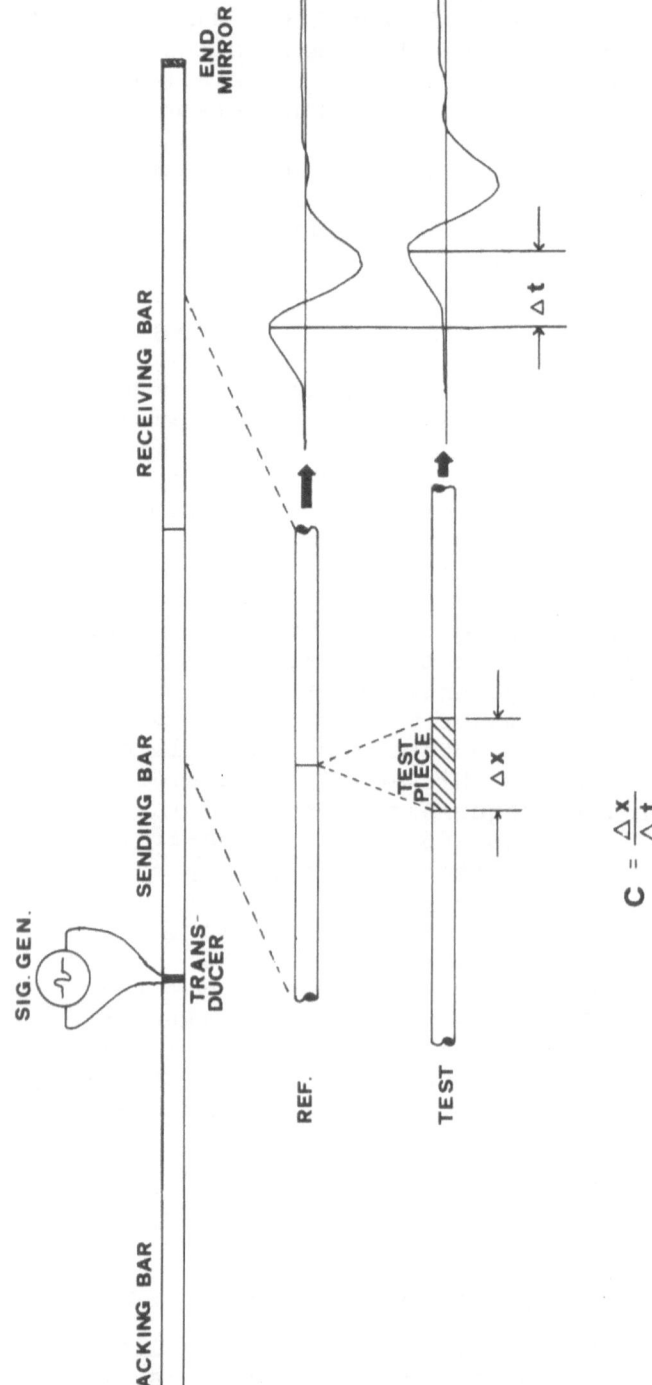

$$C = \frac{\Delta x}{\Delta t}$$

Fig. 6. Schematic Diagram of Axial Buffer Bar Design

is recorded with the aid of a stabilized Michelson interferometer as described in section 2. When the impedance of the test specimen is not sufficiently matched with those of the receiving and sending bars, internal reflections of the specimen may interfer with the primary signal. For an adequate determination of the time delay due to the specimen, however, at least the first peak and the first zero crossing of the primary signal should be free of interferences. This implies that the frequency f of a sinusoidal stress wave would have to satisfy the condition

$$f > \frac{1}{2t_f}$$
(8)

Fig. 6. Schematic Diagram of Axial Buffer Bar Design

A piezoelectric ceramic disc (Philips PXE-5) 0.2 mm in thickness and 6 mm in diameter serves as transducer and is cemented between two Pexiglas rods of 200 mm length and 6 mm diameter. Electrical excitation of this element produces a thickness vibration and thus causes axial stress waves to propagate into the sending bar on the right and into the backing bar on the left. The function of the latter is merely to provide a load for the transducer in order to increase radiation into the sending bar and to provide a delay path of sufficient length for the backward-radiated wave to avoid reflection interference with the wave radiated forward into the sending bar. The receiving bar, a Plexiglas rod 6 mm in diameter and 100 mm long, carries a small mirror at its forward end which is used as the target for the laser interferometer. To determine the axial wave speed in a test specimen the bar is operated first in the reference mode, in which the front end of the sending bar is cemented to the back end of the receiving bar, and then in the test mode, in which the specimen is cemented between the ends of the sending and receiving bars. In the test mode the axial stress waves generated by the transducer arrive at the mirror with an additional time delay due to the test piece. This time delay and the length of the test piece define the axial wave speed.

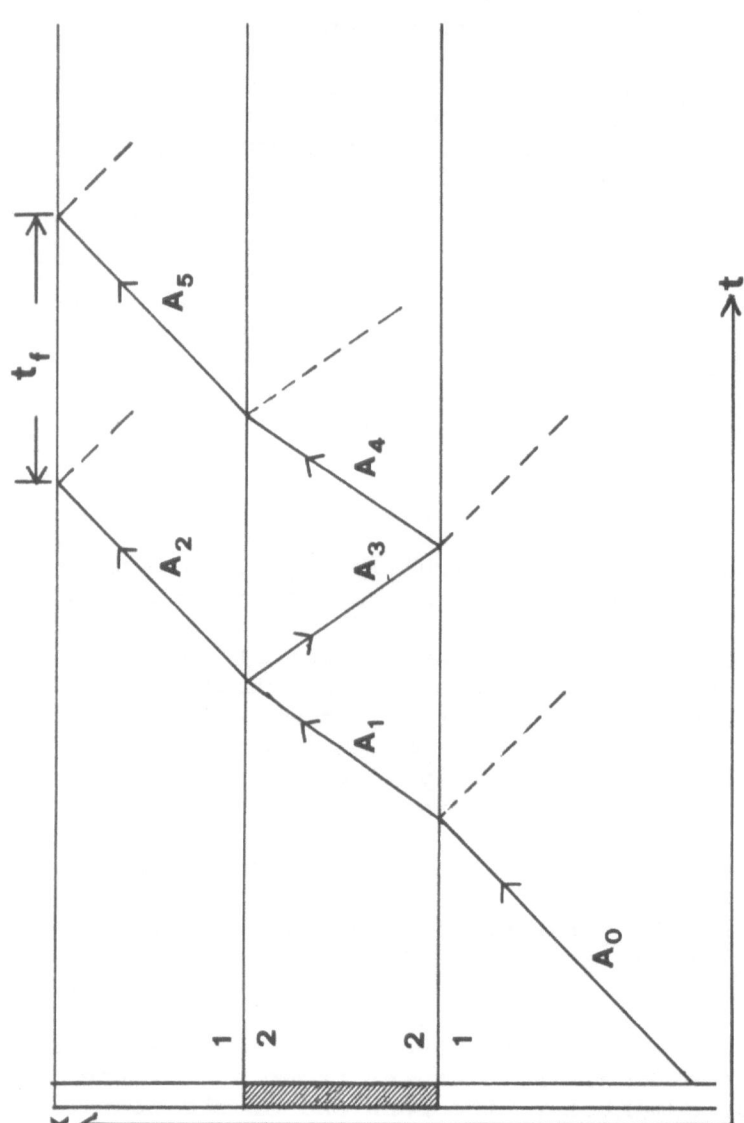

Fig. 7. Transmission of a Stress Wave through a Test Piece with Wave Impedance Different from that of the Buffer Bar

where t_f represents the round trip time of the stress wave within the specimen, as can also be deduced from Fig. 7.

Equation (8) together with the lower wavelength limit defined by intertrabecular distance and the degree of non-uniformity of the material, gives an estimate of the frequency range over which useful measurements may be made.

Based on these considerations an experiment was performed using the axial buffer bar and an aluminum test piece 6 mm in diameter and 49 mm long. Fig. 8 shows the displacement waveforms obtained. A single cycle of 50 KHz sine wave was used as an excitation signal. The time interval t_f is indicated on the recording. It may be seen that strong reflections follow the main signal. The delay times of the leading edge, the first peak and the first zero crossing yield C_A = 5320 m/s which is in excellent agreement with published values (18). From this speed, one finds t_f = 18.8 microseconds. The landmarks of the primary signal are therefore well within the reflection-free interval.

Of much importance to the accuracy of the method is also the manner in which the faces of the bars and test piece are cemented together. The glue joints must introduce negligible time delays, reflection and attenuation, and yet must be easily broken, leaving the bar ends clean and undamaged. For this purpose, zinc phosphate dental cement (De Trey's Zinc Cement) has been found ideal. It sets to a stone-like hardness within roughly fifteen minutes of preparation. Adhesion

---

Fig. 7. Transmission of a Stress Wave through a Test Piece with Wave Impedance Different from that of the Buffer Bar

The x-t diagram illustrates the propagation of a primary signal through the sending bar (A_0), the specimen (A_1) and the receiving bar (A_2). As denotes the secondary signal which arrives with a delay t_f at the mirror (end of receiving bar). During the time interval t_f the primary signal can be recorded without reflection interference.

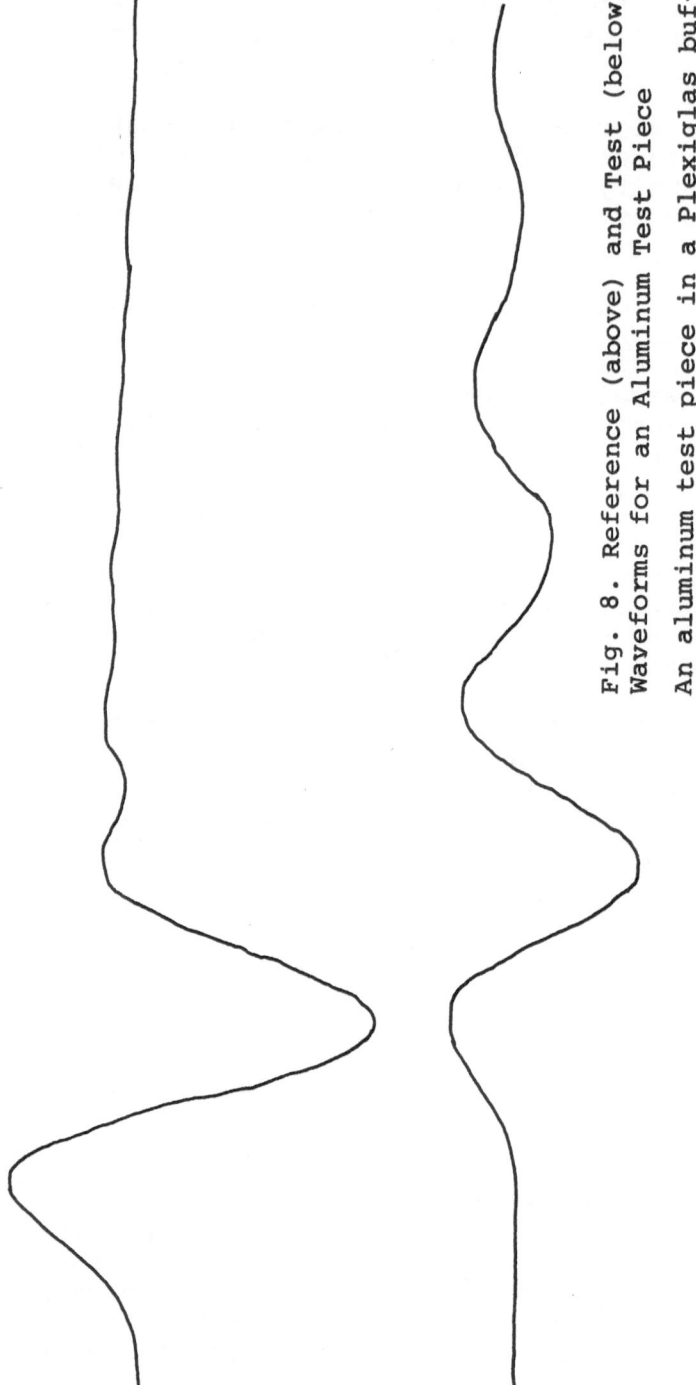

Fig. 8. Reference (above) and Test (below) Waveforms for an Aluminum Test Piece

An aluminum test piece in a Plexiglas buffer bar introduces a large wave impedance mismatch. T_f is indicated on the lower waveform. The subsequent "ringing" is due to internal reflections within the test piece. Primary stress wave is induced by exciting the transducer with one cycle of a 50 kHz oscillator.

is primarily through penetration of surface irregularities of the cemented surfaces, permitting the strength of the bond to be adjusted by grinding the bar ends with carborundum powder. Bonds of sufficient strength may be made, yet the bars are easily separated and cleaned with little surface damage.

3.2 Torsional buffer bar technique

A schematic illustration of the torsional buffer bar designed for the determination of the shear modulus of spongy bone specimens is given in Fig. 9. Basically the design is quite similar to that of the axial buffer bar. The principal differences are the type of transducer used to induce torsional waves in the bar assembly and the lateral mounting of the mirror at the end of the receiving bar for the interferometric detection of the angle of rotation.

A torsional wave generator was built according to a design published by Thurston and Andreatch (21) and shown in Fig. 10. It consists of a tube of piezoelectric ceramic (Philips PXE 21) which has its remnant polarization in the axial direction. It is split lengthwise and reassembled into a tube with the polarization of one half opposite to that of the other. The halves are cemented together with electrically conductive epoxy cement, the glue joints serving as excitation electrodes. The operating principle is illustrated in Figs. 10b,c, and d.

The small size of the mirror that could be attached to the receiving bar without creating severe problems of adjustment and stabilization required a new approach to measuring rotations with an interferometer. By utilizing the birefringence of a calcite crystal to produce two parallel beams it was possible to devise a convenient solution (11).

The operation of the torsional buffer bar, apart from the aspects described above, is in every way identical to that of the axial buffer bar. To validate the measuring procedure, series of experiments were performed with a single cycle of a 50 kHz sine wave as excitation signal, delay time measurements were made on a 41 mm long Plexiglas test piece and a 49 mm long

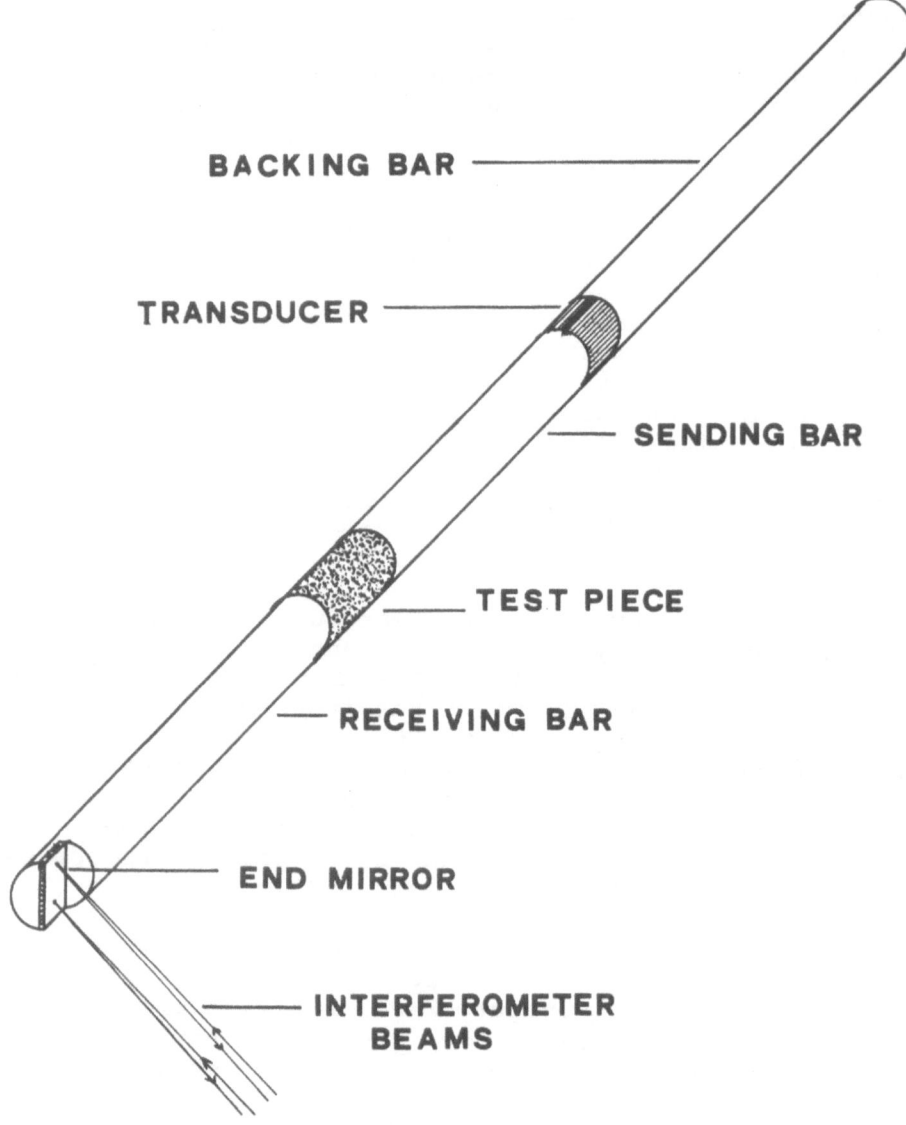

272

Fig. 9. Torsinal Buffer Bar Assembly

Detection of the rotation of the free end of the receiving bar is accomplished by means of a specially developed phase stabilized laser interferometer (11) which
is similar to the one used in the previously described
experiments. It is sensitive to rotation of the mirror
about an axis perpendicular to the plane containing the
two beams. The free end of the receiving bar is therefore fitted with a narrow mirror whose surface is parallel to and contains the longitudinal axis of the bar.

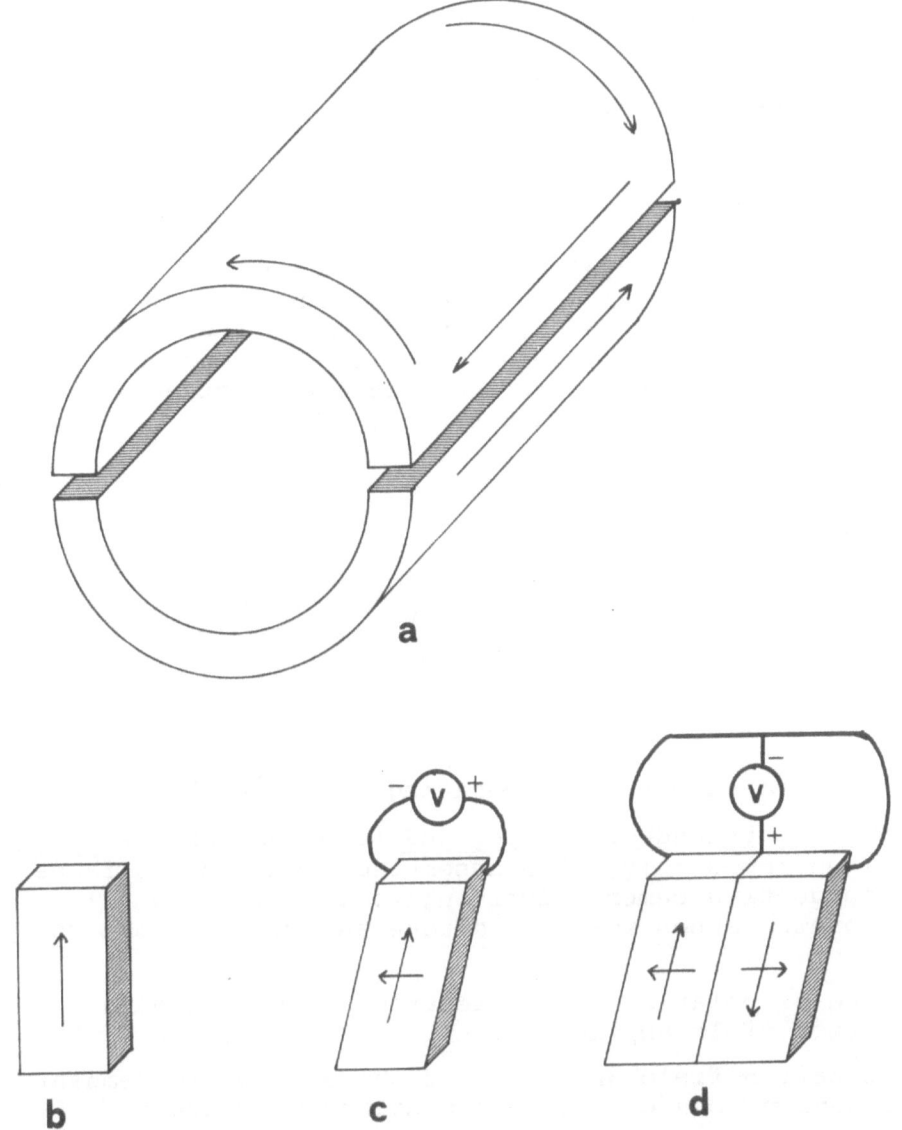

Fig. 10. Transducer for Generating Torsional Waves

aluminum test specimen. The torsional wave speed c_T obtained for the Plexiglas test piece was 1400 m/s and that for the aluminum sample 3200 m/s. As a check these values are compared with

$$c_T = \sqrt{\frac{G}{\rho}}$$ (9)

whereby the shear modulus G is computed on the basis of the observed axial wave speed and the Poisson's ratio for Plexiglas and aluminum given in the lite-rature (18,20). For $\sqrt{G/\rho}$ one finds 1350 m/s and 3200 m/s, respectively, and thus an excellent agree-ment with the measured values.

Fig. 10. Transducer for Generating Torsional Waves

a) Complete transducer. Upper and lower halves are polarized oppositely, then assembled along shaded faces with conductive cement. Exciting voltage applied to glue joints causes rotation of one end with respect to the other.

b) Plate of polarized piezoelectric ceramic with no excitation field applied

c) Excitation field applied at right angeles to remnant polarizations causes shear deformation of plate.

d) Two such plates with opposing remnant polarizations have been cemented together and connected together elec-trically so that the excitation fields are also opposite in the two plates, resulting in identical shear defor-mations of the two parts. If this last assembly is rolled up into a tube by joining its two lateral edges, one obtains the same structure as (a) above in which the shear deformation is converted into a rotation of one end of the tube with respect to the other.

3.3 Measuring procedures and estimation of errors

Preliminary experiments with spongy bone samples established that the wavelength condition for macroscopic
elastic parameters and the time requirement for a recording of the primary signal with no reflection interference before the first zero crossing after a principal
peak are satisfied in the frequency range 50 - 60 kHz.
Also, a waveform in this range is transmitted without
appreciable distortion which verifies that dispersion
is small. It was therefore decided to limit investigation to a single frequency of 50 kHz.

The procedure for performing the measurements and
evaluating the results thereof derives from the nature
of the signal processing system. A block diagram of
the measurement system is given in Fig. 11. The central
element in the system in terms of data evaluation is
the box-car detector which serves two interrelated
functions: amplification and signal-to-noise enhance-
ment of the output signal of the interferometer, and
expansion of the signal's time base. This latter
function permits reproduction of the signal on an
X-Y recorder. In order to obtain precise time of arri-
val measurements for the selected stress waveform landmarks, the details of the time transformation must be
known.

Instead of trying to predict theoretically the
expected error entailed in the measurements, the individual factors were controlled as closely as possible
and the accuracy of the system tested by means of a
series of proof experiments. The results can be summarized as follows:
1) The axial wave speed of Plexiglas as inferred
   from the round trip time in the axial wave
   buffer bar (absolute measurement) agrees to
   within 0.5 % with the wave speed inferred from
   the differential time delay introduced into
   the buffer bar by a Plexiglas test piece.
   Also, these speeds differ by less than 2 % from
   the values obtained by direct observation of
   the propagation of an axial wave in a Plexiglas
   bar as described in chapter 2.

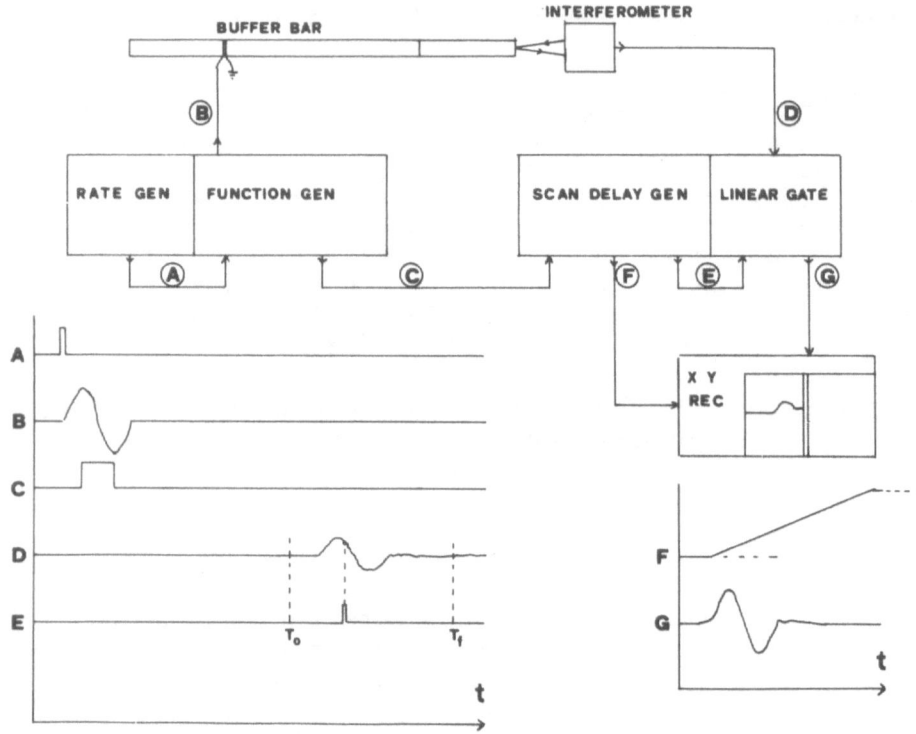

Fig. 11. Buffer Bar Instrumentation System

The rate generator periodically provides a pulse A
which triggers the function generator to excite the
buffer bar transducer with the wave form B and to produce a synchronization pulse C coincident with the
first peak of the wave form B. The sync pulse C causes
the scan delay generator to provide a sampling pulse E
at the time t, which then enables the linear gate to
sample interferometer output D. During one scan, t varies from T_0 to T_F, causing linear gate output G to
reproduce D on a stretched time base. Scan ramp voltage F is proprtional to the delay or sampling pulse
E relative to T_0 and serves as horizontal sweep for the
X-Y recorder, the vertical input of which is the linear
gate output G. The scan delay generator and linear gate
together comprise the box-car integrator.

2) The axial wave speed of 5'230 m/s measured in an aluminum test piece differs only by 2.8 % from the value (5'090 m/s) given in the literature (18).

3) Torsional wave speeds measured for Plexiglas (1'400 m/s) and aluminum (3'200 m/s) samples are also in good agreement with the speeds computed from the measured axial wave speeds and published values for Poisson's ratio as mentioned earlier.

4) Reproducibility of wave speed measurements in the Plexiglas and aluminum samples is about ±2 % over a time period of 3 months.

5) For 12 randomly chosen bone samples remounted and tested a second time at intervals of between three days and one month the reproducibility of the wave speed measurements is ±3 %. The absolute value of the difference between the two successive measurements was in all cases less than 5.6 %, in ten cases less than 2.6 %, and in four cases less than 1.5 %.

It is therefore considered highly probable that the measured values for wave speeds in spongy bone lie within 3 % of the true value. Since the computed elastic moduli are proportional to the square of the wave speed, the values of the moduli should be within 6 % of their true values.

4. ELASTIC PROPERTIES OF SPONGY BONE IN HUMAN KNEE CONDYLES

4.1 Sample Preparation

67 samples of spongy bone were excised from the knee condyles of six macerated right human femurs removed from male cadavers with age at death ranging from 21 to 83 years. The locations from which the samples were cut are shown in Fig. 12. For cutting a bone trephine was used with an inside diameter of 5.7 mm. The ends were trimmed perpendicular to the cylinder axis with the aid of a carborundum separating disc and a dental drill. If inspection showed apparent non-uniformity in density or structure near the ends of the samples, the

278

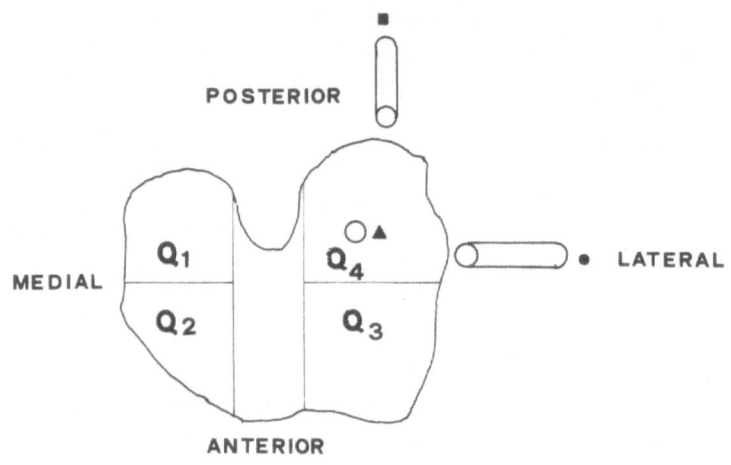

POSTERIOR

MEDIAL

Q₁ Q₄

Q₂ Q₃

ANTERIOR

LATERAL

DISTAL END VIEW

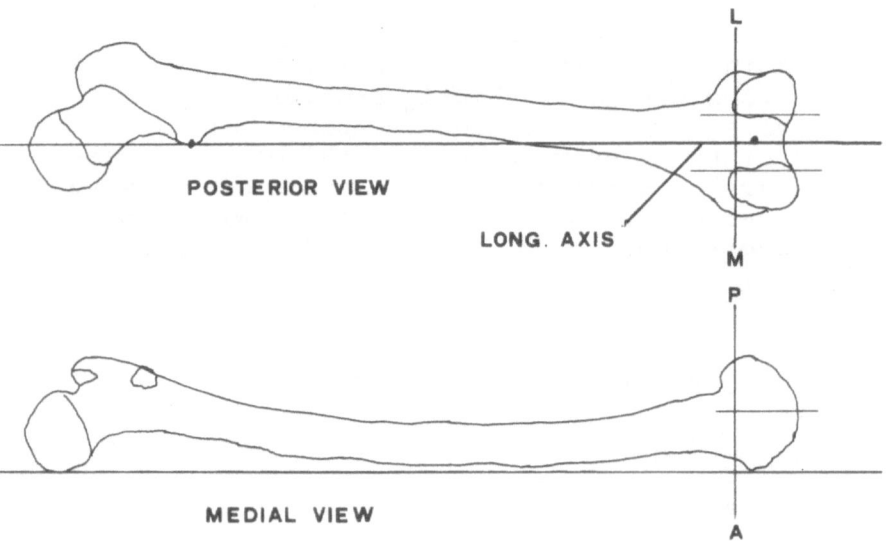

POSTERIOR VIEW

LONG. AXIS

MEDIAL VIEW

Fig. 12. Reference Axis of Femur and Locations
from which the Samples were cut

corresponding segments were cut off to render the specimens more uniform. It was found that A and B samples
whose axes are parallel to the longitudinal and ante-
rior-posterior axes of the femur, respectively, displayed a distinctly denser region of 3-5 mm thickness
near the cortex, while the C samples whose axes are
parallel to the medial-lateral axis of the femur showed
a less dense region of similar thickness. The samples
were blown free of cuttings, weighed to the nearest
3 mg and then measured in length to the nearest 0.1 mm.

Next the sample ends were capped with epoxy resin
to ensure uniform coupling of the stress waves to the
bone structure. Araldit AY 206, a fast-curing thixotropic cement was used. The thixotropic nature of the
cement ensured that it would not be drawn into the bone
structure under the influence of surface tension during
curing. The caps were applied by means of carriers of
6 mm diameter aluminum rods, the ends of which were
first coated with a film of release agent and then
with a thin layer of cement. Two coated rods with a
bone sample between them were placed in a V-block and
the ends of the rods lightly pressed against the ends
of the sample. The whole assembly was placed in an oven
at 55°C to cure the cement for one hour. After the

Fig. 12. Reference Axis of Femur and Locations
from which the Samples were cut

The reference axes are shown in relation to landmarks
on the femur which in splaced on a plane surface with
its auterior face downward. The longitudinal axis of
the femur is defined here as the projection of the
line from a point midway between the opposing faces of
the two condyles on the posterior side and the point
of the trochanter minor. The medial-lateral (M-L) axis
is obtained as the intersection of the contact plane
with a plane perpendicular to the longitudinal axis
and 3 mm distal to the more distal of the two proximal
posterior condyle faces. Finally a line perpendicular
to both, the longitudinal and the M-L axis is referred
to as the auterior-posterior (A-P) axis. In the distal
end view the quadrant designations and the 3 classes
of samples (A,B,C) are indicated. The latter are excised in such manner that their axes are either parallel
to the longitudinal axis of the femur (A), to the A-P
axis (B) or to the M-L axis (C).

280

sample had cooled to room temperature, the carrier rods
were removed, leaving thin epoxy caps on the sample.
Excess cement around the edges was ground off and the
ends of the caps roughened to improve adhesion of the
cement used in testing. The samples were at this
point ready for testing.

4.2 Results

All of the 67 spongy bone samples examined were of
cylindrical shape and had a diameter of 5.7 mm. They
were measured with regard to length (L), mass (m) and
transmission delays (Δt, Δt_T) of axial and torsion waves with a dominant frequency of 50 kHz. Densities ρ,
axial wave speeds c_A, torsion wave speeds c_T and
lengths L of these test samples varied as follows:

ρ = 0.13 to 0.60 g/cm^3

c_A = 860 to 2130 m/s

c_T = 505 to 982 m/s

L   = 10 to 32 mm

Whenever the ratio of radius r to wavelength λ satis-
fies the condition $r/\lambda \ll 1$, Young's modulus E can be
determined from

$$E = \rho c_A^2 \tag{10}$$

At a frequency of 50 kHz and a representative wave
speed $c_A = 10^3$ m/s one obtains for the test specimens
considered here r/λ = 0.14. For such a value the
error made by utilizing (10) in lieu of the wave speed
expression with the Rayleigh correction [18] is about
4 % if $c_A = 10^3$ m/s and Poisson's ratio is $1/3$. With
increasing values of c_A this error decreases. In view
of the range for c_A given above and the errors to be
expected in determining c_A and ρ one can readily justify
evaluating E on the basis of equation (10). The shear
modulus G is computed from

$$G = \rho c_T^2 \tag{11}$$

In order to estimate the degree of anisotropy of
the spongy bone samples with respect to the elastic

281

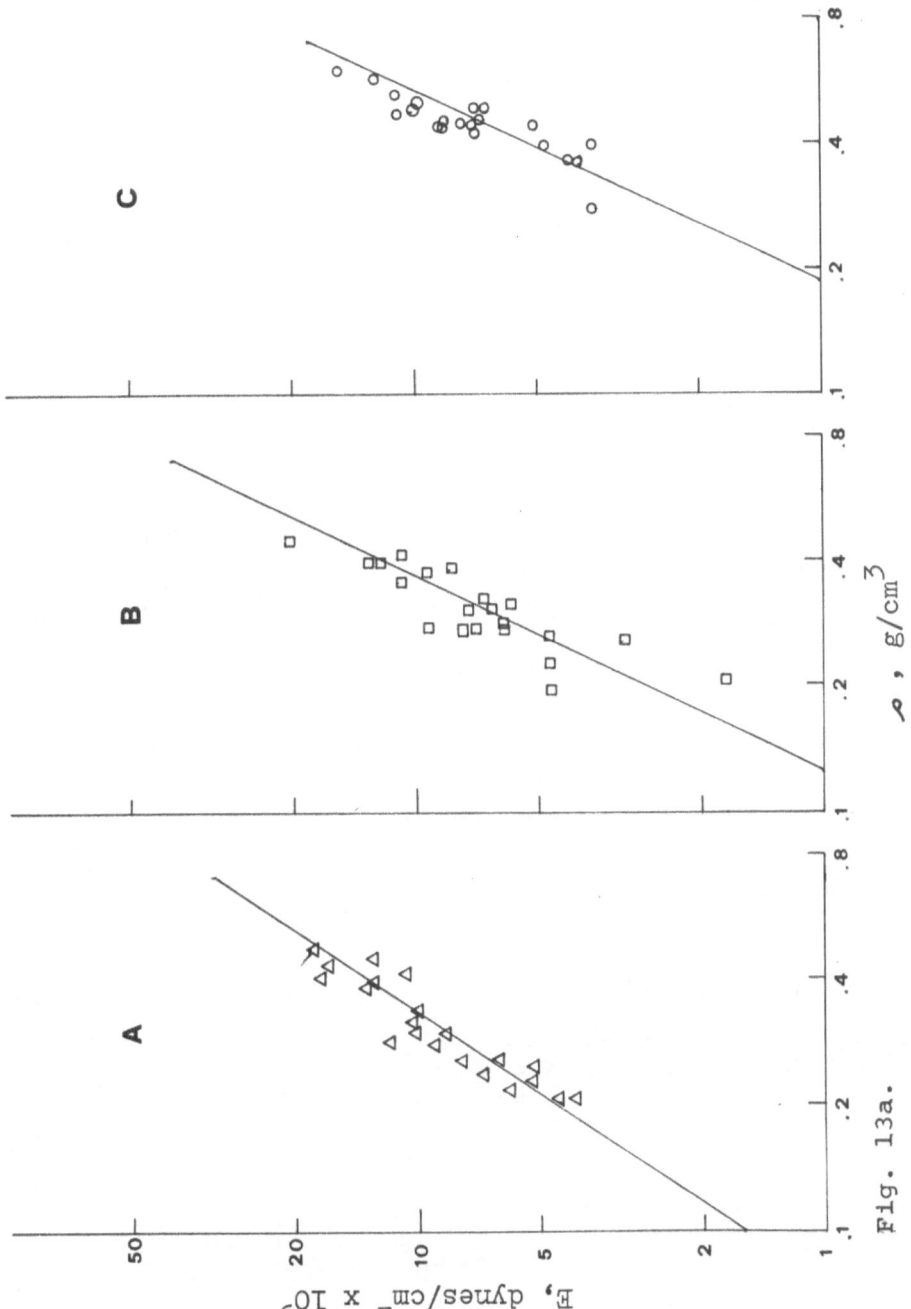

Fig. 13a.

282

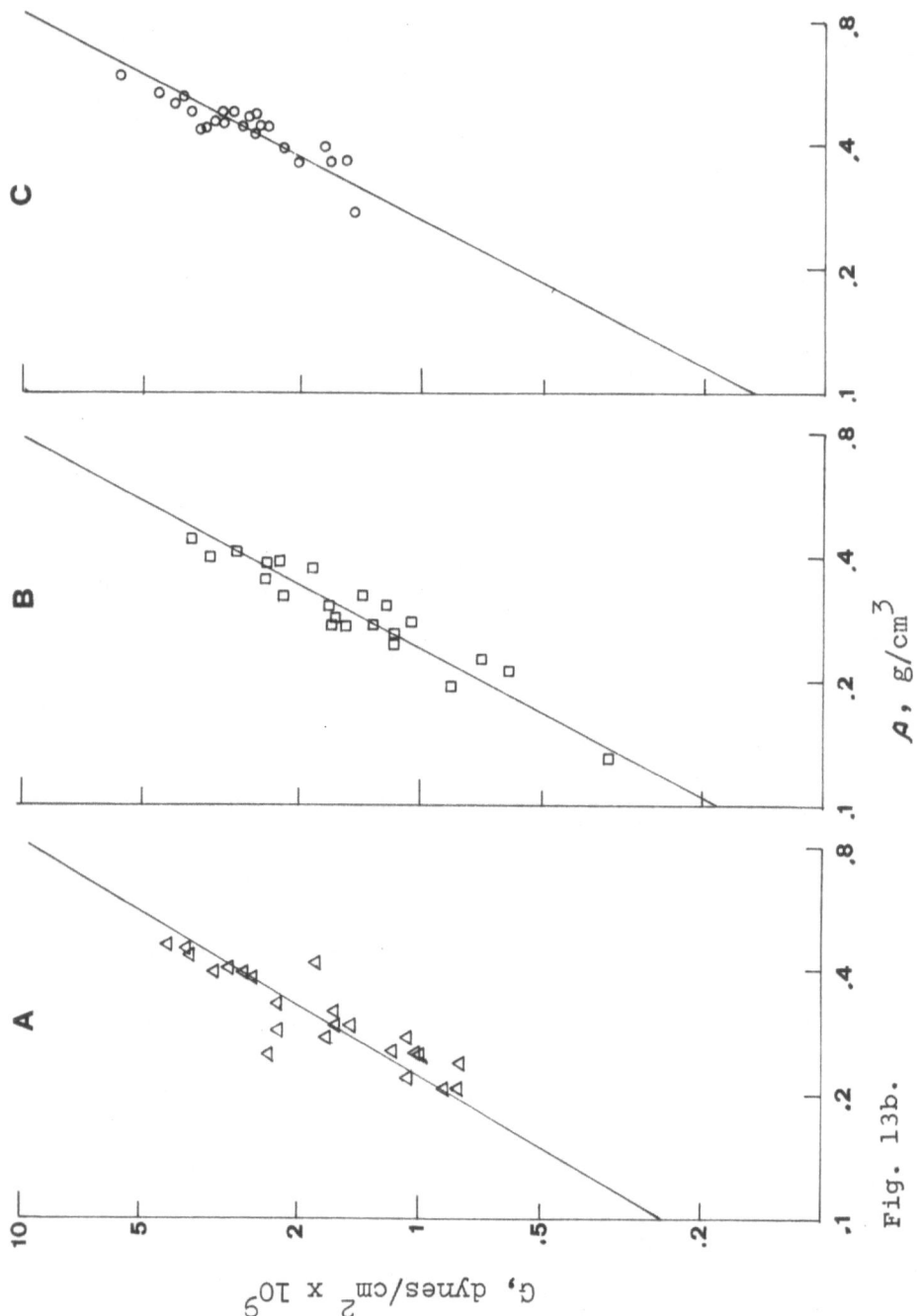

Fig. 13b.

moduli E and G, a statistical analysis was performed of the correlation between these moduli and density for each of the sample class A, B and C. For the purpose of analyzing E and G with regard to a possible power-law dependence upon density, the data were first plotted on a log-log scale. These plots are given in Figs. 13a and 13b together with the corresponding regression lines representing power law relationships. The regression line slopes at the 95 % confidence level are listed in Table 1.

The following general observations may be made concerning the data:
1) The elastic moduli correlate only moderately well with density. This is shown by the wide limits of the regression line slopes and the rather broad range of the 95 % confidence limits of the moduli.
2) The spongy bone samples are anisotropically elastic. This can be deduced from the fact, that different regression line slopes and intercepts are obtained for the different sample classes and from the clustering of the data points. Further evidence of anisotropy is given by the fact that for sample classes A and B the majority of values for Poisson's ratio ν are above the isotropic range $0 \leqslant \nu \leqslant 0.5$.
3) As one finds $(b_1)_A < (b_1)_B < (b_1)_C$ for E and G both of these two parameters appear to have the same qualitative dependence on direction.
4) All sample classes approximate to a square law dependence of elastic modulus upon density.
5) The spongy bone of the knee condyles is quite non-uniform with respect to density and the elastic moduli, a single bone displaying a wide range of values for each of these parameters.

Fig. 13a, b. Log-log Plot of E and G Versus ρ for the Three Sample Classes A, B and C

No distination is made in the data of the spongy bone samples from different quadrants of the knee condyles. The equations for the regression lines are given in Table 1.

Modulus	Sample Class	b_0	b_1	b_{1max}	b_{1min}	Equations
E	A	1.73	1.52	1.84	1.20	$E = 5.37 \times 10^{10} \rho^{1.52}$
	B	1.94	2.15	2.62	1.68	$E = 8.71 \times 10^{10} \rho^{2.15}$
	C	1.60	2.19	2.77	1.60	$E = 3.98 \times 10^{10} \rho^{2.19}$
G	A	1.14	1.76	2.19	1.34	$G = 1.38 \times 10^{10} \rho^{1.76}$
	B	1.19	1.93	2.23	1.63	$G = 1.55 \times 10^{10} \rho^{1.93}$
	C	1.15	1.99	2.45	1.53	$G = 1.41 \times 10^{10} \rho^{1.99}$

Table 1.

285

4.3 Variation of the elastic moduli with density

The broad range of trabecular geometry found within each sample class may explain to some extent the fact that the elastic parameters of spongy bone from human knee condyles correlate only moderately well with density. E and G are evidently highly dependent upon the structural configuration which may vary independently of density within spongy bone. This conclusion is supported by the work of Pugh et al. (6). Fig. 14a shows, on a log-log scale, the regression lines of $E(\rho)$ for all three sample classes of spongy bone from human knee condyles. The lower shaded area indicates the region occupied by the data points obtained from the 67 samples. The rectangular area intersected by the regression line for class C contains the range of values for E and ρ for compact bone from human femur shafts, as determined by Bundy (5). Fig. 14b is a similar plot for the shear moduli. In all cases, the regression lines for spongy bone intersect or come near to the range of values for compact bone. Furthermore the slopes of the regression lines are near the value 2.0 and thus suggest a quadratic dependence of the elastic moduli on the density.

Table 1. Linear regression coefficients and derived power law relationships based on log-log plots of E and G versus ρ

For each sample class the linear regression coefficients b_0 and b_1, in the equations

$$\log E/10^9 = b_0 + b_1 \log\rho \text{ and}$$

$$\log G/10^9 = b_0 + b_1 \log\rho$$

are given above, together with the corresponding power law relationships and limits of b_1 at the 95 % confidence level.

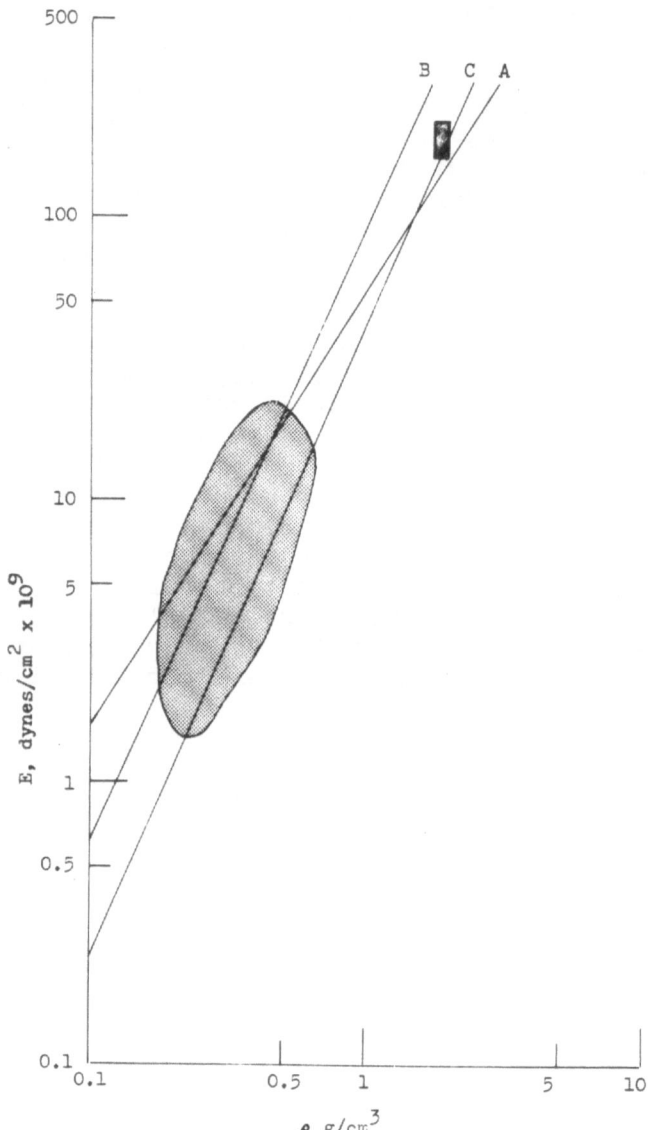

Fig. 14a.

287

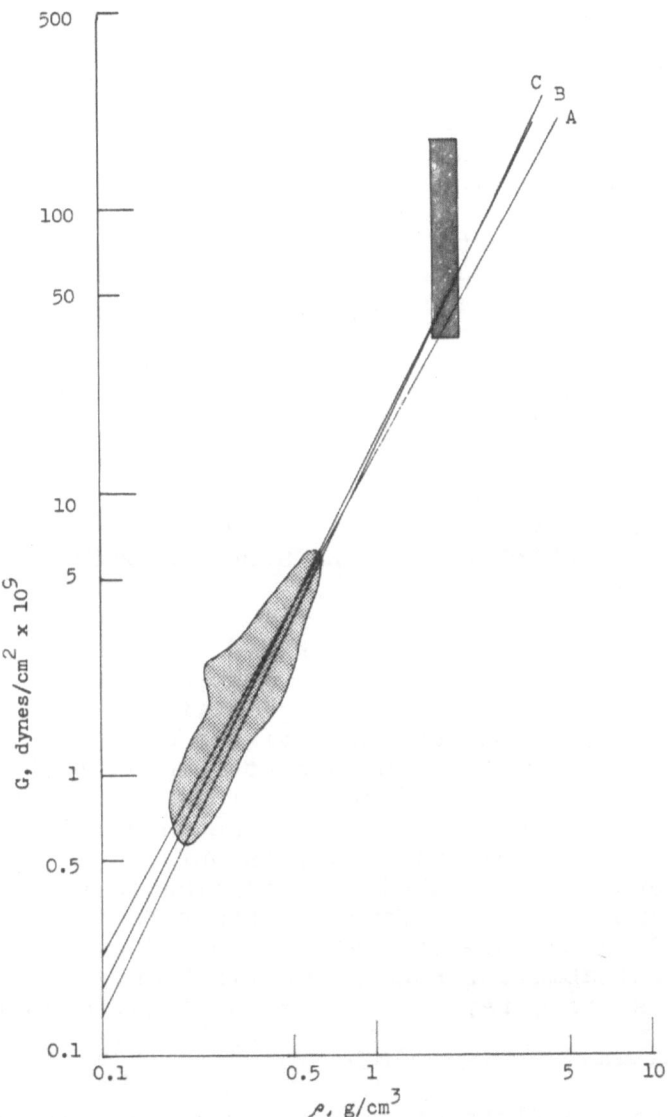

Fig. 14b. Relationship of Shear Modulus and Density for Spongy and Compact Bone

288

In view of the data presented in Figs. 14a, b
it appears that a measurement of spongy bone density
should provide estimates for the elastic moduli. Such
estimates although not highly accurate, may contribute
to the clinical evaluation of spongy bone status. It
should be stressed, however, that density measurements,
as computed tomography can provide them today in convenient form, could be misleading if a bone with normal or high density would have poor bonding of the calcium apatite crystals. But in cases of low values for
the density the elastic parameters of spongy bone are
also low and thus the inference of reduced mechanical integrity of the bone examined is amply justified. In this
sense, the measurement of spongy bone densities and
other mineralization parameters provide useful clinical
information on the mechanical status of bones.

5. MEASUREMENT OF SPONGY BONE DENSITY AND OTHER MINERALIZATION PARAMETERS BY MEANS OF COMPUTED TOMOGRAPHY (CT)

Spongy or trabecular bone show more rapid changes of
mineralization than does cortical or compact bone
(3,4,23). A method of detecting and quantifying such
changes has been developed on the basis of computed
tomography (24,25). By utilizing γ-rays from an isotope
like ^{125}I, in lieu of a x-ray tube the local radiation
exposure needed for computer tomograms which permit
an analysis of mineral distribution, is only about
5 mrem. This renders the method also applicable to
healthy human subjects (23). However, the relatively
low limited radiation intensity which can be derived
from isotopes suitable for bone mineralization studies
restricts the use of γ-ray CT to arms and legs. Measure-

Fig. 14a, b. Log-log Plots of E(ρ) and G (ρ) respectively
for Spongy and Compact Bone from Human Femurs

The regression lines of E(ρ) resp. G(ρ) for all the sample
classes A, B and C are labelled accordingly. For density
only ranges of the data points are identified rather than
their individual locations. The lower shaded areas represent the values of spongy bone whereas the rectangular
areas give the ranges for the data from compact bone.

ments made on macerated human femurs with the aid of
γ-ray CT have shown that the sensitivity of the spongiosa density parameter with reference to osteoporosis
is greater by a factor of 5 to 10 than that of the
total mineral content of the related cross section of
bone. In vivo investigations of mineralization at the
distal end of the radius of patients prompted the same
conclusion.

The principle of operation of the γ-ray CT designed
and built at the Institute for Biomedical Engineering
of the University and ETH Zurich is schematically illustrated in Fig. 15. A representative tomogram produced
with this instrument of the right forearm of a 71 y.
old male patient with moderate osteoporosis is given in
Fig. 16. Measurements made in healthy children and
adults in the age range 5 to 40 years have shown that
the mean density of the spongiosa in the radius at a
point one tenth along the ulna measured from its distal
end is, unlike other bone parameters, independent of
age and sex.

Results obtained in immobilization studies in children have shown that mineral loss as a consequence of local
immobilization principally takes the form of a reduction
of spongy bone. For example, immobilization of the arm
for 3 to 4 weeks leads to the density of the spongiosa
being reduced by 10 to 45 % in the distal region of the
forearm, whereas mineral loss in the diaphysis is only a
few percent. On remobilization the density of the spongy
bone increases again at the rate of a few percent
every week.

After γ-ray CT had been successfully applied to
short-term mineralization studies in humans, the question arose whether the equipment and the procedure
could also be used for longitudinal studies in small
animals. Preliminary measurements on hind limbs and
tails of rats verified that the instrument used on humans is also capable of micro-scans and reconstructing
images with pixels of 50 by 50 μm size. From computer
tomograms of tibias of growing rats it was possible to
quantify changes in mineralization due to weekly
growth. Hopefully this γ-ray CT will be a contributing
factor in accelerating osteoporosis research on small
animals as well as on man and in developing new thera-
pies of this widespread disease.

290

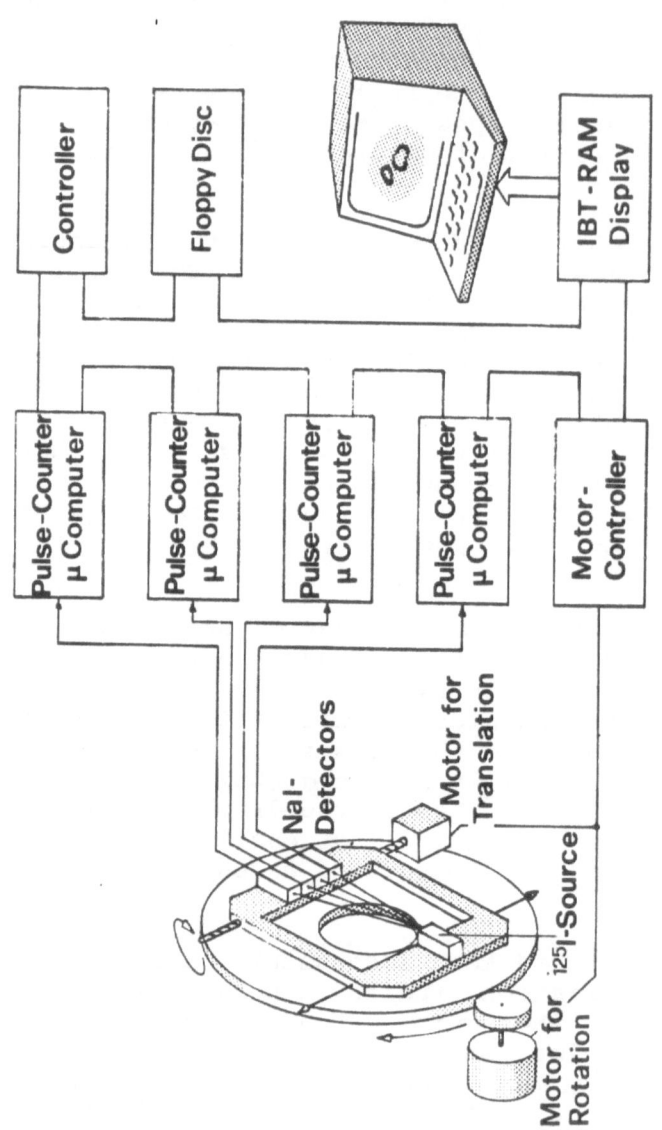

Fig. 15. Diagram of the γ-ray Computer Tomography System

Fig. 15. Diagram of the γ-ray Computer Tomography System

With the scanner illustrated, a thin section of the
forearm or the lower leg is irradiated by the linear
displacement of one or more finely collimated γ-rays
from an ^{125}I-source and the transmitted radiation, ie
the so-called shadow profile, is measured at the same
time. This scanning process is repeated N times, there
being a systematic change of the direction of radiation
by 180°/N and a reversal of the direction of the linear
displacement after each scan. The linear displacement
and the rotation are mediated by the computer-controlled
stepping motors for translational motion and rotation.
Thallium-activated NaI crystals optically coupled to
photomultipliers serve as a measuring device. On the
basis of the shadow profiles or projections generated
by the scanner an image of the cross section is re-
construced with the aid of a convolution algorithm.
The picture is defined by the linear absorption coefficients of pixels (picture elements) of the irradiated
section. For suitable visualization of this picture,
grey or colour tones are assigned to the absorption
coefficients, as may be seen in Fig. 16. With economi-
cal programming and the use of a modern microcomputer
the reconstruction of the cross-sectional picture is
also completed when the measurement is terminated. The
gradually forming picture is displayed by means of a
digital image storing unit and TV monitor during the
scanning process so that, in the event of any movement
artefacts being observed, the measurement can be discontinued and recommenced. A floppy disc is used to
store the raw data and the cross-sectional image.

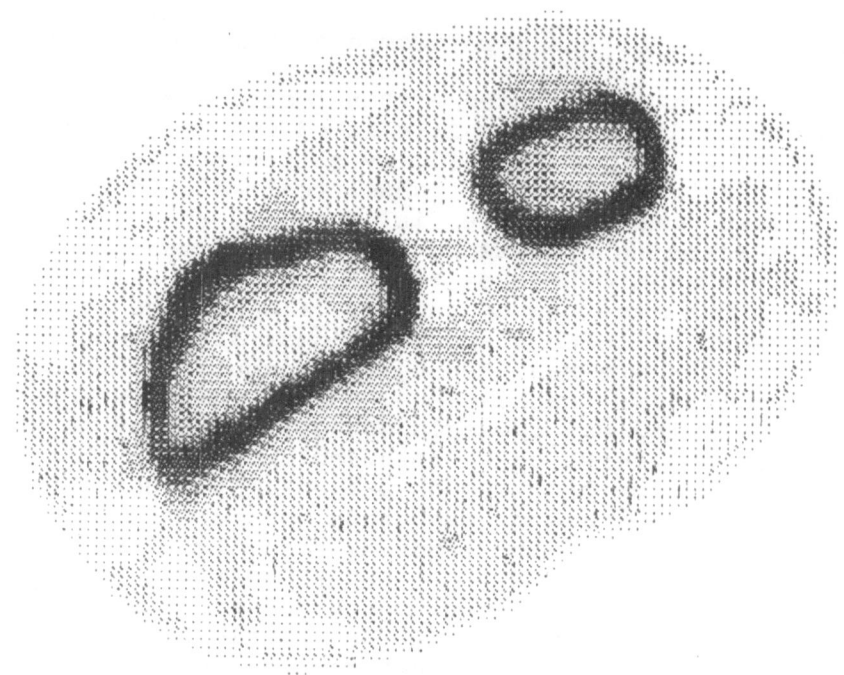

Fig. 16. Reconstructed Cross-sectional Image of the Right Forearm of a 71-year-old Test Subject

This computed tomogram corresponds to a section one-tenth of the way along the ulna from its distal end. From the distribution of the linear absorption coefficients it is possible to calculate various mineralization parameters such as the density of the spongiosa and the total mineral content of the radius. The picture was recorded by means of a Versatec plotter.

6. DISCUSSION AND CONCLUSIONS

Spongy bone material excised from knee condyles may
exhibit mechanical properties which differ from those
one would find under natural conditions. Aside from
disrupting the continuity of the trabecular bone structures by excising a cylindrical sample with relatively
small dimensions, the maceration process itself can be
expected to be responsible for some changes in the
mechanical behavior. As maceration can be achieved in
various ways, one must expect different degrees of alterations in the mechanical properties caused by different
procedures. For comparison purposes it is therefore
necessary to describe the method used for the bones for
which the results are presented here:
   1) Removal of soft tissue by immersion in 3 % anti-
      formin solution for 4-6 hours at less than
      60°C. Antiformin solution is a mixture of
      aqueous solutions of calcium chloride, sodium
      carbonate, and sodium hydroxide.
   2) Drying in air for 24-48 hours.
   3) Immersion in 3 % hydrogen peroxide solution for
      6-8 hours at less than 60°C.
   4) Air drying for 24-48 hours.
   5) Defatting with ether for 5-6 days at room tem-
      perature.
Bundy (5) has reviewed the effects of these steps on
the elastic moduli of compact bone and his findings
are considered as indicative of the changes to be expected in the spongy bone samples analyzed.

   Bundy concluded:
   1) Immersion in antiformin solution appears to have
      a negligible effect on the elastic moduli.
   2) Defatting in ether does not cause any measu-
      rable changes of the elastic moduli.
   3) Heating does not influence the elastic moduli
      as long as the temperature does not exceed
      60°C.
   4) Air drying produces a moderate increase in
      Young's modulus, reported at between 17-33 %
      by various investigators.
   5) Ratios of longitudinal to transverse Young's
      moduli and Young's to transverse shear moduli
      change by a small amount, on the order of
      3-4 % due to air drying.
Therefore the main change in the material making up

294

the trabecular framework of spongy bone during the
process of maceration could be an increase in E and G
up to about 33 %.

Pugh, Rose and Radin (6) report that no difference
could be seen between the Young's moduli of spongy bone
samples cut from the human knee condyles before and
after the removal of the marrow. Based on their studies
and their report of the work of Swanson and Freeman
(26), they assert that the intertrabecular marrow has
no influence on the elastic behavior of spongy bone in
the frequency range 0 to 300 Hz. It is difficult to
envision a large influence from marrow at 50'000 Hz.
Consequently it seems rather likely that the elastic
moduli of macerated trabecular bone given here are representative of the elastic moduli for trabecular bone
under natural conditions, with the exception of the
above-stated increase in both Young's and shear moduli
due to drying.

The frequency dependence of the Young's modulus
may be roughly estimated on the basis of the results
obtained by Pugh et al. (6). Their values for E at
frequencies between 100 and 3'000 Hz are within the
range of E values determined at 50 kHz and imply at
most a minor increase with frequency.

Eventhough the correlation of the elastic moduli
with the spongy bone density is barely acceptable, it
nevertheless reduces the need for developing a noninvasive method of measuring these parameters. In view
of the availability of computertomographic techniques
of quantifying the mineral distribution in human bones,
the bone density and accordingly also the elastic moduli
can be assessed with sufficient accuracy for most clinical purposes. Unless new reasons for direct evaluation
of the mechanical parameters can be identified, the
CT-techniques may prevail as the approach to be followed.

7. REFERENCES

1. B. Kummer, Biomechanics of Bone, in: Biomechanics, its Foundations and Objectives, Y.C. Fung, N. Perrone, M. Anliker, eds., Prentice Hall, New Jersey, 1972.
2. H.P. Vitalli, Knochenerkrankungen, Sandoz, Basel, 1970
3. P. Rüegsegger, U. Elsasser, M. Anliker, H. Gnehm, H. Kind, and A. Prader, Radiology, 121, 93, 1976.
4. M. Anliker, Triangle (Sandoz Basel), 16, No 3/4, 129, 1977.
5. K. Bundy, Experimental Studies of the Nonuniformity and Amisotropy of Human Compact Bone, Doctoral dissertation, Stanford University, 1975.
6. J.W. Pugh, R.M. Rose, and E.L. Radin, J. Biomechanics, 6, 475, 1973.
7. G.A. Thompson, Experimental Studies of Lateral and Torsional Vibrations of Intact Dog Radii, Doctoral dissertation, Stanford University, 1971.
8. D. Viano, U. Helfenstein, M. Anliker, and P. Rüegsegger, J. Biomechanics, 9, 703, 1976.
9. J.M. Jurist, and K. Kianian, J. Biomechanics, 6, 331, 1973.
10. J. Goodbread, M. Anliker, and P. Rüegsegger, J. Applied Math. and Phys. (ZAMP), 26, 735, 1975.
11. J. Goodbread, Mechanical Properties of Spongy Bone at Low Ultrasonic Frequencies, Doctoral dissertation No 5856, Swiss Fed. Inst. of Techn. Zurich, (ETHZ), 1976.
12. M. Anliker, Biomedizinische Technik in der medizinischen Praxis und Forschung, in: Forschung und Technik in der Schweiz, Haupt, Bern, 1978.
13. M. Anliker, M.B. Histand, and E. Ogden, Circulation Research, 23, 539, 1968.
14. M. Anliker, W.E. Moritz, and E. Ogden, J. Biomechanics, 1, 235, 1968.
15. S. Sizgoric, and A.A. Gundjian, Proc. IEEE, 57, 1313, 1969.
16. L.E. Nielson, Mechanical Properties of Polymers, N. Von Nostrand Reinhold, 1962.
17. W. Flügge, Handbook of Engineering Mechanics, McGraw Hill, 1962.
18. H. Kolsky, Stress Waves in Solids, Dover, N.Y., 1963.
19. J. Krautkrämer, and H. Krautkrämer, Ultrasonic Testing of Materials, Springer Verlag, Berlin, 1969.

20. H.J. McSkimin, in: Physical Acoustics, W.P. Mason ed., Plenum, New York, Vol. 1A, 1972.

21. R.N. Thurston, and P. Andreatch, cited by J.E. May, Physical Acoustics, Vol. 1A, Plenum, New York, 1972.

22. L.E. Nielson, Mechanical Properties of Polymers, N. Van Nostrand Reinhold, 1962.

23. U. Elsasser, Quantifizierung der Spongiosadichte an Röhrenknochen mittels Computertomographie, Doctoral dissertation, No. 5874, Swiss Federal Institute of Technology, Zurich, 1977.

24. G.U. Exner, E.P. Leumann, A. Prader, U. Elsasser, P. Rüegsegger, M. Anliker, to be published in British Journal of Radiology.

25. P. Rüegsegger, T. Hangartner, H.U. Keller,and T. Hinderling, Journal of Computer Assisted Tomography, 2, 184, 1978.

26. S.A.V. Swanson, and M.A.R. Freeman, Med. Biol. Engineering, 4, 433, 1966.

CONTINUUM MODELING OF HEAD INJURY

Nuri Akkaş

Department Of Civil Engineering, Middle East
Technical University, Ankara, Turkey

ABSTRACT. A review of continuum models proposed in connection
with head injuries is presented. The necessity of incorporating
the spinal cavity in future models is pointed out. Some nonlinear
aspects of head injury are discussed.

1. IMPORTANCE OF HEAD INJURY

The leading causes of death, in order of importance, are heart
disease, cancer and accidents. The first two occur at a median
age of 60 years, whereas the median age for accidental deaths is
20 years [1] . A recent study undertaken in the U.S. has revealed
that accidents are the leading cause of death between 1 and 40
years of age [2] . Among the survivors of accidents, a significant
percentage suffer some form of permanent disability. In all
accidents, the head is the leading target. In about 70% of the
people injured in motor vehicle accidents, the head is involved
[3] . The situation is even worse for children (birth through
11 years) : a frequency of 77% head injuries [4] . More than 2/3 of
the fatalities resulting from all accidents can be directly
attributed to craniocerebral trauma. This fact is evidence of the
disproportionate vulnerability of this part of the human body. In
motor vehicle accidents, the next leading cause of death is chest
injury which accounts for only 5% [5] .

 The information given above is enough to explain why the
mechanics of head injury has been the subject of an increasing
number of investigations within the last decades. Numerous
mathematical and experimental models have been developed for a
better understanding of the head injury mechanisms. This understanding

is vitally important in trying to design for vehicle impact
survival. The information to be gathered from the studies related
to the biomechanics of head injury will, hopefully, enhance the
neurosurgeon's capability to manage brain trauma.

2. SIMPLIFIED ANATOMY AND PHYSIOLOGY

In this section, some aspects of the craniospinal system, with
relation to the continuum models of head injury, are discussed.
In the preparation of this section, use has been made of the
following books and survey papers : [6-10] . A detailed presentation of the material properties of the various tissues of the
head is omitted. The "materials" aspect of head injury is discussed
in the following paper of this book.
     A cross section of the cerebral coverings is shown in Fig.1.
Note that the layer thicknesses are not in scale and the cross
section shown is not necessarily the same everywhere. The outermost
layer, the scalp, has a thickness of 5 to 10 mm. It is anisotropic
and nonhomogeneous. The scalp acts as an energy absorber and load
distributor in the transmission of the force to the brain. Its
resistance to compression increases with increasing deflection.
The thickness, firmness and mobility of the scalp are probably
important factors in guarding the skull from damage. The bony
framework of the head is termed the skull (cranium). It consists
of eight separate bones which are connected by sutures but are
immobile relative to one another. The skull is not a completely
closed system. The largest opening is the foramen magnum. The
skull thickness in the midplane shows considerable variation and
its average value is about 7 mm. The thickness increases toward
the base. The bones of the skull consist of compact inner and
outer tables and an intervening spongy middle layer called the
diploë. The cross section of a typical skull bone resembles an
engineering sandwich structure which consists of two stiff facings
separated by a low density core. The thicknesses of the bone layers
vary from place to place; however, on the average, the diploë is the
thickest. The diploë, which appears to be transversely isotropic,
consists of bone with fluid-filled interconnected cavities. It
reduces the weight of the skull without proportionately reducing
its strength and provides a material that will diminish the
transmission of vibrations.
     The next layer in Fig.1 is the dura. Under in vitro quasistatic
conditions, the mean elastic modulus of the dura mater was reported
to be about 6000 psi [11] . The in vivo experiments showed that
the dura mater is anisotropic and its circumferential and axial
Young's moduli are 3180 psi and 520 psi, respectively [10] . Its
shear modulus is about 25 psi. The dura is a tough, fibrous, dense
and relatively nonstretchable membrane. Within the cranium, it is
divided into two layers. The outer layer is firmly attached to the
inner surface of the skull bone. The inner layer forms the outermost

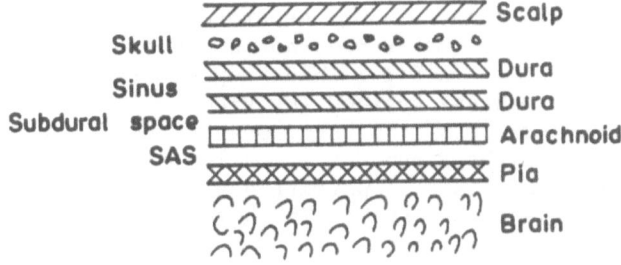

Fig. 1 Schematic view of cross section of
cerebral coverings.

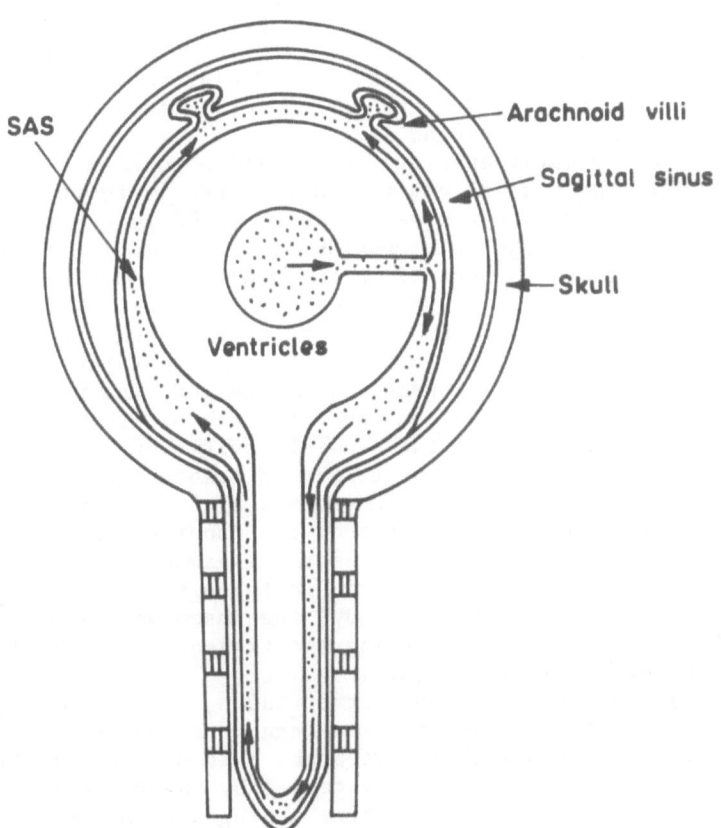

Fig. 2 Schematic view of craniospinal system
and CSF flow.

300

covering of the brain. The two **layers** of dura separate to form
the venous sinuses. The spinal dura mater does not duplicate the
intracranial arrangement, as shown in Fig.2 which represents the
mid-sagittal view of the craniospinal system. The arachnoid is
separated from the inner dura mater by the thin, noncommunicating
subdural space filled with a slight amount of lymphlike fluid. As
a result of this separation, the brain is permitted a small amount
of rotational movement relative to the skull. The arachnoid is
held to the dura by the surface tension of the subdural fluid and
it does not follow each indentation of the central nervous system
(CNS), but rather tends to bridge over the gaps. The next membrane
is the thin, delicate and highly vascular pia mater which is
separated from the arachnoid by the subarachnoid space (SAS). Fine
strands of connective tissue, the arachnoid trabeculae, bridge the
SAS. Through the interstices of the meshwork of connective tissue,
the cerebrospinal fluid (CSF) percolates. The pia adheres closely
to the surface of the brain and the spinal cord following every
indentation. Thus, several large spaces, called cisterns, are
formed in the SAS. The dura mater, the arachnoid and the pia mater
are collectively called the meninges.

The brain is the greatly enlarged and modified portion of the
CNS. It nearly fills the cranial cavity and is approximately
spherical. The average adult brain weighs about 1,400 gm and it is
about 1,200 cm^3 in volume. The bulk modulus of the brain in vitro
is 300,000 psi, very close to that of water. Its shear modulus is
much lower. The brain consists of 78% water, 10-12% phospholipids,
8% protein and small amounts of other substances. A freshly excised
brain creeps under its weight. It is in relative hydrostatic
equilibrium in the buoyant medium provided by the CSF. The weight
of the brain in the CSF envelope is about one-tenth of its actual
weight. The brain is suspended in the cranial cavity very effectively
by the blood vessels, nerve roots and arachnoid trabeculae.

The boundary conditions for head movements are represented
by the neck structure. The neck consists of the upper seven
vertebrae of the vertebral column, muscles and ligaments of various
sorts. In untensed condition, the neck can go through a 120^0 motion.
When a dynamic load is applied to the body, the muscular state of
the neck is an important factor affecting the trajectory of the head
and, hence, the severity of head injury.

There is a cylindrical column of nerve tissue, continuous
with the brain, extending from the foramen magnum to the level
between the first and second lumbar vertebrae. This portion of the
CNS, the spinal cord, is enclosed and protected by the vertebral
column. The cord is surrounded by the three meninges also; however,
now there is only one layer of the dura mater as shown in Fig.2.
The SAS extends below the level of the spinal cord.

There are two fluids circulating in the cranial and spinal
cavities. These are the blood and the CSF. The blood is a non-
Newtonian fluid consisting of plasma and cellular elements. The
CNS has a very rich blood supply. For the whole brain of an adult

human, the cerebral blood flow (CBF) is roughly 800 ml/min. At any
moment, there is 75 ml of blood present in the brain. The blood
supply to the brain is basically derived from the internal carotid
arteries and the vertebral arteries. The venous drainage from the
brain basically occurs through the internal jugular veins, the
paravertebral veins to the spinal cord and the emissary vessels
through the skull. Most of the venous blood of the brain drains
into the dural sinuses, located between the two layers of the dura
mater, and from there to the base of the skull. Some of the blood
in the dural sinuses may also flow into the veins in the scalp
through the emissary veins through the skull. The emissary veins
act as pressure valves; hence, they are probably effective in
assisting to regulate, at least locally, the sudden changes in the
intracranial pressure (ICP). Autoregulatory control of the CBF
also has an effect on regulating the ICP. The blood vessels are
more or less elastic thin-walled tubes showing large deformation
capability. There are smooth muscles within the vessels. When the
pressure outside the vessel is greater than the blood pressure,
which corresponds to, for instance, a drop in blood pressure, the
smooth muscles relax and the vessels dilate. When the case is
reversed, for instance an increase in blood pressure, the muscles
contract and the vessels constrict.

Within the brain tissue, there is a series of interconnecting
cavities called the ventricular system. The CSF, for the most part,
is formed in the ventricles. It is a clear, colorless and nearly
Newtonian liquid consisting of water, protein, gases in solution
and organic constituents. The specific gravity of the CSF is about
1.007. The ventricles, the central canal of the spinal cord and
the SAS are all filled with this fluid. The total CSF volume in a
normal adult is approximately 140 ml of which about 80 ml is in
the ventricles and the rest in the SAS. On an average, 500 ml of
CSF is formed daily. The pressure generated by the CSF secretion
results in the flow of the fluid. The choroid plexuses in the
ventricular systems can be considered to act as a faucet. As shown
in Fig.2, the CSF produced by this faucet enters the ventricles
and flowing through certain foramina empties first into the
subarachnoid cisterns which communicate freely with the SAS
enveloping the CNS. Thus, the CSF slowly circulates through the
SAS. The drainage of the CSF out of the SAS is considered to be
through the arachnoid villi into the dural venous sinuses, Fig.2.
The villi could be considered fingerlike herniations of the
arachnoid into the dura. The CSF inside the villi passes into the
blood, probably through the mesh work of channels which has a
valve-like role. When the CSF pressure in the SAS is larger by a
certain amount than the venous pressure in the dural sinus, the
"valves" open and permit the CSF to flow into the venous blood.
When the venous pressure is larger than the CSF pressure, the tubes
in the arachnoid villi collapse and the "valve" closes, Fig.3. Thus,
the blood can not flow into the SAS. The "valves" open when the
pressure difference is of the order of 25-50 mm saline [7] . It is

302

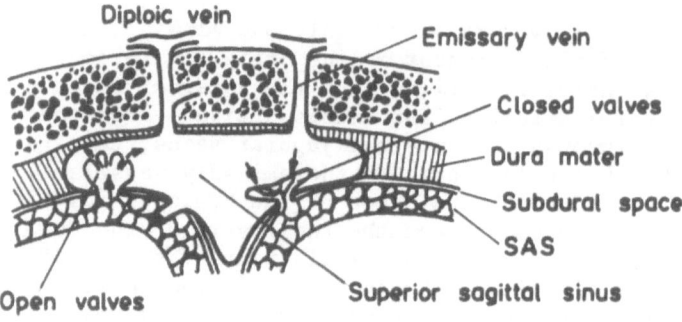

Fig. 3   CSF flow into venous blood

generally accepted that the CSF system, together with the autoregulatory control system of the CBF, very likely plays an
important role in protection of the brain against injury.

3. PROPOSED MECHANISMS OF HEAD INJURY

In this section, head injury is broadly defined as the externally
produced temporary or permanent damage to the cranial vault and
to the CNS. Head injuries produced by static loading are not
discussed. Moreover, it is assumed that dynamic loading, which may
lead to brain injury, leaves the dura intact in which case it is
called a closed brain injury. Impacts by sharp objects such as
bullets, shell fragments, etc., that usually penetrate the skull
and dura are not considered.
      With the limitations given above, there are roughly two
possible ways of dynamic load application which may lead to head
injuries. In a direct loading case (A of Fig.4), the head collides
with another object. The head of the occupant striking the windshield in head-on car collisions is subjected to this type of
loading. In an indirect loading case (B of Fig.4), the head is not
in direct contact with any object. It is the torso which undergoes
sudden changes in its motion. The loading which occurs as the result
of rear end automobile impacts is of this second type. The extent
of head injury depends upon the type of loading as well as its
magnitude, duration, location and direction. Generally speaking,
head injuries can be grouped into four categories [9] : scalp
damage, skull fracture, extracerebral bleeding or hematoma, and
brain damage. The first three are invariably generated by a direct
impact, whereas a direct impact or an indirect loading can cause
brain injury which is the most serious type. To be able to understand the bases of the proposed mechanisms of brain damage, it is
in order to discuss the possible response of the head-neck system
shown in Fig.4 under either type of loading.

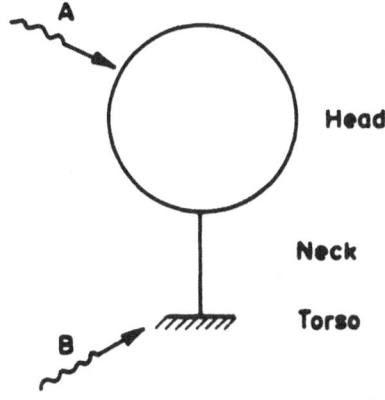

Fig. 4   Load   application   to   head

A blow to the head initiates stress waves which propagate
from the site of the blow through the scalp and the skull into
the intracranial contents. The waves propagating in the medium
filling the cranial cavity eventually encompass the entire volume
and reflect internally. Along with those through the central region,
stress waves propagate around the skull also. There is a strong
tendency for geometrical convergence of these waves near the antipole.
The distortion of the skull around the impact pole by the blow is
called "contact phenomenon". At the contact point the skull is first
forced inward, then it rebounds to its normal position and probably
a little beyond for a brief instant, and in the meantime, producing
additional waves. The characteristic transit time required for a
wave to travel across the head either along the skull or through
the brain is of the order of 0.1-0.2 msec.

A free-floating body subjected to an external force will
accelerate. If the resultant force passes through the center of
mass of the body, the acceleration will be purely translational.
Otherwise, a rotational acceleration will also be imparted. It is
extremely unusual that the resultant force of a direct impact passes
through the center of mass of the head. Moreover, the head is not
a free-floating body but it is pivoted to the neck. Therefore, a
direct impact, even if it is assumed that its resultant passes
through the center of mass of the head, will cause both translation
and rotation of the head. In the case of an indirect loading, both
motions will definitely occur. If the head is given a translational
acceleration, the intracranial contents, having a rigidity less
than that of the skull, lag behind the skull. A pressure gradient
develops across the skull. If the head is imparted a rotational
acceleration, the brain, although connected to the skull by numerous

blood vessels and nerves, still lags behind it.

If the duration of the loading is, at most, of the same order as the characteristic transit time, the response of the head is dominated by the wave propagation effects and, for all practical purposes, the constraint of the neck can be ignored. For impacts with longer durations, translational and rotational motions dominate the response of the head. In this case, the constraining effects of the neck should not be ignored in the response analysis. If the load duration is much longer than the transit time, it is reasonable to ignore the stress wave propagation [9,12] .

The following major injury mechanisms have been proposed by various investigators over the past few decades to clarify trauma of the CNS [9,10] :

a. Injury mechanism associated with translational acceleration: Large pressure gradients are initiated in the brain. The propagation of stress waves, their geometric focusing and the relative linear displacement of the brain with respect to the skull are the possible causes of these gradients. In certain regions of the brain, the ICP is considerably reduced. This underpressure may be sufficient to rupture the capillary walls. The transcapillary pressure is normally only a few mm Hg. A sudden decrease in the surrounding tissue pressure causes a sudden increase in the pressure differential across the capillary wall. The regulatory system is slow in providing an equilibrium state. If the transcapillary pressure acts over a sufficiently long period of time, the capillaries will rupture. At some points within the brain, the rarefaction pressure may be reduced to near its vapor pressure. In this case, cavitation bubbles may be formed. Their subsequent violent collapse could produce trauma. In addition to capillary rupturing and bubble collapse, the separation of the brain from the cranial wall at the antipole and neurovascular friction may be other possible causes of brain damage.

b. Injury mechanism associated with rotational acceleration: The relative angular motion between the skull and its contents produces sizable shear strains in the brain matter. The bulk modulus of brain tissue is considerably larger than its shear modulus. The local stresses will, therefore, be approximately proportional to the shear strain. Accordingly, the shear strain, rather than the compressional effects, can be regarded as being responsible for the rupturing of the cerebral blood vessels, axons and the tissue [13] . Contusions and lacerations of the soft tissue can be caused also by the rough protuberances on the inner surface of the skull during the angular motion of the brain. Shear strains in the brain tissue can be produced by the translational acceleration of the head as well. However, according to Holburn [13], they could be neglected compared to the shear strains produced by the rotational acceleration.

c. Injury mechanism associated with cranial volume change: The ICP changes in head impact are caused by the change in cranial volume also. The local distortion of the skull by the blow and the vibration of the entire skull are the possible causes of this volume change. If there is an increase in the cranial volume, the

CSF may start flowing in to fill up the extra space. However, the inflow is much slower than the volume increase. In the process, cavitation bubbles may be formed. This view has been named the structural, as opposed to the wave propagation, theory of cavitation [14].

d. Injury mechanism associated with brain stem : At the region of craniocervical junction, tissue has a tendency to be extruded or sucked in when the head is subjected to an external blow. This probably results in the development of high shear stresses and/or pressure gradients in the brain stem which may produce trauma. The existence of pressure gradients of this type has been validated experimentally by various investigators [15].

e. Injury mechanism associated with cervical cord and neck : During a bending, twisting or other rotation of the head on the neck, the upper cervical cord undergoes flexion-extension and/or bending. If neck motion exceeds tolerable limits, the cervico-spinal components are distorted excessively. This may lead to damage of ligaments, nerve roots, intervertebral disks, blood vessels and the spinal cord itself.

There appears to be no reason why the mechanisms cited above, all together or in combinations, can not be effective in producing brain injury. These proposed mechanisms are probably the extremes among which all sorts of intermediate actions are possible. The characteristics of the impact and its location are the factors to be taken into account in deciding which mechanism predominates the injury.

4. CONTINUUM MODELS

The first mathematical treatment of continuum type head injury models apparently goes back to 1943 [16]. Except one published in 1950 [17], there appears to be no other pertinent work contained in the literature for more than two decades. Goldsmith's paper [18] seems to have provided the impetus for the sudden increase in the number of the mathematical head injury models. More than 30 mathematical models have been developed since then. A detailed classification of mathematical models of the head impact is given by King and Chou [19]. This classification, in a modified and updated form, is given in Table 1. The lumped parameter models and the investigations dealing only with steady state solutions are not included. An overall study of Table 1 reveals that the models can be grouped in more or less the same manner as the major head injury mechanisms discussed previously. The mathematical difficulties associated with modelling the complex geometry of the head are circumvented by using spherical or cylindrical shapes. In the models which simulate more closely the actual skull and brain geometry, numerical discretization techniques, especially finite elements, are used. In none of the models given in Table 1, is the spinal cord included; although some finite element models contain the foramen magnum.

306

Table 1. Classification of continuum models of head impact

		Shell	Core	Reference
Translation	Cylind. tube	Rigid	Fluid	Hayashi [20], Liu and Chandran [21], Liu [22]
		Elastic	Fluid	Kopecky and Ripperger [23]
	Spherical	Rigid	Fluid	Anzelius [16], Güttinger [17], Liu and Chandran [24]
			Pseudo elastic	Chandran et al. [25]
			Maxwell fluid	Chandran et al. [26]
		Elastic	Fluid	Engin [34], Engin and Roberts [39], Kenner and Goldsmith [35], Liu et al. [37], Akkaş [28], Benedict et al. [31], Chan and Liu [33], Merchant and Crispino [36], Gordon et al. [27], Khalil and Hubbard [30], Shugar and Katona [29], Lee and Advani [32]
			Elastic	Advani and Owings [46]
		Viscoel.	Viscoelastic	Hickling and Wenner [48], Chan [49]
	Nonspherical	Elastic	Fluid	Merchant and Crispino [36], Khalil and Hubbard [30]
		Viscoel.	Viscoelastic	Chan [49]
Rotation	Spherical	Rigid	Elastic	Lee and Advani [51], ByCroft [52], Liu and Chandran [53], Liu et al. [54]
			Viscoelastic	Lee and Advani [51], Ljung [50], ByCroft [52], Liu et al. [54], Chandran et al. [26]
Translation and Rotation	Spherical	Elastic	Fluid	Landkof et al. [12]
	Actual Geometry (FEM)	Rigid	Elastic	Ward and Thompson [56]
		Elastic	Fluid and Elastic and Viscoelastic	Shugar and Katona [29], Shugar [64]

4.1 Translation

Cylindrical tube. The one-dimensional model proposed by Hayashi
[20] is the simplest continuum model by which the brain injury
mechanism associated with translational acceleration can be studied.
The Hayashi model consists of a rigid-walled but massless cylindrical
tube filled with an inviscid, compressible fluid and padded by a
spring k. The model was improved later by Liu and Chandran [21]
by taking the mass m of the rigid tube into consideration and also
adding a dashpot d into the system (Fig. 5a). The spring and dashpot
combination represents the elastic and dissipative properties of
the biological components plus any protective cover. The cylinder
and the fluid represent the skull and the intracranial contents,
respectively. When the vessel strikes a rigid barrier with velocity
v , a direct loading case, a pressure variation along the direction
of impact occurs. The response is governed by the spatially one-
dimensional wave equation with appropriate boundary and initial
conditions. Hayashi obtained an infinite series solution to the
massless problem without the damper, utilizing a separation of
variables technique. Liu [22] obtained a finite series solution to
the same problem using Laplace transform techniques. Later, Liu
and Chandran [21] presented a finite series solution to the improved
version of the problem also. The Hayashi model has obvious shortcomings. Since the cylinder is rigid-walled, the skull deformation
and, hence its effects on the ICP, can not be investigated. In
spite of its shortcomings, the study of this simple model shed some
light on the cavitation theory of brain injury. According to the
results given in Liu [22], the pressure distribution (relative to
ambient conditions) along the cylinder is skew-symmetric about the
center. The pressure fields in the container at various times are
shown schematically in Fig. 5b. The wave-propagation nature of the
problem is obvious. The maximum negative pressure always occurs at
the antipole. If the pressure at this point drops below the vapor
pressure, cavitation bubbles are presumably formed.

In a similar vein, Kopecky and Ripperger [23] computed pressures
developed in a fluid-filled elastic cylindrical tube with rigid ends
during constant acceleration along its longitudinal axis. The
undeformed and exaggerated deformed configurations of the model are
shown in Fig.6a. The unknowns in the problem are the pressure at
the top of the shell and the deformed shell configuration. The
shell deflection can be expressed in terms of the unknown pressure
using appropriate linear shell equations. To determine the unknown
pressure the idea of conservation of mass for the fluid is introduced.
The results indicate that a negative pressure develops at the top
end of the cylinder and it is linearly proportional to acceleration.
At a given acceleration, the negative pressure varies nonlinearly
with both shell stiffness and fluid bulk modulus. As shown in Fig.6b,
the pressure distribution along the tube is linear. The point of
zero pressure change can occur anywhere along the axis, its location
being dependent on the shell stiffness. The results of this model

308

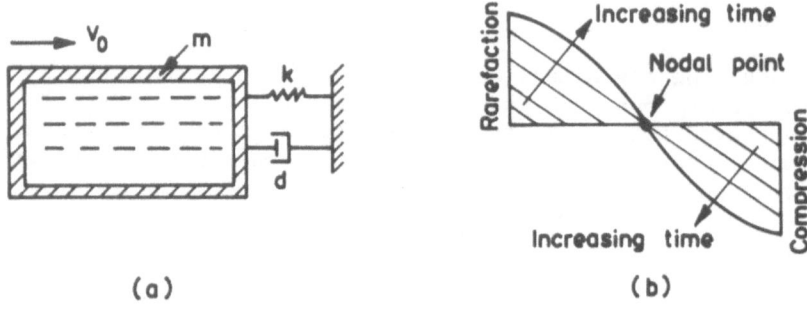

(a)   (b)

Fig. 5   (a) Improved   Hayashi   model   and   (b) pressure
fields   in   container

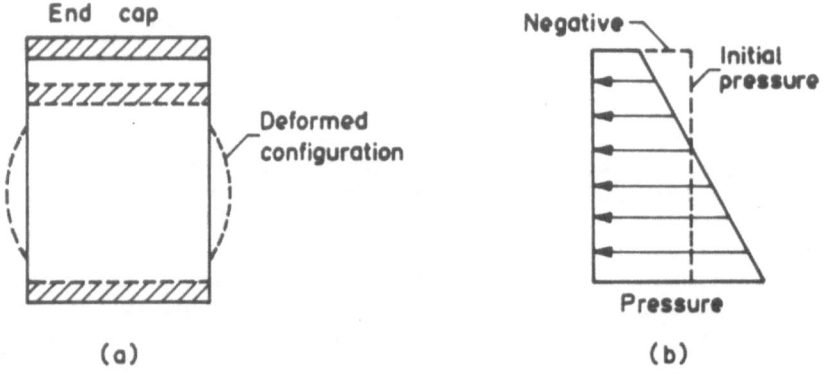

(a)   (b)

Fig. 6 (a) Kopecky – Ripperger   model   and   (b) pressure
distribution   due   to   acceleration , [23].

show that cavitation is possible in an indirect loading case also.
    Rigid spherical shell. Spherical models obviously approximate
the shape of the human head better than cylindrical models. The
first mathematical models of craniocerebral trauma were fluid-filled
rigid spherical shells. Anzelius [16] and later Güttinger [17]
stuied the pressure wave propagation in the fluid when its rigid
spherical container is subjected to a sudden impulse load. The
fluid is inviscid and compressible. In [16], the container, initially
traveling with constant translational velocity, is brought to a
sudden stop. Güttinger [17] studied the case in which the container
is initially at rest and it is suddenly accelerated to a prescribed
constant velocity. The two problems differ primarily in the form of
the initial conditions. The coupling between the fluid and the shell
is eliminated because of the rigid shell assumption. Thus, the
problem is reduced to an axisymmetric solution of the classical wave
equation in spherical coordinates. Utilizing a separation of
variables technique, both Anzelius and Güttinger obtained an infinite

series solution to the wave equation for their appropriate boundary and initial conditions. Recently, Liu and Chandaran [24] presented a finite series solution of the problem. The conclusions obtained from numerical evaluation of these models can be summarized as follows. An initial compression wave is generated at the point of impact. As a consequence of the assumption of a rigid container, a tension wave is simultaneously emitted from the antipole. The two waves propagate toward the center of the sphere and they eventually collide. Thus, at this point, a situation is produced in which the pressure is zero but the pressure gradients are large. The negative pressure and the large pressure gradients may be considered to be causes of brain trauma.

A possible way of extending the Anzelius-Güttinger model is to simulate the brain as an elastic or viscoelastic medium but keeping the rigid shell assumption. Chandran et al. [25,26] considered this modified model. In [25], the rigid spherical shell contains an elastic core with a very low modulus. This assumption is essentially the same as assuming that the medium is incompressible and, hence, has an infinite bulk wave speed. Accordingly, no pressure wave propagation is possible within the shell. Translational acceleration of the container induces shear waves only. This situation is exactly the opposite of that in the acoustic core model of Anzelius and Güttinger, in which only pressure wave propagation is possible. Chandran et al. [25] conclude that a model with at least a Maxwell fluid in the container is needed in order to yield both pressure and shear stress variations. Such a model, which consists of a rigid spherical shell filled with Maxwell fluid, is analyzed in [26]. According to the results presented in [26], brain matter may get damaged by the induced shear stress well before the negative pressure can cause cavitation, even though the acceleration is purely translational. The shear stress values are comparable with, sometimes even larger than, the pressure values. In [26], the very high bulk modulus of the brain is excluded in the constitutive equation; hence, the pressure is of very low magnitude. The general conclusion of these two works [25,26] is that the contents of the intracranial cavity should be modeled neither as an acoustic fluid only nor as a Maxwell fluid only, if a better simulation of the pressure and shear stress distribution is desired.

Elastic shell-fluid core. The obvious necessity of modeling the skull as an elastic shell has been pointed out by Goldsmith [18]. The possible locations of skull fracture and the effect of the skull vibration on the ICP can be analyzed by such a model only. The investigations in which the head is modeled as a spherical elastic shell filled with an inviscid and compressible fluid are many, as shown in Table 1. The main differences among these investigations are due either to the type and duration of loading considered or to the shell theory used. In Gordon et al. [27], Akkaş [28] and Shugar and Katona [29], the skull is modeled as a three- layered sandwich shell. In Khalil and Hubbard [30], the scalp is also considered, so the shell has four layers. In the other references cited, the skull is assumed to be homogeneous.

Except for Benedict et al. [31] who use extensional shell theory
only, both extensional and bending effects of the shell are included
in the investigations. Lee and Advani [32] and Chan and Liu [33],
in addition to membrane and bending effects, consider rotatory
inertia and shear deformation effects also. Thus, their analyses
are valid for moderately thick shells. In the following, a discussion
of some of the investigations cited will be presented in more detail.
However, the emphasis will be on those results of the analyses
which are related to brain injury rather than to skull fracture.

Consider an elastic, homogeneous, spherical shell filled with
an inviscid, irrotational and compressible fluid (Fig.7). The shell
is subjected to an axisymmetric arbitrary time-dependent pressure
pulse over a given cap angle. The linear equations governing the
response of this shell-fluid system can be written in the following
symbolic form :

$$L_{11}u + L_{12}w + A_1\ddot{u} = 0 , \tag{1}$$

$$L_{21}u + L_{22}w + A_2\ddot{w} = A_3 p_e + A_4 p_f \quad (r=a), \tag{2}$$

$$\frac{1}{r^2} \frac{\partial}{\partial r} \left(r^2 \frac{\partial \Phi}{\partial r}\right) + \frac{1}{r^2 \text{Sin}\phi} \frac{\partial}{\partial \phi} \left(\text{Sin}\phi \frac{\partial \Phi}{\partial \phi}\right) = \frac{1}{c_f^2} \ddot{\Phi} , \tag{3}$$

in which u and w are the meridional and radial displacements of the
shell, respectively. Φ is the velocity potential and c_f is the speed
of sound in the fluid. The external pressure, which is a function
of meridional angle ϕ and time t, is denoted by p_e. Equation (3) is
the classical axisymmetric wave equation. A_i (i=1,...,4) are constants
depending upon the modulus of elasticity E, Poisson ratio ν and the
density ρ_s of the shell material, the radius a and the thickness h
of the shell, and the density ρ_f of the fluid. L_{ij} (i,j=1,2) are
differential operators containing derivatives with respect to ϕ and
the parameters a, h and ν. Finally, dots denote derivatives with
respect to time. Equations (1) − (3) have been developed and solved
analytically first by Engin [34] for the Dirac-delta pulse. Additional
equations for the shell behavior are needed if it is desired to use
the sandwich shell theory [28] or the one in which rotatory inertia
and shear deformation effects are included [32,33]. The formulation
of the problem is completed by ascribing the appropriate boundary
and initial conditions. One of them is the kinematic boundary condition which states that the radial velocities of the shell and the
fluid at the interface are equal for all ϕ and t, and it is given by

$$\dot{w}(\phi,t) = \frac{\partial \Phi}{\partial r} (a,\phi,t). \tag{4}$$

A slip interface condition is assumed in the meridional direction.
Finally, the pressure in the fluid is given by

$$p_f = -\rho_f \dot{\Phi} . \tag{5}$$

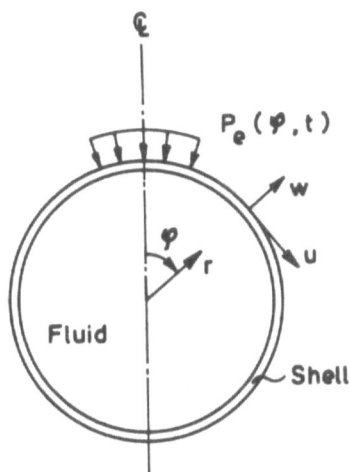

Fig. 7 Axisymmetric elastic shell - fluid core model

The solution to the coupled shell-fluid equations can be obtained
through analytical means [34,35] , finite difference techniques
[28,31,36] or the finite element method [29,30].

In their analyses, Benedict et al. [31] and Akkaş [28] use
the same axisymmetric forcing function which is

$$p_e = 2500 \exp \{-4.73 \ (\tfrac{t}{T})^2\} \ \mathrm{Sin}(\tfrac{\pi t}{T}) \ \mathrm{Cos}(5\phi) \ \mathrm{psi}, \qquad (6)$$

in which T is the duration of the load and it is assumed to be
1 msec. Benedict et al. [31] use extensional shell theory, whereas
Akkaş [28] uses sandwich shell theory in which both membrane and
bending effects are included. Considering both bending and membrane
effects, the author obtained the corresponding solution for a
homogeneous shell also. The pertinent shell and fluid properties
used in these investigations are comparable. In all three of the
solutions, finite difference techniques are used. Therefore, to
make a comparison of the numerical results would be reasonable.
However, the finite differencing schemes used in approximating the
time derivatives are not the same. In addition, the spatial mesh
sizes and the time increments are also different. Figure 8 gives
the impact pole pressure as a function of time for the three different
shell theories investigated. The purpose of presenting this figure
is to show not the effect of using different shell theories on the
ICP but, rather, that the curves are alike. Thus, the conclusions
obtained are in agreement and they can be summarized as follows.
The pressure fluctuations are greatest near the skull-brain interface. They are damped as the geometrical center is approached. The
impact pole pressure, which is initially compressive, becomes tensile
as the skull snaps back. The counterpole pressure is always tensile.
These regions of negative pressure are conceivable sources of brain

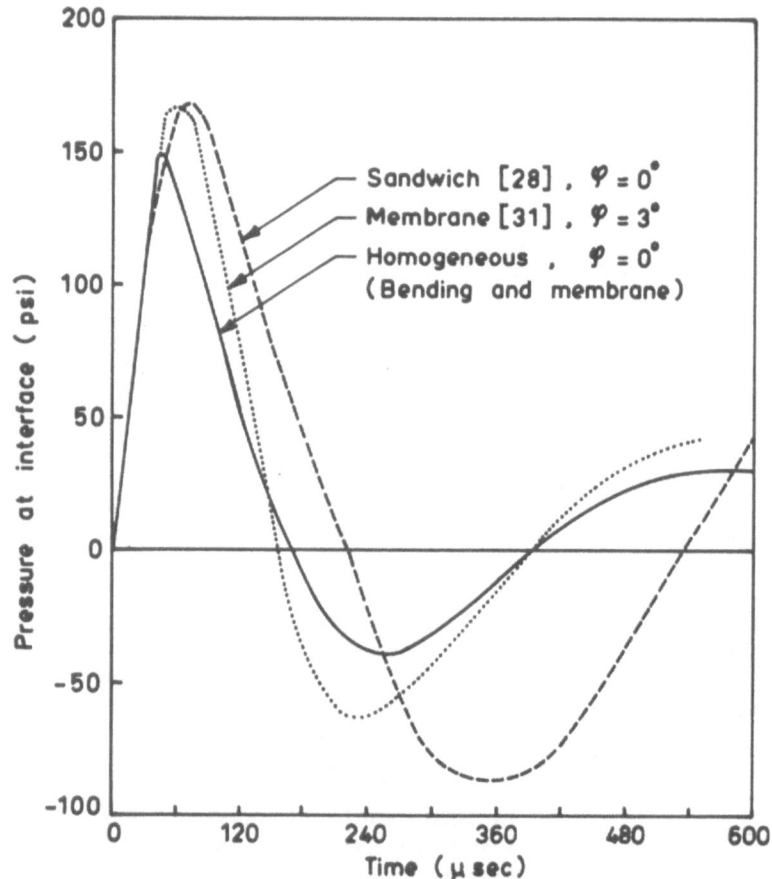

Fig. 8 Impact pole pressure as a function of time.

damage. The negative pressure at the impact point, which is highly localized, is greater in magnitude than that at the counterpole, which is more diffuse. If one is interested in the ICP variations only, use of extensional shell theory is sufficient to obtain the needed qualitative information. However, for a better understanding of the stress distribution in the skull, it is necessary to use a higher-order shell theory.

The duration of the impact has a significant effect in determining the type, location and severity of brain damage. A Dirac-delta type impulse represents an extreme case. This type of loading has been used by Engin [34] and Chan and Liu [33]. In both, the impulsive load has a constant magnitude of 546.5 psi on a polar cap angle of 15^0. In [33], there is also a constant tangential traction acting over the same area. Since the fluid core is inviscid, the rotation of the shell due to the asymmetric loading does not influence the core directly. Engin's results on the pressure in the fluid indicate that high regions of negative pressure occur near the quarter positions along the axis of symmetry, rather than at the poles. The negative pressure occuring at approximately halfway between the center and the antipole is larger; hence, there is a strong possibility of an "intermediate coup" at this location. The negative pressure at this point is more than 3000 psi, but it is highly localized. Chan and Liu's findings support Engin's results; however, the addition of the tangential traction shifts the location of the maximum negative pressure closer to the geometric center. If one defines the amplification factor as the ratio of the maximum negative pressure to the intensity of the external pressure, this factor is about five in [33,34,37] for the Dirac-delta type impulse. The same mathematical model has been analyzed by Kenner and Goldsmith [35] and Merchant and Crispino [36] for the case of an impact load of finite duration. In the first, the pulse durations considered vary between 50 μsec and 600 μsec. In the second, the duration is 61.4 μsec. The numerical results indicate that the amplification factor is less than one. The results of [36], which are obtained via an explicit finite difference technique, are confirmed by Shugar and Katona [29] using the finite element method (FEM). The maximum rarefactions in the models of these studies did not occur at the points identified by Engin [34] but occurred near the impact point. The results of Kenner and Goldsmith [35], Merchant and Crispino [36], Benedict et al. [31] and Akkaş [28], which are for finite time pulses, are all in qualitative agreement in spite of the differences in the approaches and the pulse durations.

The pulse durations used in the investigations cited in the previous paragraph are all equal to or less than 1 msec. On the other hand, Khalil and Hubbard [30], in their parametric study of head injury modeled as a free-floating body, select a pulse duration of 4 msec. In addition to the effect of the shape of the shell on the response, they also study the effects of loading duration by varying the period of load from 2 to 12 msec for one of their models. Their numerical results, which are obtained via the FEM, indicate that the model response may be regarded as a vibrational motion of the shell superimposed on a rigid body motion of the shell-fluid system. The fluid pressure (the stresses in the shell also) versus time curves follow closely the external load history. In other words, the system response is governed by its inertial characteristics. It should be noted that, as stated in the previous section, for impacts with long durations, the constraining effect of the neck, which is not considered in [30], should not be ignored in the response analysis. According to the conclusions of [30], the fluid pressure distributions along the impact axis are almost linear with the compressive components near the impact pole changing to tensile at the antipole. The back of the skull pulls away from the brain and thus produces negative pressure as required by the cavitation hypothesis of brain damage. At the antipole site, the rarefaction pressures developed in another model comprised of segments of two spheres and a cone are higher in magnitude than those developed in the spherical models. This is stated to be largely due to the longer pole-to-pole distance of the sphere-cone-sphere model. A similar conclusion has been obtained by Merchant and Crispino [36].

In 36 , the head is modeled as an elastic spherical fluid-filled shell and also as a prolate ellipsoid of revolution. The numerical results given are very suitable for a comparative study of the effects of the shell shape on the ICP. The duration of the rectangular pulse used is 61.4 μsec for both models and its magnitude is 540 psi. The fluid pressure versus time curves for the impact pole are shown in Fig.9 for both the spherical and ellipsoidal models. There is no amplification of the input pulse pressure. The maximum rarefactions in both models occur near the point of application, at the same time and at the same distance from the loading point. Therefore, the geometry of the model does not affect the location nor the time of occurrence of the critical negative pressure. However, the magnitude of the rarefaction pressure in the ellipsoidal model is about 1.5 times as large as that in the spherical model. In a similar vein, Talhouni and DiMaggio [38] model the head as an elastic prolate spheroidal shell enclosing an acoustic medium. A uniform step pressure is suddenly applied over the whole shell surface, a loading case which is not common in head injury analysis.

The ICP variations in a fluid-filled elastic spherical shell, having a uniform velocity for t< 0 and brought to a sudden stop at t=0, have been investigated by Engin and Roberts [39]. This is a loading mechanism similar to the one used by Anzelius [16] and Güttinger [17] in their rigid shell models. The spherical shell equations include both membrane and bending effects. The governing equations of the shell-fluid system have the same form as Equations (1-3), but now the initial conditions are different. The analytical solution shows that in the equatorial plane, which is perpendicular to the direction of impulse, pressure is zero at all times, as was the case for the Anzelius-Güttinger model. The pressures at the points located symmetrically with respect to the equatorial plane have the same magnitude but opposite sign. The maximum negative pressures occur at the poles. Engin and Roberts [39] obtain the pressure variations in a rigid shell also. Their comparative results indicate that the pressure in the brain is reduced considerably when the elasticity of the shell is taken into acount.

Before closing this section on the elastic shell-acoustic core head models subjected to translational acceleration, it should be mentioned that the effects of pulse shape [40,35,41], pulse duration [42,43,44,30], head size [45,43,30], local radial load contact angle [30] and skull bending stiffness [30,41] on the ICP distributions have also been investigated.However, a discussion of these aspects is left out for the sake of brevity.

Elastic or viscoelastic core. An obvious improvement of the elastic shell-fluid core models of the head would be to treat the

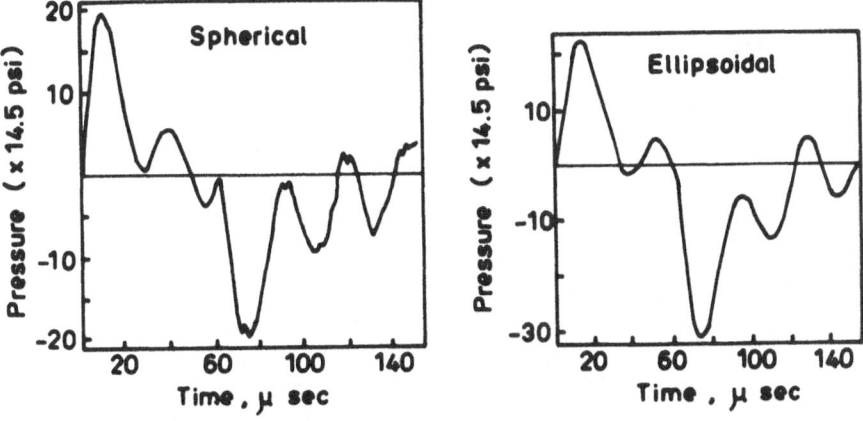

Fig. 9 Impact pole pressure - time history in spherical and ellipsoidal models , [36].

brain as an elastic or viscoelastic medium. Shear stresses will also develop in such a core when the head is subjected to an axisymmetric impact causing translational acceleration only.

Advani and Owings [46] model the head as an elastic, free-floating spherical shell containing an elastic core. The boundary conditions used require the continuity of the radial and meridional displacements and radial and shear tractions at the interface. Although such an interface condition is probably more realistic than the slip interface condition used in the fluid-core models, apparently it is "severe", since it is known that the brain can have a small amount of relative meridional displacement with respect to the skull. The head is subjected to an axisymmetric, local radial load with a te^{-t} variation in time. Since the skull bones and the brain tissue are assumed to be linear, isotropic and homogeneous, the motion of the model is governed by Navier's equations of elastodynamics. Using the modal acceleration method, Advani and Owings obtain an infinite series solution to the governing equations. The numerical results are presented for a peak head acceleration of 150g and impact duration of 20 msec. This duration is much longer than the characteristic transit time and, hence, not considering the constraining effect of the neck is unreasonable. Moreover, for such a pulse duration, it should be possible to ignore the stress wave propagation. As seen in [46], the response is governed by the inertial characteristics of the system. The displacement and stress histories are similar to the load history, with small amplitude free vibrations superimposed. Essentially for the same reason, it is not surprising to find out that no rarefaction occurs at the impact pole and cavitation is possible at the antipole only. From their results on the brain shear elastic response, Advani and Owings conclude that brain damage at the midbrain region due to high shear strains is very likely for the load considered.

As a problem of interest in theoretical mechanics, rather than head injury biomechanics, Valanis and Sun [47] studied the axisymmetric wave propagation in a viscoelastic sphere, without a shell, subjected to diametral loads. If the viscoelastic sphere is bonded to viscoelastic shell, then the system can be considered as a head injury model. Hickling and Wenner [48] study the response of this model subjected to an axisymmetric impact. In their formulation, they use the three-dimensional equations of linear isotropic viscoelasticity to describe the behavior of both the brain and the skull. At the interface, it is assumed that the brain and the skull do not become separated, but no shearing stress is maintained between them. This is similar to the slip interface condition of the fluid -core models. The input pulse, distributed over a polar cap angle of 15^0, has a triangular shape in time. The problem was solved by a Fourier synthesis of steady state solutions. Numerical results were obtained for pulse durations from 2 to 6 msec and also for "large" and "small" heads. The model predicts that significant negative pressures are developed at the antipole only, supporting the cavitation theory of brain damage. The greatest negative pressure at the antipole occurs for the shortest pulse duration considered. The same conclusion is also valid for the maximum shear strain in the brain which occurs at a point near the impact pole. The figures showing the variations in the peak negative pressure and the maximum shearing strain in the brain of the "large" head with pulse duration are reproduced in Fig.10. The trend of the curves given in this figure does not agree with the generally accepted view that the short loading pulses are less damaging. However, Hickling and Wenner claim that increasing the damping in the system would reverse this trend.

The conclusion of another related study is not in agreement with that of [48] on the cavitation being possible only at the antipole. Chan [49] investigated the transient response of the viscoelastic shell-core model subjected to an axisymmetric pulse. The pulse duration varied from 1 to 5 msec. Chan's results show that the peak antipole negative pressures are less than those at the impact pole which is also a possible region of cavitation. In [49], an axisymmetric ellipsoidal shell model has also been studied for comparative purposes.

4.2 Rotation

The transient response of an elastic or viscoelastic core bonded to a rigid shell and suddenly rotated about its axis has been studied by various investigators. It is suggested that such a model simulates rotational impacts of the head such as those resulting in whiplash. Thus, useful information on the rotational acceleration theory of brain damage can be deduced from its study. Not surprisingly the most common shape of shell is spherical. An infinitely long

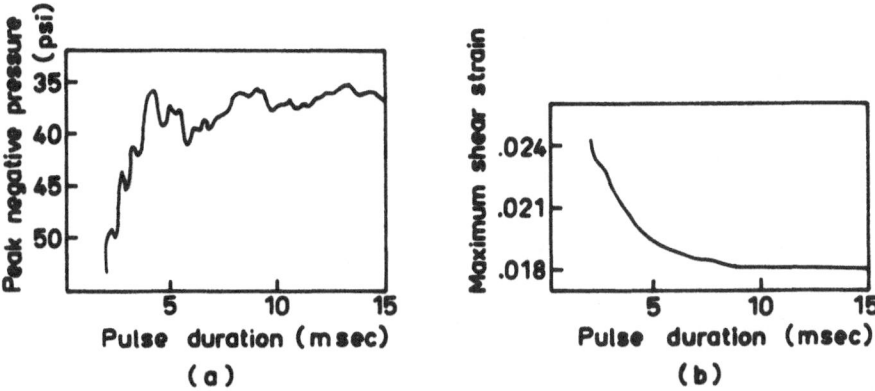

Fig. 10   Variation in (a) peak negative pressure (b) maximum
shear strain in brain with pulse duration [48]

cylindrical shell and a semi-infinite cylindrical shell terminated
at one end by a plane wall have also been used [50].

The first two-dimensional continuum model in this category
was proposed by Lee and Advani [51]. The brain matter is assumed
to be elastic or viscoelastic. It is firmly bonded to a rigid
spherical shell. The core is suddenly rotated about a diametral
axis, but the shell remains stationary. The angular acceleration
imparted to the core is in the form of a step function in time.
As a consequence of the no-slip condition assumed, the torsional
displacement of the core at the interface is zero at all times.
The disturbance originating at the interface propagates towards
the center as a shear wave. The maximum angular displacement occurs
approximately halfway between the center and the shell, slightly
towards the former. At a given time, the shear stress decreases
with radius, and at the origin it is zero at all times. ByCroft
[52] treats essentially the same problem, but now the shell, rather
than the core, is imparted an angular acceleration consisting of
a single sine wave pulse. The no-slip interface condition induces
the subsequent brain motion. The results show that the shear strain
decreases rapidly towards the center. In both these works, the
response of an elastic sphere was obtained first and then viscoelastic solutions were deduced by the correspondence principle.
In [51], the solution was obtained by the method of mode-super-
position; whereas ByCroft [52] obtained the solution via Laplace
transformation. In both, the results are in the form of an infinite
series. On the other hand, Liu and Chandran [53] express the results
in terms of a finite series, and they also discuss the difficulties
associated with the slow convergence of the infinite series for
small values of time.

The motion of a viscoelastic material contained in a rigid spherical shell has been investigated by Ljung [50] and Liu et al. [54] also. In both, it is the rigid shell which is subjected to a sudden rotation about its axis. In [50], a step angular velocity is used, whereas Liu et al. [54] use a step angular acceleration. The only non-vanishing component of the displacement vector is the angular displacement v. Hence, the Navier-Stoke's equation of motion in the axisymmetric spherical coordinate system will read

$$\ddot{v} = (\frac{\mu'}{\rho} \frac{\partial}{\partial t} + \frac{\mu}{\rho})(\frac{\partial^2 v}{\partial r^2} + \frac{2}{r} \frac{\partial v}{\partial r}$$

$$+ \frac{1}{r^2} \frac{\partial^2 v}{\partial \theta^2} + \frac{\cot\theta}{r^2} \frac{\partial v}{\partial \theta} - \frac{v}{r^2 \sin^2\theta}) , \qquad (7)$$

in which ρ is the mass density of the viscoelastic material, and μ and μ' are its shear modulus and viscosity coefficient, respectively. Ljung employs Hankel transformation technique to obtain the solution for the governing equation and the results are expressed in the form of an infinite series. As far as the mathematical aspects are concerned, the emphasis in [50] is on the fact that it is possible to use a cylindrical model to get a fair description of the solution in the spherical one. However, for a reasonable agreement, the radius of the corresponding cylinder has to be smaller than that of the sphere. In [54], a finite difference scheme is employed and the results are given for both the viscoelastic and elastic cases for comparative purposes. Figure 11 gives the maximum shear stress in the core as a function of the nondimensional time for both cases and for two different values of the nondimensional radius. The numerical results for the viscoelastic case are for the nondimensional viscoelastic parameter $\varepsilon = \mu'/(a \sqrt{\rho\mu}) = 0.122$. The conclusions obtained from the results of [54] can be summarized as follows. In the case of the viscoelastic material, the shear stress is greatly attenuated before it reaches the geometric center of the sphere; whereas, in the elastic case, the shear stress takes significant values even near the center. Therefore, under the assumption that the brain material is viscoelastic, a rotational acceleration input to the head will possibly result in subdural and subarachnoid injuries without subcortical involvement. In [54], the effect of pulse duration on shear stress distribution is also studied. The results show that the maximum shear stress always occurs at the surface of the sphere in the viscoelastic case; whereas the location of the maximum shear stress depends on the pulse duration in the elastic case, being closer to the center for short durations.

4.3 Translation and rotation

If the head model considered has a point symmetry as in the case of free-floating spherical models, it is possible to impart a combined translational and rotational acceleration to the model by an oblique impact only. Moreover, if the governing equations are linear, then the effects of the two accelerations on the stress distribution can be studied separately and the results can be superposed. This approach has been used by Chandran et al [26] in the analysis of their rigid spherical shell-viscoelastic core model. However, what is meant in the present work by a combined translation and rotation is not the case described above, but rather, it is the case in which the combined motion is aroused by the unsymmetry of the model or by the consideration of the head-neck junction.

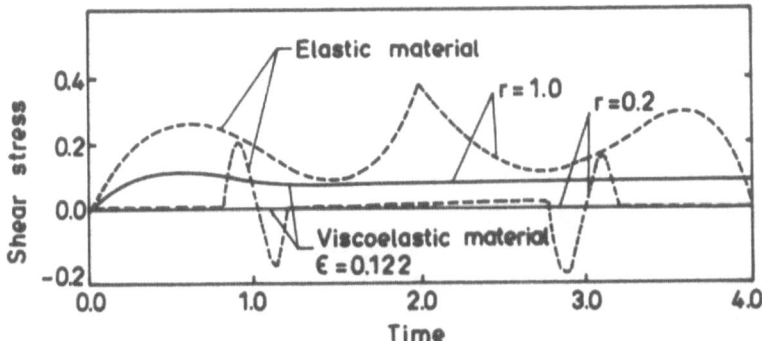

Fig. 11 Comparison of maximum shear stress between elastic and viscoelastic material [54]

A much less investigated phase of the continuum modeling of head injury involves studies of the effects of the neck. Studies in this area have generally been restricted to the lumped parameter modeling. Landkof et al. [12] are apparently the first who dealt with an analytical (and also experimental) study of a continuum model of the head-neck structure. The model consists of a fluid-filled elastic spherical shell representing the head constrained by a viscoelastic neck, as shown in Fig.12. The purpose of this investigation was to determine the effect of the head-neck junction on the motion of the head subjected to a long duration impact loading. The impact pulse, applied uniformly over a polar cap, has a sinusoidal shape in time with its duration being 2.5 msec. The direction of the resultant passes through the center of the shell. The constraint exerted by the head-neck junction turns the problem into a three-dimensional one in space. The spherical shell is considered as a rigid body in order to determine the interaction forces and moments at the junction. In determining these forces and moments, it is assumed that the angle of rotation of the shell with respect to the initial axis of the viscoelastic beam is small and that the beam is connected rigidly to the shell. The interaction forces and moments obtained via the "rigid shell" analysis are then applied over the

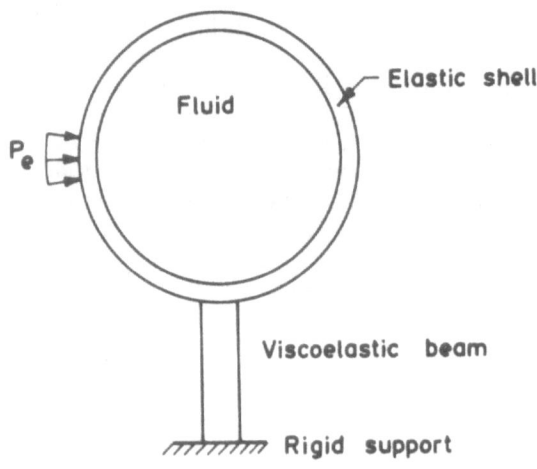

Fig. 12 Head - neck model used by
Landkof et al. [12].

bottom polar cap of the elastic shell. In this second part of the
investigation, both membrane and bending effects of the shell are
included. In the solution of the resulting linear coupled, partial
differential equations, the laplace transform method together with
a separation of variables is used. The solution is expressed in
terms of infinite series in the transformed space and the inversion
is performed numerically. The principal conclusions of [12] related
to brain injury are as follows. During the impact period, positive
and negative pressures develop in the loaded and distal hemispheres,
respectively. Beyond the end of the loading period, negative pressures
appear in the frontal hemisphere also. The antipole rarefaction
pressure is low in magnitude. The maximum negative pressures occur
at two locations in the distal hemisphere. The first one develops
close to the moment when the impact force reaches its maximum and
at the nondimensional radius equal to -0.27. The second one,
occurring approximately halfway between the center and the antipole,
develops during the deceleration period and it has a much longer
duration. Therefore, the potential location of the most severe
brain injury will be at this intermediate coup position. It should
be recalled that, in free-floating spherical shell-fluid models
subjected to such long duration impact forces [30], the antipole,
rather than an intermediate point, was potentially vulnerable for
brain injury. This shift in the location is apparently due to the
influence of the neck constraint. In 12 , the shell participates
in both translational and rotational motions. However, since the
fluid core is inviscid, it is not influenced directly by any

rotation of the shell. Although the neck is included in the model, the shell is still a completely closed vessel. Hence, the effect of intracranial flows through the foramen magnum on the ICP can not be studied with this model. In passing, it should be mentioned that Landkof et al. [12] make also an experimental study of the problem described. Goldsmith et al. [55] replace the spherical shell with a water-filled human cadaver skull in their more recent experiments. However, these are beyond the scope of the present work.

When the actual skull geometry is used in a model, the impact, whether direct or indirect, will generally produce rotation and translation of the brain. In the study of such models which are capable of simulating more closely. the actual geometry, it becomes necessary to resort to the numerical methods of the finite element type. Ward and Thompson [56] formulate a finite element model of the brain. The model was revised later and also experimentally derived head injury data are correlated with model dynamic response [57,58]. In the model, the actual three-dimensional geometry of the brain, with its various membranes and fluid-filled cavities, is approximated. The soft brain tissue and contained fluids are simulated with isoparametric brick elements. Membrane elements represent the internal folds of dura. Measured head rotational and translational accelerations and rotational velocities are input to the model instead of forces. The dynamic response is calculated by using a modified version of the general purpose finite element program SAPV. The response time considered is around 10 msec. The response is excited purely by the translational and rotational motion of the head. In other words, the propagation of pressure waves generated by skull deformation is not considered. The finite element model used in [56,57,58] does not include the spinal cavity; hence, the CSF flow into and out of the cranial cavity can not be simulated. However, Ward and her co-workers introduce the promising concept of an effective bulk modulus for the intracranial domain. A high bulk modulus would cause large stresses to develop due to small changes in volume. As will be discussed in the following section, this is actually not the case. The vascular and CSF systems provide pressure relase mechanisms. According to Ward et al. an effective low bulk modulus can account for these mechanisms. In those regions near the large arteries and near the foramen magnum, an effective bulk modulus, which is about 20 times smaller in magnitude than that of the remaining domain, is used [58]. The fact that the pressure release mechanisms (for instance, the "valves" mentioned in the previous section) may become active only after the local ICP reaches a certain value is not considered. The numerical results obtained from the finite element brain models of a monkey, a baboon and a human indicate that no simple scaling relationship exists between the models. A conclusion, similar in principle, has been obtained from the simpler axisymmetric shell-fluid model also [45]. Other conclusions of [56,57,58] obtained from the numerical analyses can be summarized as follows : The ICPs are of short-time duration

and the response is highly damped. High positive and negative
pressures develop in the cerebrum and cerebellum due to head motion.
The skull-brain relative displacements at the interface are small.
The internal folds of dura affect the dynamic response of the brain
significantly. The brain response is also affected by the geometric
shape.

In a similar vein, Shugar and Katona[29] present some
preliminary results of their continuing research aimed at validating
a dynamic three-dimensional finite element head injury model. They
use an axisymmetric, fluid-filled spherical shell model and a
plane strain model. The first one undergoes a translational motion
only. The plane strain model simulates the geometry of a unit slice
in the midsagittal plane of the skull. The fact that the skull
bone consists of three layers with different properties is taken
into consideration. The brain is represented as an acoustic fluid
in the first part of the investigation. The results are presented
for a uniform pressure with a time variation in the form of a haversine
function. The loading duration used is 10 msec. In the numerical
integration of the governing finite element equations, the time
increment used is 0.4 msec which is apparently too large to obtain
high frequency fluctuations due to wave propagation in the core.
Large rigid body motions of the head are restrained by providing
the model with supports at the base of the skull near the foramen
magnum. Although the plane strain model is not realistic as far as
the actual three-dimensional shape of the head is concerned, the
results are useful in an understanding of the effect of the skull
shape on the ICP. The numerical results presented indicate that the
stresses in the fluid emanate from the impact pole and the antipole,
and that the location of the maximum tensile pressure occurs near
the back and top of the brain. The maximum positive pressure occurs
near the impact pole. Moreover, the magnitudes of the maximum
positive and negative pressures are of the same order. Shugar and
Katona emphasize that the ICP variation depends strongly on the
restraints employed at the head-neck junction. They also investigate
the effect of modeling the brain as an elastic or viscoelastic
medium on the ICP. Figure 13 gives the ratio of the computed
compressive stress to the applied pressure in the core element
nearest the load as a function of time for the three different core
materials considered. The loading is the same as before. There is
no amplification of the pressure in the brain. For the elastic
and viscoelastic cases, stresses in the brain are attenuated
continuously. In constrast to the results obtained from the fluid-
core model, in the case of an elastic or viscoelastic core, stresses
emanate from the base. Shugar and Katona conclude that, as far as
the indication of contrecoup brain injury is concerned, the fluid
is a better characterization of brain matter.

In a recent report, Shugar[64] presents the results of a
head injury model development program. The head injury model
developed is fully three-dimensional. In the analysis, the FEM is
used. The computer code is referred to as the HIM code (Head Injury

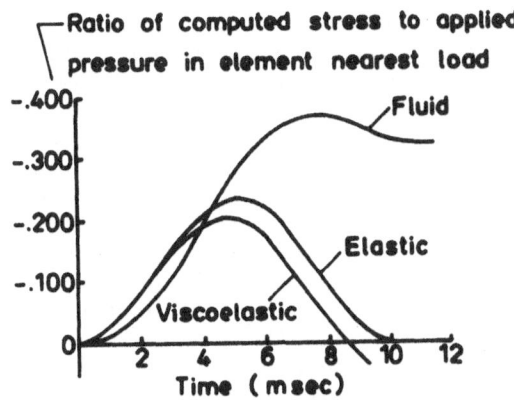

Fig. 13 Influence of material properties
on intracranial response [29]

Model). The model is applicable to closed brain injury. Neck-related
trauma and skull bone injury are not considered. The foramen magnum
can be included in the model. The numerical results indicate that
this inclusion causes a posterior shift in the null point of the
pressure distribution. The brain is simulated as being isolated
from the cranial wall by representing the SAS as a different layer.
By assigning a smaller bulk modulus to the SAS, it is possible to
observe the brain slosh mechanisms in the model's response.
According to Shugar, the stress in the brain is somewhat alleviated
by the relative displacement between the skull and the brain, but
only up to a point. As the relative motion tends to increase, it is
prevented by constraints at the skull-brain interface causing strain
at the brain's surface. As of today, it appears that the HIM code
and the one developed by Ward [56] are the most sophisticated codes
in the field. It is believed that the conclusions to be obtained
from the future investigations based on these codes will contribute
a lot to the progress in the field of head injury biomechanics.

5. FURTHER CONSIDERATIONS

The material-filled closed shell models discussed in the previous
section can be named as the first generation of continuum models
of head injury. Recent investigations have revealed that the events
taking place in the craniospinal cavity of an impacted head are
apparently more complex than those that can be described by the
first generation models. Although the discussion to be presented in
the following is limited to the cases quasi-static in nature, it is
hoped that it will shed some light on the dynamic nature of the head
injury problem as well.

Assume that the wall of the craniospinal cavity is rigid and
the fluid in the cavity has a bulk modulus B = 21000 kg/cm². With
these assumptions, a 1% decrease (increase) in the cavity volume
will produce a 210 kg/cm² (=155100 mm Hg) pressure increase
(decrease) in the fluid. The pressure changes recorded by Löfgren
et al. [59,60] are much lower than this value. They determined the
CSF pressure-volume (p-v) curve in dogs by measuring the pressure
response to rapid injection of fluid into the cisterna magna by
means of a constant flow infusion pump. The pressures were measured
in the lateral ventricle, the cisterna magna and the lumbar SAS.
Usually, an injection rate of 0.25 ml/sec was employed, because
it was fast enough so that the CSF inflow from the choroid plexus
and its drainage via the arachnoid villi were negligible and it
was slow enough so that a uniform "hydrostatic" rise was achieved
in the pressure in the system. Löfgren and Zwetnow [60] were able
to resolve the composite CSF p-v curve into a cranial and a spinal
component by using a spinal block at the level of the first cervical
vertebra. The results are presented in Fig.14. The conclusions of
[59,60] can be summarized as follows : The CSF p-v relationship is
nonlinear. The curves consist of three distinct parts : Two high
elastance parts connected by an intermediate low elastance part;
the term elastance being defined as the slope dp/dv of the CSF p-v
curve. In the interval of pressures usually encountered clinically,
the low elastance and the upper high elastance parts of the p-v
curve can each be approximated by a straight line. The slope of the
steep ascending part of the composite curve, which is essentially
constant, is, on the average, about 20 times greater than the slope
of the intermediate region. The range of variation in volume is
the smallest in the case of the cranial curve. At the low pressure
end, 70% of the total variation in volume takes place in the spinal
compartment. The ICP and volume changes are moderated by the spinal
compartment which essentially acts as a nonlinear expansion vessel.

The effect of the spinal cavity on the ICP can be investigated
mathematically only if a vessel representing this cavity is included
in the model of the head. Such a model may approximately be considered
as the next generation of continuum models of head injury. Liu [10]
performs a simple quasi-static analysis of this improved model. The
skull is idealized as a rigid spherical shell with an opening
simulating the foramen magnum. A thin-walled cylindrical shell, made
of Hookean material and modeling the spinal dura mater, is fitted
to this opening. The system is filled with an incompressible fluid.
Using the equations of the classical shell theory, Liu [10] obtains
the elastance of the system. Since the resulting p-v relationship
is linear, it is not possible to differentiate between low and high
pressure elastance in such an analysis. Moreover, the elastance
obtained by Liu from his simple model is two orders of magnitude
larger than that obtained by Löfgren and Zwetnow [60]. Rather than
presenting Liu's numerical results, here it is preferred to present
the solution of the problem associated with a similar but, in a sense,
improved model.

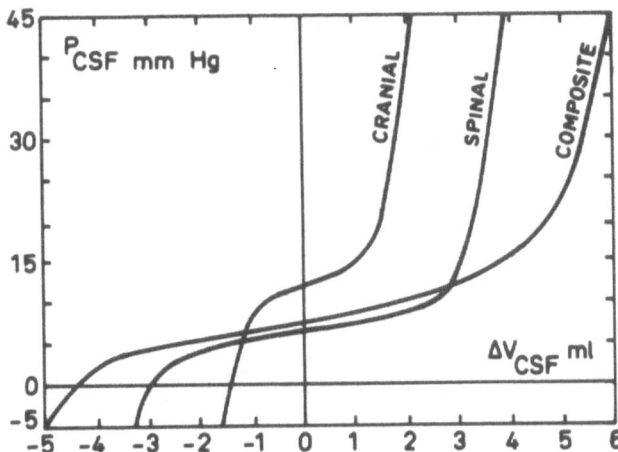

Fig. 14 P - V curves recorded by Löfgren and Zwetnow [60].

The skull is modeled as a rigid spherical shell and it is connected to a smaller elastic spherical shell which models the spinal dura mater, as shown in Fig.15. The cranial dura mater is assumed to be bonded to the skull. The connection between the shells is such a hypothetical one that the system is nothing more than two separate complete spherical shells in which the pressures are the same. Obviously, the spinal compartment is not spherical in shape, so the results to be presented should be considered as qualitative only. The values used for dimensions and materials are given below. It should be noted that, since the results are qualitative in nature, the use of other, possibly more realistic, values should not change our conclusions. Volume of the rigid shell, V_s = 1470 cm^3. Volume of the elastic shell when the internal pressure is zero, V_{mi} = 15 cm^3 with corresponding radius, R_{mi}=1.53 cm. Bulk modulus of the fluid, B = 20000 kg/cm^2. Modulus of elasticity for the spinal dura, E_d = 220 kg/cm^2 [10]. Poisson ratio for the spinal dura, ν = 0.5. Thickness of the spinal dura, t = 0.01 cm [10].

If it is assumed that the elastic shell is made of Hookean material, then, using the classical thin shell theory, one obtains

$$w = (1-\nu)R_{mi}^2 \ p_f/(2E_d t), \qquad (8)$$

in which w is the radial deflection of the shell and p_f is the internal pressure. Let ΔV_s denote an increase in the skull volume. Under the assumption of small deflection for the elastic shell, the total volume change ΔV of the two-shell system is

326

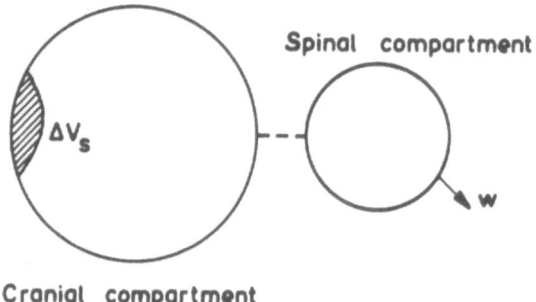

Spinal compartment

Cranial compartment

Fig. 15   Two - shell   model   of   craniospinal   system

$$\Delta V = \Delta V_s + 4\pi R_{mi}^2 .w \ . \tag{9}$$

Making use of the definition of the bulk modulus, the resulting pressure in the system is obtained as

$$p_f = - \frac{B\Delta V_s}{(V_s + V_{mi})} \left\{ 1 + \frac{3(1-\nu)R_{mi}.BV_{mi}}{2E_d t(V_s + V_{mi})} \right\}^{-1} \tag{10}$$

Since the shell theory used is linear, p_f is a linear function of ΔV_s and it is given as curve I in Fig. 16 for the values cited above. For a given ΔV_s, it is seen from equation (10) that p_f is a non-linear function of the other quantities. A parametric study of the variation of p_f with these quantities might yield some interesting results; however, this is beyond the scope of this work.

Löfgren et al [59,60] inject fluid into the craniospinal system from outside, whereas, in the above formulation, the fluid mass remains constant but the system volume is changed. The two approaches are similar in principle. The p-v curve recorded by Löfgren et al. is nonlinear. It was known at the beginning that the mathematical formulation presented above would not yield a nonlinear p-v relationship. The nonlinearity can be incorporated in the system if we assume that the elastic shell material is not of the Hookean type, but rather that it shows a nonlinear behavior. Indeed, it is well known that biological soft tissues do not generally have a linear stress-strain relationship. Representation of the spinal dura mater as a nonlinear elastic material in the formulation will probably be more realistic. Accordingly, here it is assumed that the dura is of the Mooney material type, which is not necessarily the best representation of living tissues but is sufficient for our purposes. The improvedmodel now consists of a rigid spherical shell and an elastic spherical shell made of Mooney material, the two shells being connected hypothetically as before. Making use of the equations

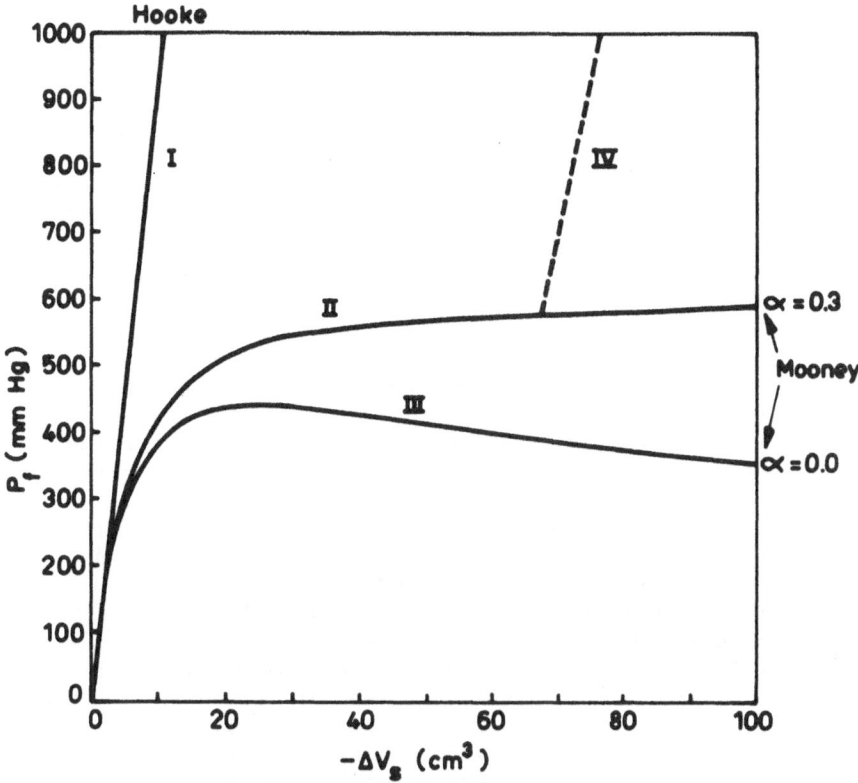

Fig. 16   ICP as a function of decrease in cranial volume

given by Akkaş [61], it can be shown that the quasistatic behavior of the model is governed by the following equations :

$$V_{mf} = V_{mi} - \Delta V_s - (V_s + V_{mi})p_f/B \ , \tag{11}$$

$$p_f = 4C_1 t(4\pi/3)^{1/3} V_{mf}^{-1/3}(1-V_{mi}^2 V_{mf}^{-2})(1+\alpha V_{mi}^{-2/3} V_{mf}^{2/3}) \ , \tag{12}$$

in which V_{mf} is the final volume of the elastic membrane, $\alpha = C_2/C_1$, and C_1 and C_2 are constants of the Mooney material. The others are the same as before. Since, for small strains, the Mooney material is expected to behave as the corresponding Hookean material, it can be shown that $C_1 + C_2 = E_d/6$, [62]. Equations (11) and (12) are two coupled nonlinear equations with p_f and V_{mf} being the unknowns. In the numerical solution, the same values as those of the previous linear formulation are used. The variation of p_f with the decrease in the skull volume $(-\Delta V_s)$ is presented in Fig.16 as curves II and III for $\alpha = 0.3$ and $\alpha = 0.0$, respectively. A comparison of Figs.14

and 16 reveals that the low elastance portion of the experimental
results has been recovered. Indeed, it is, in principle, possible
to obtain the exact low-pressure elastance recorded by Löfgren
et al. [59] by selecting appropriate values for the dimensions
and/or material properties. This parametric study is not within
the scope of the present work.

The use of the Mooney material is not, all by itself, sufficient
to recover the upper high elastance portion of the curves given in
Fig.14. For this, other considerations are needed. For instance, it
can be suggested that, when V_{mf} reaches a specified value, the
spinal dura will be in full distension and tight against the
vertebral column. From then on, the spinal compartment should be
modeled as a linear elastic shell and, hence, any further decrease
in the skull volume would result in a linear p-v relationship
similar to curve IV of Fig. 16. Or, it could be assumed from the
beginning that the spinal dura were resting on springs with forces
nonlinearly proportional to V_{mf}, in which case the discontinuity
of the slope at the intersection point of curves II and IV of
Fig.16 would also be eliminated. As seen from Fig.14, the cranial
component of the p-v curve is also nonlinear. In other words, as
opposed to what has been assumed in the above formulation, the
cranial dura mater is apparently not tight against the skull at
low pressures. In the light of the results and the discussion
presented so far, here it is suggested that the following model of
the craniospinal system may be promising: Two fluid-filled, interconnected nonlinear elastic shells resting on nonlinear springs
with different constants or behaving as linear elastic shells above
some specific, but different; pressure values. As a start, the cranial
and spinal compartments may be modeled as spherical and cylindrical
shells, respectively. The equations governing the quasistatic behavior
of such a model and their solution should not be much more complex
than those of the simpler model discussed above. However, it should
be emphasized that the formulations of this section are all limited
to quasistatic analyses. A dynamic analysis of the improved model
subjected to an impact will, very likely, be an extremely complicated
one. The problem is essentially three-dimensional in space, it is
nonlinear as far as both deformations and material properties are
concerned, and finally it is time-dependent. Apparently, one will
have to resort to the numerical techniques of the finite difference
or the finite element for its solution.

Even the two-shell nonlinear model discussed above is not
sufficient to account for all the events taking place in an impacted
skull. There seem to be other mechanisms serving to protect the CNS
from potentially lethal changes in the ICP. For instance, an increase
in the ICP results not only in a distension of the meningeal membranes
but also in a reflex increase in blood pressure and in a consequent
reduction in the volume of cerebral veins. Moreover, the CBF is
coupled with the CSF system. Changes in the CSF pressure are directly
related to changes associated with the heartbeat and the respiratory
cycle. ICP changes affect the CSF displacement to and from the spinal
compartment and also its efflux into the blood via the arachnoid

villi. Changes in CSF volume in the cranial cavity are usually compensated by reciprocal changes in the intracranial blood volume. These have been mentioned here shortly only for the purpose of emphasizing the complexity of the events occuring in the CNS. It may be said that such events, which take place over a relatively long time, will not have any effect on the transient response of the system. However, it is also very likely that some of the events mentioned may start taking place before the impact occurs, thus compensating for the time differences. As an example, we can mention the known fact that the hormones of the adrenal medulla tend to rally the body to situations of emergency, as in the case of a traffic accident. One of these hormones, adrenaline, causes an increase in the heart rate, an increase in blood pressure and an increased blood flow by dilating the blood vessels. Accordingly, it should not be too presumptuous to state that the transient ICP variations in an individual will be different depending upon whether the impact is expected or unexpected. The development of a mathematical model in which some or all such factors are taken into consideration will be a very challenging task.

The present work will be concluded by mentioning shortly two other nonlinear aspects of brain injury. They are essentially related to the cavitation theory discussed previously. According to this theory, if the negative pressure at some location within the brain reaches a critical value, the capillary walls may rupture and cavitation bubbles may be formed. Rupturing of capillaries and expansion and subsequent collapse of bubbles are both nonlinear, time-dependent problems. Indeed, Akkaş [61,63] has shown that they are both essentially dynamic instability problems. Modeling the capillaries as thin-walled tubes made of Hookean material and then estimating the critical pressure using an appropriate linear shell theory would be to oversimplify. As far as cavitation is concerned, the critical negative pressure is a function of the size of the microbubbles present in the fluid medium. Are there such microbubbles present in the brain substance and the CSF ? If so, what is the range of their sizes ? What are the instability pressures for rupturing and cavitation? The answers to these questions will hopefully shed some new light on the cavitation theory of brain injury.

REFERENCES

1. N. Perrone, Dynamic response of biomechanical systems, ed. by N. Perrone, ASME, New York, 1970, 1-22.
2. Anonymous, Accident facts, National Safety Council, Illinois, 1974.
3. J.K. Kihlberg, Impact injury and crash protection, Thomas, Springfield, 1970, 5-24.
4. J.O. Moore, B. Tourin, J.W. Garrett and R. Lilienfeld, Traffic Safety Res. Rev. (4), 1959, 16-21.

330

5. R.A. McFarland, Proc. 13th STAPP Car Crash Conf., 1969, 1-17.
6. C.R. Noback and R.J. Demarest, The Human Nervous System,
    McGraw-Hill, New York, 1975.
7. H. Davson, A Textbook of General Physiology, J. and A.
    Churchill, London, 1970.
8. C. Eyzaguirre and S.J. Fidone, Physiology of the Nervous
    System, Year Book Medical Publ., Chicago, 1975.
9. W. Goldsmith, Biomechanics - its foundations and objectives,
    ed. by Y.C. Fung, N. Perrone and M. Anliker, Prentice-Hall,
    New Jersey, 1972, 585-634.
10. Y.K. Liu, ASCE J. Engng. Mech. Div., 1978.
11. J.H. McElhaney, J.W. Melvin, V.L. Roberts and H. Portnoy,
    Persp. in Biomed. Engng., MacMillan, London, 1972, 215-222.
12. B. Landkof, W. Goldsmith and J.L. Sackman, J. Biomechanics
    (9), 1976.
13. A.H.S. Holbourn, Lancet, 1943, 438-441.
14. R.E. Nickell and P.V. Marcal, ASME J. Engng. for Industry,
    1974, 490-494.
15. S. Lindgren and L. Rinder, Acta Physiol. Scand. (76), 1969,
    340-351.
16. A. Anzelius, Acta Patho. Microbio. Scand. (48), 1943, 153-159.
17. W. Güttinger, Zeits. für Naturf. (5A), 1950, 622-628.
18. W. Goldsmith, Head Injury Conference Proceedings, ed. by
    W.F. Caveness and A.E. Walker, J.B. Lippincott, Philadelphia,
    1966, 350-382.
19. A.I. King and C.C. Chou, J. Biomech. (9), 1976, 301-317.
20. T. Hayashi, J. Fac. of Engng. Univ. Tokyo (30B), 1969, 59-72,
    117-124.
21. Y.K. Liu and K.B. Chandran, ASME J. Appl. Mech. (42), 1975,
    541-546.
22. Y.K. Liu, Symp. Biodyn. Models and Their Applic., Dayton, Ohio,
    1971, 701-736.
23. J.A. Kopecky and E.A. Ripperger, J. Biomech. (2),1969, 29-34.
24. Y.K. Liu and K.B. Chandran, Math. Biosci. (24), 1975, 1-16.
25. K.B. Chandran, Y.K. Liu and D.U. von Rosenberg, ASME J. Appl.
    Mech. (42), 1975, 759-762.
26. K.B. Chandran, Y.K. Liu and D.U. von Rosenberg, J. Sound and
    Vibr. (47), 1976, 107-114.
27. S.L. Gordon, G.D. Moskowitz and R.K. Byers, ASME, Paper No.
    73-DET-113, 1973.
28. N. Akkas, J. Biomech. (8), 1975, 275-284.
29. T.A. Shugar and M.G. Katona, ASCE J. Engng. Mech. Div. (101),
    1975, 223-239.
30. T.B. Khalil and R.P. Hubbard, J. Biomech. (10), 1977, 119-132.
31. J.V. Benedict, E.H. Harris and D.U. von Rosenberg, ASME J.
    Basic Engng. (92), 1970, 597-603.
32. Y.C. Lee and S.H. Advani, 5th Southeast Conf. on Theor. and
    Appl. Mech., 1970.
33. H.S. Chan and Y.K.Liu, J. Biomech. (7), 1974, 43-59.
34. A.E. Engin, J. Biomech. (2), 1969, 325-341.

35. V.H. Kenner and W. Goldsmith, Int. J. Mech. Sci. (14), 1972, 557-568.
36. H.C. Merchant and A.J. Crispino, J. Biomech. (7), 1974, 295-301.
37. Y.K. Liu, H.S. Chan and J. Nelson, Proc. Summer Computer Simulation Conf., Boston, 1971, 984-994.
38. O. Talhouni and F. Dimaggio, J. Biomech. (8), 1975, 219-228.
39. A.E. Engin and V.L. Roberts, Biodyn. Models and Their Applic., Ohio, 1971, 877-903.
40. J.V. Benedict, Symp. Biodyn. Models and Their Applic. Ohio, 1971, 123-139.
41. V.H. Kenner and W. Goldsmith, J. Biomech. (6), 1973, 1-11.
42. N. Akkaş, ASCE J. Engng. Mech. Div. (103), 1977, 35-49.
43. A.E. Engin and N. Akkaş, Aviation, Space and Env. Medicine, Jan. 1978, 120-124.
44. N. Akkaş, METU J. Pure and Appl. Sci., Special Bioengng. Issue, 1977, 71-94.
45. N. Akkaş, METU J. Pure and Appl. Sci. (9), 1976, 349-365.
46. S.H. Advani and R.P. Owings, ASCE J. Engng. Mech. Div. (101), 1975, 257-266.
47. K.C. Valanis and C.T. Sun, Int. J. Engng. Sci. (5), 1967, 939-956.
48. R. Hickling and M.L. Wenner, J. Biomech. (6), 1973, 115-132.
49. H.S. Chan, Proc. 18th STAPP Car Crash Conf., 1974, 557-578.
50. C. Ljung, J. Biomech. (8), 1975, 263-274.
51. Y.C. Lee and S.H. Advani, Math. Biosci. (6), 1970, 473-486.
52. G.N. ByCroft, J. Biomech. (6), 1973, 487-495.
53. Y.K. Liu and K.B. Chandran, Recent Dev. in Engng. and Sci. (7), 1976, 255-264.
54. Y.K. Liu, K.B. Chandran and D.U. von Rosenberg, J. Biomech, (8), 1975, 285-292.
55. W. Goldsmith, J.L. Sackman, G. Ouligian and M. Kabo, ASME J. Biomech. Engng. (100), 1978, 25-33.
56. C.C. Ward and R.B. Thompson, 19th STAPP Car Crash Conf., San Diego, 1975, 641-674.
57. C.C. Ward, P.E. Nikravesh and R.B. Thompson, J. Avia. Space and Env. Med., 1978.
58. A.M. Nahum, R. Smith and C.C. Ward, 21st STAPP Car Crash Conf., 1977.
59. J. Löfgren, C. von Essen and N.N. Zwetnow, Acta Neurol.Scand. (49), 1973, 557-574.
60. J. Löfgren and N.N. Zwetnow, Acta Neurol. Scand. (49), 1973, 575-585.
61. N. Akkaş, Int. J. Nonl. Mech., 1978, in press.
62. H. Alexander, Int. J. Engng. Sci. (6), 1968, 549-563.
63. N. Akkaş, J. Appl. Math. Phys. (ZAMP) (29), 1978, 92-99.
64. T.A. Shugar, CEL, Naval Construction Battalion Center, Ca., Technical Report R854, July 1977.

SOME ASPECTS OF HEAD AND NECK INJURY AND PROTECTION

Werner Goldsmith

Department of Mechanical Engineering, University of
California, Berkeley, California, U.S.A.

ABSTRACT. A survey on head and neck injury is presented which
covers the experimental and certain phases of the analytical treatment of the subject. The anatomy of the system and the mechanical
properties of its components are described, types and mechanisms of
damage are detailed, and the epidemiology of the injuries is cata-
logued. Head injury models involve, on the analytical side, rigid-
body, lumped and distributed parameter, and continuum representations of the structure; the last approach, covered in a previous
summary, is not discussed here. Experimental models involve volunteers, human cadavers, animals, and inanimate replicas subjected
to impact and impulsive loading. Tolerance levels for head and
neck injury are indicated, and the use and efficacy of protective
devices are described.

1. INTRODUCTION

During the last two decades, the subject of head injury--defined
as damage to the brain and its covers--has received an enormous
amount of attention from both biological and physiological scientists and their professional counterparts, physicians and engineers
who have attempted to document and explain the physiological and
physical alterations resulting from traumatic mechanical loading
of this structure. Head injuries result from either direct contact
or from inertial loading of some other part of the body, such as
the change of motion associated with a rear-end vehicular collision; however, in both instances, some part of the head trauma depends upon the character of the motion of the cervical region
which, in itself, is frequently injured either independently or
concurrently. Thus, it seems logical here to consider the effects

of force or inertial loading on a system composed of both head
and neck, with an essentially stationary reference denoted by a
plane through one of the upper thoracic vertebrae. In some cases,
such as the penetration of the calvarium by a high-velocity small
missile, the neck motion will not play a role in the deficit; however, in most instances, the joint consideration of these two major
anatomical regions appears to be justified in examining the physiological damage and its mechanical causation.

Studies of the subject can be divided according to the primary
purpose (or viewpoint) of the investigator: (1) the epidemiologist
is primarily interested in the environment and de facto causation
of the injury, (2) the biomechanician attempts to delineate the
physical processes causing the trauma and considers the event in
terms of a mechanical and mathematical model that permits prediction of response from a knowledge of the system parameters and the
loading function; this requires a determination of all relevant
geometrical and constitutive properties of the system, (3) the
physiologist or biophysicist who can gage the effect of mechanical
input on cellular or anatomical regional output, and (4) the prac-
ticing physician faced with the need to interpret and act upon a
set of physiological (or, in extreme cases, pathological) symptoms.
The interaction of these practitioners supposedly is designed to
prevent or mitigate injuries, by development of better protective
environments, and to improve diagnosis and treatment including
creation of superior replacement parts. However, it is inevitable
that significant compartmentalization in these various specialties
has been and will continue to be retained. Thus, the sources of
published information on head and neck injury, i.e., books, proceedings of symposia, and periodicals, can generally be classified
as belonging either to the biomechanical or the medical/biological
camp. Typical examples in the first category involving major concentration of the subject include [1-5], the ASME Applied Mechanics
Division Symposia on Biomechanics, the Journal of Biomechanics,
the Journal of Biomechanical Engineering, and the Proceedings of
the Stapp Car Crash Conferences and Automotive Engineering Congresses; representative publications in the second class include
[6-12] and a large number of medical journals. Refs. [13-15] provide a mixture of both viewpoints; this may also be found in some
other periodicals such as the Proceedings of the Alliance for Engineering in Medicine and Biology, Proceedings of the International
Congresses of Bioengineering, the Journal of Aviation Medicine,
Aerospace Medicine, and many other publications, although these
are not devoted exclusively to head and neck problems.

The present author has presented two previous summaries
concerned with the biomechanics of head injury, devoted to a description of the system, material properties of the components of
the head, a catalogue of the types and mechanisms of head injury,
analytical representations of closed-brain injuries, a brief

description of related experiments and human tolerance and protective devices [16-17]. Other reviews of the biomechanics of head injuries have also been published [18-20]. While some overlap with these publications is inevitable, a major effort has been exerted here to minimize such duplication and to focus attention on experimental and protective aspects of the topic of impact and impulsive loading of the head and the neck and their interaction. The subdivisions of this paper will include a brief description of structure and anatomy, epidemiology, injury mechanisms, experiments, modelling, tolerance levels, and the effects of helmets and other protective devices.

2. ANATOMY OF THE HEAD AND NECK

The human head-neck system shown in Fig. 1 is usually divided into three separate entities consisting of the identifying bony structure and surrounding softer tissues: (1) the skull (cranium), (2) the face, and (3) the neck (cervical region). The cranium consists of hair and scalp overlying the skull, two interior membranes, the dura and pia-arachnoid enveloping the brain, vessels carrying blood, and the cerebrospinal fluid (CSF). The scalp is a multilayered anisotropic cover varying in thickness from 6.5 to 13 mm. The skull consists of an outer and inner table of solid bone separated by a trabecular domain (diploë) with a total thickness

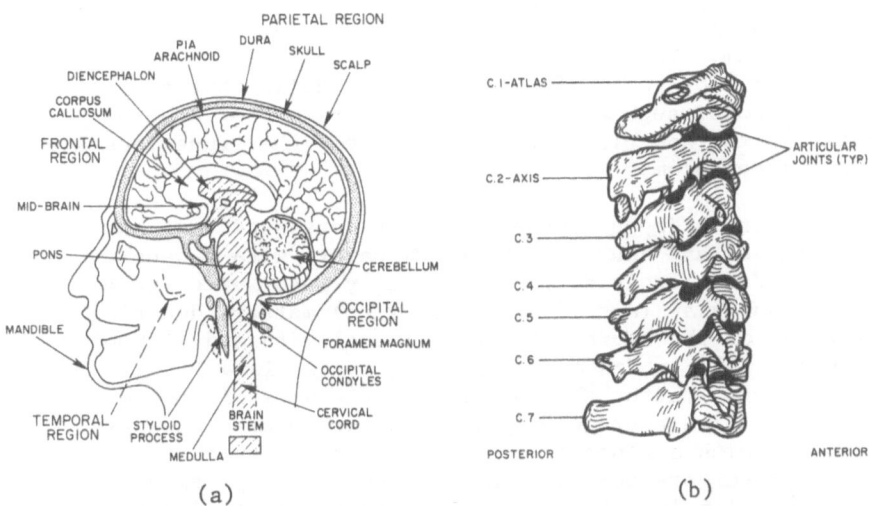

(a)   (b)

Fig. 1. Human (a) head, sagittal plane; (b) neck vertebrae.

ranging from 6.5 to 7.9 mm; the vault is of non-uniform spheroidal shape with smooth surfaces closed at the bottom by a base containing three irregular compartments (fossa). Although eight separate bones form the skull, their junction in an adult is so calcified that it cŏmposes a single structural unit containing several holes (foramen) through which blood vessels and the brain stem enter the cranium. The dura represents the interior lining of the skull; it is a tough, fibrous, anisotropic, dense, relatively inelastic two-layered membrane whose inner layer separates from the outer and then partitions both the two cerebral and the two cerebellar hemispheres as well as horizontally compartmentalizing the cerebral occipital lobes and the upper cerebellar surface. The pia-arachnoid is a gossamer tissue whose strength characteristics may be ignored. It is separated from the dura by a closed capillary labelled the subdural space which contains a lymph-like fluid and also forms a series of compartments occupied by the CSF, a clear, colorless, nearly Newtonian fluid with a specific gravity of 1.004-1.008. This liquid also invests the four ventricles of the brain, the central canal of the spinal cord, and the perivascular spaces.

The brain consists of the two convoluted hemispheres of the cerebrum, the two foliated hemispheres and a central region of the cerebellum, the midbrain, and the medulla that connects to the spinal cord. Each cerebral hemisphere is also divided by superficial grooves (fissures and sulci) into frontal, parietal, temporal, occipital, limbic, and insula lobes. The brain stem consists of the diencephalon, the midbrain (or mesencephalon), the pons and the medulla which passes into the cervical cavity through the foramen magnum. The reticular formation which relates to consciousness envelops most of the pons and medulla that control the lower functions, such as respiration and vasomotor control (heart rate, rhythm and blood pressure). The higher functions are located in the cerebrum.

The human brain is egg-shaped, has the consistency of an extremely soft gel and contains about 78% water, with a density of about 1.16 g/cc. It is divided texturally into white (specific gravity 1.10) and gray (specific gravity 1.20) matter, denoting conglomerations of the neural elements (axons) with and without fatty sheaths (myelin), respectively. The cortex is a 1.5-3.5 mm thick layer of gray matter that covers the fissures of the cerebral hemisphere. The average weight of the brain of a Caucasian male is 1500 g (with a range of 1000-1700 g) and its length and transverse diameter are about 165 mm and 140 mm, respectively [21]. The brain is heavily infested with large and small blood vessels connecting to the scalp and dura and to the neck structures, with diameters ranging from 1-2 mm to micron size. The vessels are elastic tubes consisting either of a single layer of endothelial cells or, for the larger sizes, of additional layers of connective tissue. A series of neuroglial cells forms a barrier between blood and brain permitting interchange of only a few selected materials. The rheology of blood, a highly non-Newtonian fluid, is extremely complex; a thorough review of its characteristics is given in [22]. "Head injury" is biomechanically and medically defined as damage to any of the components listed above, and has been investigated extensively.

The facial bones that are integrally connected to the skull include the orbit (eyeball sockets), the cheekbones (zygomatic bone), a portion of which forms the zygomatic arch, and the upper jaw (maxilla); the lower jaw, or mandible, is hinged to the immovable portion of the skull. Both jawbones embed the teeth, bonelike structures. The face also contains substantial cartilage, i.e., nose, ears, muscles, other connective tissue, and skin. Relatively few biomechanical investigations of facial injury have been conducted, perhaps because of the generally non-lethal and frequently reversible effects encountered.

The neck consists of the first seven vertebrae, C1-C7, of the spinal column and adjacent tissue; occasionally, the first two vertebrae of the thoracic region are included in the biomechanical analysis of neck response. The cervical spine is an agglomeration of functional units consisting of two vertebral bodies and an anterior (forward) interspersed disk that consists of a cartilage container enclosing a mucopolysaccharide gel initially containing about 80% water, but dehydrating with age, that serves as a shock absorber. The hole formed by the arches of the vertebral body accommodates the spinal cord and its accessories. The posterior portion of this unit, except for C1 and C2, consists of two vertebral arches, one central and two transverse spinous processes (projections), and two symmetric lubricated (synovial) jointed surfaces called the articular facets. The integrity of the system including the synovial joints and avoidance of damaging movements are maintained by the vertebrally joined disk cartilages and by numerous stiff ligaments. The size of the vertebral bodies and projections increases downward. The atlas, C1, has no spinous process; its superior synovial articular surface bears against the occipital condyles of the skull permitting forward or backward "nodding" (flexion or extension) relative motion of skull and neck, the combination forming the occipital-atlantic unit. Rotation of the head occurs principally between C1 and C2 (the axis) about the odontoid process (or pivot) of the axis, although some flexion-extension can also occur there. Both rotation and flexion, forward and sideways, can take place between C2 and C7; the latter functions as a thoracic vertebra, and thus neck motion is primarily confined to the region between C2 and C6 [23-24]. These motions are portrayed in Fig. 2 [24].

Stresses generated in the neck are borne principally by muscles and ligaments, and primarily by the latter when the former

338

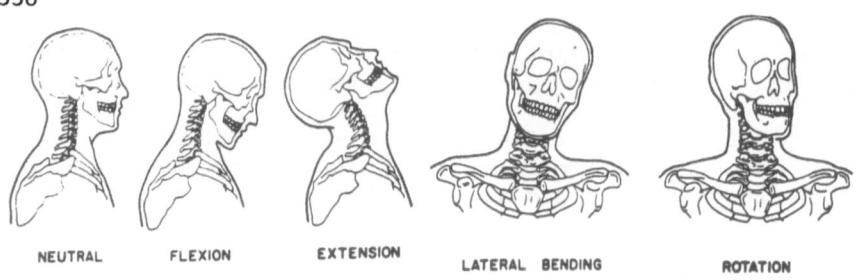

NEUTRAL   FLEXION   EXTENSION   LATERAL BENDING   ROTATION

Fig. 2. Relative head/neck displacements.

are fatigued. The stability of all cervical joints, but particularly that of the occipital-atlantic and atlantoaxial junctions
is maintained by ligaments. Neck articulation is accomplished
through muscle pairs attached to the skull, individual vertebrae
and the torso, symmetrically located relative to the midsagittal
plane. Muscle pairs can be functionally divided into those that
flex and extend the head, and those that flex and extend the spine,
or, alternatively, those that provide resistance to neck extension
and rearward rotation (longus capitis and colli, anterior rectus
capitis and scalenus, hyoids, sternothyroid and sternocleido-
mastoid—attached to the mastoid process slightly below and behind
occipital condyles), and those preventing neck flexion and forward
head rotation that are located posterior to vertebral bodies
(trapezius, levator scapulae, splenius, longissimus and semispinalis
capitis, splenius and semispinalis cervicis, obliquus capitis in-
ferior and superior, and rectus capitis posterior major and minor).
The total area of the postvertebral muscles is larger and the cen-
troid of their skull attachment is much further from the occipital
condyles than for the prevertebral muscles, implying that the head
should be able to resist greater flexing than extending moments
[24-25]. Additional structural elements of the neck include the
two major arteries, carotid and vertebral, the jugular veins, and
surrounding connective tissue and skin. However, the spinal cord
and emanating nerves attached to vertebral bodies through canals
or foramina represent the major source of potential trauma and
require suitable protection. While numerous theoretical and experimental investigations have been conducted with respect to the response of the entire spine to impulsive loading, those specifically
limited to the neck are much less frequent. Mass distributions of
the head and neck are presented in [26-27]; the head/neck combination ranges in mass from about 4.7 to more than 6 kg (or 7-9% of
total body weight) and evidences a specific gravity from 1.07-1.13.
The mass moment of inertia about the transverse axis is of the
order of 0.1 kg-m^2. Data on resistive moments under voluntary
static hyperextension and maximum extensions for forced motion of
cadavers are given in [24,28].

3. MECHANICAL PROPERTIES OF HEAD AND NECK TISSUES

Much information is available on the mechanical properties of various human and animal head tissues obtained under various biopsy and/or autopsy conditions [13,17,29-31]. The protective effect of massed human hair under compressive loading does not appear to have been studied; the maximum tensile strength of a single strand, 22-23 MPa, with an elongation of around 40% occurs for persons in their twenties. Scalp, a highly viscoelastic substance, exhibits a strain-rate sensitive initially concave-upward stress-strain curve with a zero-strain tangent modulus of 0.5 KPa (compared to a value of 1.5 KPa for monkeys); the ultimate tensile strength and elongation for humans were found to average 0.46 MPa and 54%, respectively, with a reported bulk modulus $K = 2$ GPa [13,30-31].

The properties of skull differ depending upon whether the sample consists of compact bone, the diploë, or the composite (dry-weight specific gravity 1.4), and in what condition (biopsy, autopsy, frozen, embalmed) it is tested [31]; no specimen exhibited significant strain-rate sensitivity. Properties reported by various investigators vary widely and appear to depend on particular location for a given skull specimen. For unembalmed compact skull bone, a more or less isotropic material, average values (with sizeable deviations) of the tensile and compressive modulus were 14 MPa, with tensile and compressive strengths of about 70 and 165 MPa, respectively; the tensile failure strain amounted to 0.55-0.7%, but an increase of only 40% in tensile failure stress was found upon increasing the strain rate by 4-1/2 decades [32-33]. Compressive strength of the diploë averaged 34 MPa, with values as low as 9 MPa reported. Composite samples presumably are transversely isotropic; depending upon sample condition, radial and tangential compression moduli range from 0.4-2.6 and 2.6-5.6 GPa with a Poisson's ratio of 0.19 and 0.22, respectively, while the modulus in tangential tension ranged from 5.4-8.8 GPa. Values of ultimate strengths for the various samples of the composite were given as 71-145 MPa in radial compression, 50-97 MPa in tangential compression, and 43 MPa in tangential tension. In examining the flexural characteristics of layered cranial bone [34], the bending stiffness was found to be about 2.75 $N-m^2$, corresponding to a structural Young's modulus of 10.2 GPa. The equivalent shear modulus varied from 138-745 MPa for the composite and from 138-690 MPa for the core.

As a basis for comparison, the values for the constitutive parameters of long bones, modelled as transversely isotropic elastic solids, were found to be $E' = 17$ GPa , $E = 11.5$ GPa , $G' = 3.28$ GPa , $v' = 0.46$, and $v = 0.58$, with primes denoting axial and unprimed values denoting transverse directions [35], and with E , G , and v denoting the quasi-elastic Young's and shear moduli and Poisson's ratios, respectively. The corresponding ultimate strengths were found to be 133 and 51 MPa for tension in the axial and transverse direction, respectively, and 193 and 133 MPa for compression in these directions; torsion about the longitudinal axis yielded an ultimate strength of 68 MPa. Repeated loading of bone caused progressive loss of stiffness and ultimate tensile strength.

Fracture mechanics has also been applied to crack propagation in bone [36-38], with fracture energies of 1.85 and 7 KN-m evaluated for the anthropoid in the transverse and longitudinal directions of the bone, respectively. Critical stress intensity factors K_c were found to vary with bone density, ρ, with a value of $K_c = 4.0$ MN/m$^{3/2}$ observed for a dry bone density of 2, that corresponds to a strain energy release rate of about 1600 N-m/m^2. Fractures in intact human heads produced by falls on hard surfaces required 45-100 N-m of energy, whereas such fractures were initiated by a ten-fold lower energy level when the scalp was removed. Vibrational modes in living humans have been found at about 300 (antiresonance), 600 and 900 Hz (resonance), with some variability depending on location of the driving force and topography of the individual [13,39]. Below 200 Hz, the skull moves as a rigid body and will so respond to impacts of more than 5 ms duration.

Values of 42 MPa and 2.3 MPa have been published for the quasi-static elastic modulus and ultimate shear strength of dura [40]. Its complex Young's modulus, $E^* = E_1^* + i\,E_2^*$ has been determined as $E^* = 32.8 + 3.45i$ MPa from free vibration tests at 22 Hz [30,41].

Brain, a highly viscoelastic material, has a bulk modulus of 2 GPa, nearly that of water, and a compressive modulus of the order of 65 KPa (with values as low as 10 KPa reported for both animal and human samples). The complex modulus for direct shear at 10 Hz has been found to range from 550-1100 and 225-655 Pa for G_1^* and G_2^*, respectively, while the corresponding domains for torsion tests executed from 2-400 Hz were 827-137,900 and 345-82,700 Pa, respectively [17,41]. The concave-upward variation of modulus with applied load is mirrored by the true stress-strain curve which can be expressed by the relation

$$\ln\left(\bar{\sigma}/\dot{\bar{\epsilon}}\right) = 3.45 + 5.4\ln t , \qquad (3.1)$$

with true stress $\bar{\sigma}$ in KPa and time t and true strain rate $\dot{\bar{\epsilon}}$ expressed in units of seconds. Other investigations have found a mechanical shear strain failure level of 0.035 rad at 10 Hz, representation of storage and shear loss moduli G_1^* and G_2^* by an empirical exponential relation, linear viscoelastic behavior in shear, and Bingham plastic comportment with non-linear hardening in compression [31].

Animal tests indicate a decrease in modulus with time after
death, while fixation increases it without altering its behavior
with applied stress [42]. Data from confined in vitro human brain
indicate a linear relation between volume and the logarithm of the
applied pressure p ; the slope, representing the amount of volume
required to raise the CSF pressure by a factor of 10, was found to
be 31.6 ml over the range from 2.5-118 mm Hg [43]. Completely
different values have been obtained by various investigators for
the viscosity of brain, ranging from 0.46-50 poises at normal body
temperature; the differences have been attributed to the method of
measurement, with a likely value of around 40 poises near 20°C.

Blood vessels of the brain appear to be non-linearly elastic.
The ultimate tensile strength of the carotid artery is 115 KPa
with an ultimate elongation of 86% for the 20-29 age group, both
values decreasing with age [40,44].

Virtually no information exists concerning the mechanical
properties of human soft and hard facial tissues; a model of the
mandible utilized values of E = 17.9 GPa and   G = 6.9 GPa for
the cortical bone and a set of lower moduli for partially cancellous
bone scaled according to the percentage of solid bone present [45].

Physical property data on the human neck is also sparse; most
of the available information, categorized by age, is contained in
[40]. Average ultimate tensile strength and ultimate elongations
for cervical vertebrae are quoted as 0.33 MPa and 0.8%, only
slightly in excess of other spinal regions; ultimate compressive
strength and contraction for C1-C7 were found to be 1.1 MPa and 8%,
substantially higher than for other vertebrae, all values decreasing
with age. Stress-strain curves for vertebrae, disks, and skeletal
muscle all exhibit concave-upward trends. The ultimate tensile
strength and elongation of the cervical disks are 0.3 MPa and 77%,
while the ultimate torsional strength and angle of twist average
at 0.48 MPa and 34°. The ultimate tensile strength of nerves was
found to be about 1.32 MPa with an ultimate elongation of 18%.

The tensile strength of skin for the head appears to be around
0.5 MPa with an elongation ranging from 44-70%, whereas the values
for the neck are quoted as 1.2 MPa and 93%. The ultimate strength
of unembalmed tendons in extremal regions was found to be 28.7 MPa
[46]. A variety of constitutive models have been proposed for the
various tissues; in particular, a three-element description has
been given for muscle with viscoelastic passive elements that includes a contractile unit behaving as a sacromere [47]. Additional
mechanical and geometric properties for components of the neck are
presented in [48-49], with dimensional parameters of vertebrae obtained from direct autopsy skeletal and in vivo X-ray measurements,
or else by extrapolation from dimensions obtained from the thoracic
or lumbar regions.

4. TYPES AND MECHANISMS OF HEAD AND NECK INJURY

The standard macroscopic classification of head injury differentiates between blunt and penetrating blows as well as tissue types
as follows: (1) Scalp damage: (a) bruises (subgaleal hematoma);
(b) abrasion; (c) laceration or avulsion (peeling) [50]. (2) Skull
fracture: (a) depressed due to (i) high-speed projectile, producing
bone perforation and comminution, (ii) lower-speed bullet, yielding
perforation and fragmentation, (iii) slow-speed partial piercing
by a pointed object with small skull deformation; (b) linear or
stellar, produced by a slowly moving blunt body; (c) indented,
usually occurring in small children; and (d) crushed, due to static
loading [9,13,51]. (3) Extracerebral bleeding: (a) clot in epidural
space; (b) subdural clot in arachnoid space. (4) Brain damage:
(a) concussion, or immediate and transient impairment of neural
functions such as alteration of consciousness, response loss to external stimuli, breathing or heart rate irregularities, and loss
of reflexes and voluntary movements; (b) contusion (or bruising)
without a break in the surface or deeper tissues, but rupture of
small vessels; (c) rupture of large brain vessels (cerebral hematoma); and (d) laceration, or tearing of neural tissue. Various
methods have been employed to index the severity of the brain
damage, primarily based on the duration of the irregularities and/or
reversibility of the injury [52-57].

A review of the biomechanics of experimental central nervous
system (CNS) trauma, the mechanisms involved and correlation with
physical, physiologic and pathologic data is given in [58]. Classi-
cally, three different, relatively independent hypotheses have been
suggested as biomechanical mechanisms for neurological damage;
since no direct verification can be obtained from data on living
humans, their validity must be determined indirectly by a combination of analytical models and tests on physical replicas, on living
and in vitro animals, and on human cadavers. These theories involve [17]: (1) generation of large pressure gradients primarily
resulting from translational acceleration of the head, that produce damage due to both absolute motion of the brain and relative
motion with respect to the skull, or also from either cavitation
collapse after generation of negative pressures or else damage due
to shear strains in the brain stem induced by large intercranial
flows through the foramen magnum; (2) flexion/extension of the
upper cervical cord; and (3) the simultaneous actions of skull deformation due to local indentation or vibration of the entire shell,
and rotational acceleration with concomitant production of sizeable shear stresses. Clinical and experimental evidence exists to
counter the cavitation theory of contrecoup brain damage [58].
Contusions and hemorrhages have been found at temporal and fronto-
orbital regions regardless of the temporal or occipital locations
of the impact. Most cases of fatal fall show contrecoup, but no
coup lesions, while death from blows to the head manifests coup

damage. The first instance involves the stopping of the head by
an immovable object, resulting in diffuse load distribution with
high linear and angular accelerations, and consequent large shear
strains. In the second event, the relatively large head mass is
struck by a smaller mass, evidencing more focal damage and lower
accelerations that could only produce shear-strain injury near the
impact point.

The last mechanism was first proposed by Holbourn [59] and
is backed by a sizeable body of experimental evidence as well as
by the pathological findings just cited. Recently, a different
categorization of the relationship between mechanical loading and
biological response has been proposed. Here, the damage to the
CNS is characterized by four direct and two consequential results
of the application of tensile, compressive, bending or shear
stresses produced either by static, impulsive, or impact loading
[54]. The direct consequences are focal (or zonally restricted)
or cerebral (diffuse) concussion, primary brain lesions involving
visible structural disruption of neural tissue, and skull fracture;
these deficits may produce secondary lesions and/or post-traumatic
sequelae. It is proposed that cerebral concussion--where an adequate amount of data is available for testing the damage mechanism--
be defined as "a graded set of clinical syndromes following head
injury wherein increasing severity of disturbance in level and
content of consciousness is caused by mechanically induced strains
affecting the brain in a centripetal sequence of disruptive effects
on function and structure," always initiated at the surface and
extending inward towards the midbrain in the most severe cases.
This theory is supported by experimental, clinical and pathological
observations, and concurs with the conclusions of [60].

Virtually no biomechanical data exists on damage to the facial
region; bruises and lacerations of the skin as well as fracture
of the bone structure, including removal of teeth, are generally
caused by direct blows rather than by impulsive loading. Both of
these mechanisms, however, can cause serious or even fatal injuries in the cervical region [61]. The former occur by direct
contact with the environment or those involving helmet or restraint
harnesses; the latter involve sudden deceleration of the torso,
but in both cases the most frequent cause of trauma results from
automobile accidents.

Injury to the cervical spine involves both fractures and
dislocations; extension/tension fractures occur due to forceful
hyperextension and fixation of the head while the body moves fur-
thur forward, by "whiplash," the excessive extension of the head/
neck system generated by a rear-end vehicular collision, that also
is associated with cerebral concussion [62] or else by a head extension while the body moves down and forward, or "submarines"
[24,63]. The first two cases are converses, where tension is

exerted on the anterior spina ligament that chips the bone of the forward interior surface of a vertebra (teardrop fracture). The third situation arises when the face is arrested by an interior object, such as a steering wheel, during an automobile collision while the body submarines, causing an avulsion of the neural arch of the axis and a subsequent anterior dislocation of C2 on C3. This phenomenon is identical to what occurs in judicial hangings and is, therefore, known as "Hangman's Fracture"; it is prevented by use of a shoulder belt.

Extension/compression fractures include that of the arch of C1 when the forehead or upper face is struck, throwing the head/ neck system into forced extension, and loading the spine in compression. Such an impact may also cause posterior dislocation of C6 on C7. Flexion/compression fractures occur due to head impact at, or posterior to, its vertex, resulting in flexion and, if eccentric, in lateral bending and rotation, producing fractures of the lower three cervical segments; this can also produce teardrop fracture of vertebral bodies and/or anterior dislocations. Fracture of the odontoid process of the axis has been attributed to shear generated by impact to the mid- or lower facial region, particularly when extreme flexion, extension or rotation of the cervical region is involved. For each of these mechanisms of neck damage, the force trajectory can be established by examination of the deformation pattern and the position of the impact or impulsive loading [63]. In addition, the motion limiting function of the arterial facets in caudocephalad acceleration has been demonstrated; this can serve as a source of injury in some spinal regions [64-65].

5. EPIDEMIOLOGY

In order to prevent trauma, one of the functions of biomechanics, it is necessary to be aware of the causes of disabilities. Head and neck injuries are frequently accompanied by damage to other regions and occur as the result of motor vehicle collisions (which are often fatal), industrial or domestic accidents and falls, recreational and sports activities, suicide, assault, and war. The approximately 50-60 million annual injuries in the U.S. can be divided into the following categories: vehicular accidents, 6.7%; work-related events, 20%; home accidents, 43.6%; and other categories, 35.6% [55,57]. The annual death rate from head injury is 112,000 due to accidents, of which about 35,000 involve one or more vehicles and thus represent the largest single fatal category at 47 per billion passenger miles, whereas 21,000 result from suicide and 12,000 from homicide [13,66]. In Britain, 44% of adult head injuries are due to road accidents that claim from 4500-9000 annual fatalities; the number of hospital admissions is about 140,000 per year for all head trauma causes, with a corresponding death rate of about 5000 [10,67]. Statistics of vehicular mortality rate during the 1950's in the BDR show a decrease from 26 to 17 per 1000 accidents from the beginning to the end of the decade [68]. Relatively little information is available for industrial and home accidents, presumably because trained observers generally cannot appear as rapidly as in vehicular cases. In the sports injury area, football and boxing have received the most attention, the former exhibiting an average of 25 annual fatalities, mostly in the high school and sandlot arena in the U.S., or 2 per 100,000 participants, with head and spinal injuries accounting for nearly 80% of the deaths [69]. Boxing, an international activity, is not so readily subjected to statistics although head injury and even death are frequent; some data on this subject and other sports, notably the martial arts, soccer, rugby, basketball, baseball, track and field events, wrestling, skiing, ice-skating, sledding, ice hockey, and surfing, together with an extensive bibliography are presented in [70]. Motions of participants in team sports have been recorded by cinematography which has shed some light on injury potential (cf. [71]). A fatal injury for a swimmer has even been attributed to shock waves generated by the proximate explosion of a firecracker [72].

By contrast, the incidence of American combat casualties including the efficacy of protective devices has been exhaustively documented [73-77]. Here, a significant difference relating to head injury is represented by the comparatively high incidence of penetrating wounds--a subject that has not attracted biomechanical studies--as compared to blunt head trauma in non-assault situations. A study during the Vietnam War of 120 casualties with a 50% survival rate indicated the much greater lethality of bullets relative to fragments, and a very poor prognosis for either multiple lobe injury or brain penetration [73]. Of the 4065 casualties aboard aircraft examined from this war, wounds accounted for 32% of the fatal and 77.8% of the non-fatal cases, yielding 5200 and 14,000 flying hours per non-fatal and fatal injury, respectively; the head and neck accounted for 14.2% of the total and 53% of the fatal wounds [74]. Data on American naval aviators in the early 1960's showed about 7000 individuals to be subjected to accidents involving ejection, bail out and collisions with ground or water, of whom 89% were exposed to crash accelerations; 70% of propeller and 88% of fatal jet accidents were collisions with water for a total number of 226 deaths, while only 22% of all jet and 51% of all propeller plane accidents involved collisions with water [76]. In 1967, 228 naval aviators were killed or missing due to all causes, combat or otherwise. It is hypothesized that a frequent cause of such accidents is drowning associated with impulsively produced concussion, perhaps due to neck stretch.

Cervical flexion and extension injuries are produced in 55% of the accidents involving two or more vehicles; mortality from hyperextension is 2.5 in urban and 18.5 in rural areas per 10,000

cases, while that due to hyperflexion is 185 and 22 per 10,000
incidents in the two environments, respectively [13]. In a representative British study of 206 hospital cases involving neural
spinal injuries [78], 58% of which resulted from traffic accidents,
43% involved the cervical region, and of those about half had associated head injuries. This ratio is confirmed by an American study
of 55 cervical spine injury victims from automobile accidents [63].
Thus, impact head injury frequently induces cervical spine syndromes, and excessive motion of the cranial region often causes
concussive effects.

6. HEAD AND NECK INJURY MODELS

The most crucial biomechanical aspect of head/neck injury investigation is the appropriate analytical or experimental modelling of
the phenomenon; in addition to the actual or replicated anatomical
component, the restraint or protective device must be properly
delineated. The theoretical development may involve representation
of the system by lumped-parameter mass-spring-dashpots, by discrete
parameter models of a basic anatomical unit encompassing the mechanical behavior of a combination of elements, or by a continuum;
solutions have been obtained in closed form (or quadrature) or by
standard numerical finite-difference or finite-element methods.
Continuum models form the subject of a concurrent paper and will
not be pursued further. Experiments have been executed on human
volunteers, cadavers, living animals (usually anesthetized), and
inanimate replicas such as the heads and necks developed for anthropometric dummies. Each of these systems has advantages and disadvantages. Volunteers must be subjected to loads considerably
below the danger (or tolerance) level and may vitiate normal response by anticipatory reflex action; repeatability from subject
to subject is likely to be difficult. Cadavers can be subjected
to loads beyond the onset of serious trauma, but their properties
may differ from that of the living human, particularly when pre-
servatives have been used on the sample. Animals, while perhaps
somewhat more similar structurally within a given species, do not
exhibit some of the same critical anatomical features and mass as
humans, particularly in the head/neck area. The scaling of data
from animals to man has thus far only been treated in terms of the
angular acceleration $\ddot{\theta}$ required to produce cerebral concussion
in the model (M) relative to the prototype (P), based on brain
mass m [58-59,79]:

$$\ddot{\theta}_P = (m_M/m_P)^{2/3} \ddot{\theta}_M .$$

(6.1)

The use of any inanimate device raises questions as to its equivalent physical response in the absence of the corresponding physiologic reaction to a given loading. It is necessary to perform

cross-correlations and extrapolations among these various methods, a task that has just been barely initiated and requires considerable further effort.

To supplement the earlier discourse on head injury biomechanics [17] and the encyclopedic compilation of the results of cadaveric, animal and inanimate model tests given in [13], a recent review has discussed the state of the art of human biodynamic response, including an enormous bibliography, that isolates, among others, the head/neck region [80]. Other surveys have addressed the question of the efficacy of the mathematical modelling process of actual human response to dynamic loading [81-82]. A catalogue of available head models subjected to both impact and impulsive loading is presented that, in addition to the difference in discrete- or continuum-parameter representation, differentiates in terms of the dimensional character of the model, its geometry, permitted kinematics, the number of components and their constitutive representation, and the type of applied loading. Lumped, discrete-parameter and continuum models of the spine are also so categorized, with particular reference to successive inclusion of axial compression, bending, spinal curvature and the existence of a second load path through the facets. Two- and three-dimensional gross motion simulators, represented by lumped-parameter systems designed to primarily ascertain the effects of various restraint systems, have been extensively developed. It is concluded that while the results from most simulations agreed reasonably well with each other, their accuracy in replicating test data was generally poor, and was not resolved by inclusion of additional articulation [82]. The principal reason for these discrepancies was given as the absence of precise input data, including mechanical and geometric properties, particularly for animated experimental models.

Many analytical representations, including almost all early versions, consider the head as a rigid body, so that linear and angular accelerations are calculated from Newton's law and the moment-angular momentum relation. This concept has also been utilized to portray the forces F and moments M transmitted to the head, which has mass m and centroidal moment of inertia I_{CG}, by the neck at the occipital condyles for sagittal-plane motion, as defined in Fig. 3 with axes fixed in the head. Thus, for extension and flexion, respectively, the governing equations are

$$\sum F_x = S_o = ma_x \; ; \qquad \sum F_y = A_o + mg = ma_y$$

$$\sum M_{CG} = A_o d_A + S_o d_s + T_o = I_{CG}\alpha \qquad (6.2)$$

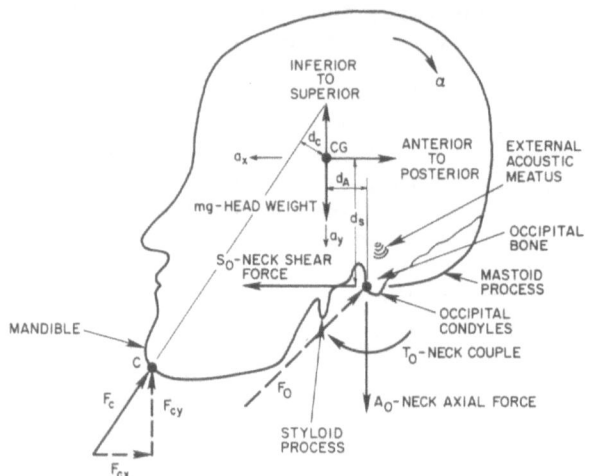

Fig. 3. Forces and moments on head in sagittal-plane motion.

$$\sum F_x = S_o - F_{cx} = ma_x \; ; \quad \sum F_y = A_o + mg - F_{cy} = ma_y$$

$$\sum M_{CG} = A_o d_A + S_o d_s + T_o - F_c d_c = I_{CG} \alpha \qquad (6.3)$$

where the latter must incorporate an additional chin contact force F_c, and g is the acceleration of gravity [24,28]. However, since the head actually deforms significantly, it is reasonable to apply the general maxim that, on the average, any energy (or work) imparted to the system is divided approximately equally into kinetic and potential energy; the average rigid-body acceleration of the head for a specified force input is then only about half that predicted by Newton's law.

Lumped-parameter models of the head have been used, in part, to define very simple criteria for brain injury tolerance. The system consists of either one or two masses (the latter segregating the parietal sector mass m_1 from that of the brain and other bones, m_2), preceded or interconnected by a parallel linear spring and dashpot of constant k and c that portray skull stiffness and soft tissue viscosity, respectively. It is acted upon either by a time-dependent force F(t) or an acceleration a(t) . The equation of forced motion for both situations is given by [83-86]

$$\ddot{x} + (c/m_1)\dot{x} + (k/m_1)x = -a(t) \qquad (6.4)$$

where $m_1 = m$ for a single mass and $m_1 = m_2$ for the two-mass system. The equation of free vibration of frequency ω and the mechanical system impedance   Z   for the second system are given by

$$\ddot{x} + [1 + (m_2/m_1)][c/m_2]\dot{x} + [1 + (m_2/m_1)][k/m_2]x = 0 \qquad (6.5)$$

and

$$Z = i\omega(m_1 + m_2) \left[\frac{1 - [\omega^2 m_1 m_2/k(m_1 + m_2)] + [i\omega c/k]}{1 - [\omega^2 m_2/k] + [i\omega c/k]} \right] \qquad (6.6)$$

Other lumped-parameter systems have been employed to obtain
the response of various anatomical regions or of the whole body
(the latter usually in the presence of restraint systems) to impact or impulsive loading. The computer solutions employed are
generally of the finite-difference type. Head/neck motion has been
studied in [49,87-92], the effect of air bag protection on the neck
is given in [93], discrete and lumped-parameter models of the spine
have been examined in [64,94-98], while whole body response is
treated in [99-105].

Continuum models of head or head/neck impact, including those
initiated by the present author [106-107] that were correlated
with the results of inanimate system replicas, have been summarized in [17,81]. These analyses involve fluid-filled thin shells,
either spherical or ellipsoidal and either single- or multilayered, subjected to radial or tangential impact, with or without
the constraints presented by the head/neck junction. Solid components are generally considered to be elastic, with the brain
represented either by a Newtonian fluid or a linear viscoelastic
material, and radial loading is most frequently applied over a
finite area. Solutions are obtained by transform and series expansion techniques, with the eventual result obtained by means of
digital calculators.

Head impact on a structural component has also been modelled
by rigid body dynamics with a deformable head and an exponentially
decaying applied force to derive effective accelerations, contact
stresses and durations [31]. It is shown here that brain shear
distortion is a significant trauma mode. Recent three-dimensional
finite-element analyses of head impact comprise another type of
continuum approach for the phenomenon [108-110].

Initial continuum models of the spine consisted of straight
homogeneous elastic rods, linear or otherwise, with or without
an attached mass to represent the head [111-113]. Curvature effects, eccentric inertial loading and rotational inertia and shear,
as well as the effects of musculature were introduced subsequently
and solutions were obtained by a variety of techniques; however,
no analysis was specifically concerned only with the cervical
region.

350

The biodynamic study of impact to the head and impulsive loading for the head/neck system has been carried out systematically only during the last 40 years [114]. Early qualitative low-force level information was obtained from volunteers running into obstacles to test helmets. However, most quantitative data for living humans subjected to such loading conditions have been acquired either by sled or other types of deceleration tests, notably the pioneering work of Col. J. Stapp, or by the attachment of transducers to athletes and the transmission and recording of signals representing the histories of stress, acceleration and/or physiological outputs under field conditions. In some instances, tests on volunteers have been replicated with cadavers, but under more severe loading conditions. Living humans have involuntarily served to advance the biomechanical studies of physical cause and physiological end-effect, both under recoverable and fatal conditions, by serving as source material in the analysis of accidents when sufficient data concerning mechanical parameters could be extracted from the event a posteriori. Such studies have involved not only comprehensive and long-term data acquisition and interpretation of vehicular collisions*, but also an analysis and simulation of free falls [115].

A complete catalogue of the extensive tests on volunteers conducted to anticipate the effects of landing of the Apollo vehicle, involving forward ($-G_x$), backward ($+G_x$), right side ($+G_y$), left side ($-G_y$), upward ($+G_z$) and downward ($-G_z$) acceleration, including the magnitude, duration and rate of onset of the acceleration as well as the physiological response is given in [116]. A more recent and more completely instrumented series of tests has been conducted on volunteers subjected to accelerations from 3-15 ($-G_x$) for various durations and rates of onset and for identical initial angular and linear positioning of the head and the first thoracic vertebra [61,117-122]. The acceleration histories at the mouth between various subjects subjected to comparable loading appeared to exhibit many similarities but were substantially greater (by a factor from 2-4) than the measured sled accelerations; peak angular velocities of 30 rad/s at the mouth and head/neck flexion angles ranging from 60-80° for 10 ($-G_x$) were observed. An increase of either the neck or the head angle was found to produce a significant reduction in peak angular velocity and acceleration [121]. The data correlated well with the numerical predictions of both two- and three-dimensional distributed parameter computational schemes [92,123-124] and also permitted the construction of a predictive type of model for this motion [125]; however, it exhibited significant differences when compared to the response under the same loading of an artificial head/neck system (Hybrid II) prescribed by the U.S. Federal Motor Vehicle Safety Standard 208

* Such as conducted at Wayne State University by L. E. Patrick and at the University of Heidelberg by E. Gögler.

[104]. Whiplash tests in automotive collision simulations at
16 km/hr revealed peak angular acceleration of 500 and 200 rad/s^2
for volunteers and cadavers with the latter increased to 700 rad/s^2
at 37 km/hr [126]. The kinematics of various landmarks over the
entire body of volunteers subjected to 8 ($-G_x$) acceleration is
given in [127].

Voluntary static human neck torque levels developed at the
occipital condyles resisting flexion or extension have been measured as 31.9 and 14.2 N-m for the normal neck position, as 33.9
and 23.7 N-m for an extended neck, and as 35.2 and 16.9 N-m for the
flexed neck [28]. Maximum static shear and axial (anteroposterior)
forces in the sagittal plane at this position were 845 N and 1110 N,
respectively. Under dynamic loading of 4.2 ($-G_x$) with muscles relaxed, the equivalent moment about this point was found to be 16.3
N-m, while that at 6.8 g with tensed muscles was about 28.5 N-m,
corresponding to axial peak forces of 280 N and 410 N, respectively;
the moments include the effect of the chin reaction on the chest
and those exerted by the soft tissue.

Instrumentation has been attached to the head and to the
helmets of athletes engaging in American football, with an FM
transmitter sending the head acceleration and EEG histories to a
nearby recording station [128-132]. For one season, 650 impacts
were measured for one player; 50 of these exhibited peak accelerations ranging from 150-450 g with most durations from 300-350 ms,
with one concussion resulting from these blows. However, the data
of [132] that cites measured peak accelerations for two different
offensive backs in excess of 1000 g is suspect on the basis that
these values apply to the accelerometer mounted on a strap around
the head, but not necessarily to the point under the head directly
below the transducer. From accelerometers attached to the heads
of amateur boxers using 12 oz gloves, the majority of recorded
blows exhibited amplitudes between 0 and 5 g, with a few accelerations extending to 25 g; it is estimated that the magnitude of
these blows would have been doubled if professional gloves weighing
16 oz had been used [133]. Blows within voluntary limits were
also directed at a human volunteer up to a peak head acceleration
of 14 g (corresponding to a striking velocity of 1.4 m/s directed
by a 6 oz boxing glove on a wooden fist backed by a 4.5 kg additional mass). This was related to impacts on a physical head model
whose frequency was correlated to that of the human head, executed
with peak accelerations up to 40 g; the results indicate substantial excess of safe tolerance limits for the head [134].

The function of cadaver tests in head injury studies has been
to delineate the mechanisms of impact or impulsive load damage, to
determine tolerance limits, to evaluate mechanical properties of
head/neck tissues, and to ascertain the effectiveness of protective and/or crash-ameliorating devices, using either separate skulls

or entire corpses [17]. Changes in volume, deformation patterns
and variations in intracranial pressure in skulls subjected to
blows are discussed extensively in [13,50]; the distribution of
the peak pressure was found to be linear up to levels of 75 g and
reasonably predicted by a simple static model [135]. A recent
study on bare skulls and those covered with a simulated scalp indicated substantial differences in pressure distribution for frontal
as opposed to occipital impacts in the former, but not the latter,
case, and a substantial reduction of fluid pressure as opposed to
that found in acrylic thin shells struck in a similar manner [136],
attributed to the layering effect of the biological system relative
to its homogeneous replica. Other pressure measurements have been
compared with data on inanimate physical models [137]. Accelerometers, strain gages and brittle lacquer techniques have been utilized to define the deformation and failure characteristics of the
cranium, including studies to assess the effect of the presence of
the scalp [13].

Cadavers have been employed to study the effect of restraint
systems, collapsible steering wheels, padded dashboards, air bags,
or windshields [138-140] in vehicular crash environments, using
either free fall or sled techniques. This type of investigation
has led to better design and the use of improved materials, such
as laminated windshields with plastic interlayers.

Cadaver studies have also provided information on head/neck
motion under dynamic loading and static and dynamic strengths of
the system, primarily supplementing and extending data from human
volunteers [24,28], although cadaveric response differs from that
of the living human, especially under high acceleration. Torques
of 190 N-m and axial forces in the sagittal plane of 2090 N did not
produce damage to the cervical spine as determined by X-rays;
torque-angular deformation plots are considered to be an excellent
indicator of neck strength [25]. Studies of spinal motion have
attempted to examine the mechanisms and locations of fracture
[141-142], particularly in reference to pilot ejection [64,98,143]
or head-on and rear-end vehicular collisions [144]. Tests up to
20 ($+G_z$) indicated a somewhat non-linear relation between acceleration and cervical vertebrae strain [141], the compressive strain
in this region increasing with enhanced amplitude of the movement
of head and thorax. The facets carry both compressive and tensile
loads, and in greater proportion the lower the acceleration, suggesting they also carry some of the static load [64]. It is proposed that one of the major causes of ejection vertebral fracture
is the dynamic reaction of the column under this acceleration in
the presence of improper restraint [143]. The vehicular simulated
impact tests were carried out at speeds up to 30 km/hr with maximum
head and cranial accelerations of 1-6 g and 20-36 g, respectively,
and restraint forces of 40-250 N, with the head rotating about C1.
Most common and serious failure was found at C6, indicating that

restraint systems should be designed to avoid this damage, such as by devices limiting antiflexion of the head [144]. The model description for this case regarded the neck as an elastic bar with joints at C6 and C1.

Although the use of experimental animals for the assessment of medical, surgical, and even pharmacological treatments has a history of many centuries, their systematic and fully documented use in biomechanical studies appears to have been initiated during and subsequent to World War II. Since then, however, a plethora of such investigations has been published, and only a few selected results can be cited in the present limited space. A substantial accounting of such findings is given in [13], with shorter summaries available in [17,20]. The advantage of using a live animal is that it permits the measurement of both physical and physiological response parameters under controlled dynamic loading conditions ranging in severity from minor to fatal, as well as subsequent pathological examination for the correlation of the observed deficit with input and damage mechanisms. However, the extremely complicated problem of scaling such data to the living human, while addressed, has not been adequately resolved due to the variability of the specimens, the differences in concussive effects, divergences in reflexes, and the presence of anesthesia.

Types of animals employed have included rats, cats, dogs, rabbits, and various types of monkeys, with the Macaca mulatta, the squirrel monkey and the chimpanzee as favorite specimens in view of their closer similarity (compared to other species) to man. They have been subjected to a variety of impact and impulsive loading conditions using free fall, sleds, or pendulum-type mechanisms while instrumented to record kinematic variables, pressure, stress, electrophysical, reflex, respiration and heart rate, and while monitored by ordinary and/or flash X-ray cinematography in one or two orthogonal planes.

One of the main thrusts of animal experiments has been an attempt to resolve the questions as to whether linear or rotational acceleration resulting from dynamic loading is the main contributor to brain damage. The enormous destructive potential of relative motion between brain and skull under impact was graphically demonstrated in classical experiments [145], since repeated [58] where a portion of a monkey skull was replaced by a Lucite calvarium to permit direct photography of the movement of the cranial contents. This question has been addressed by many investigators who subjected both cats and primates to linear accelerations produced by sled arrest or to angular acceleration by means of a pendulum in which the head was either free to move or fixed relative to the head [54,58,79,146-153]. Monkeys with larger heads and deeper implanted electrodes appeared to be easier to concuss [133]. While the controversy concerning the relative damaging

effects of the two mechanisms has not by any means been resolved--
since deficits have been demonstrated to occur when each mechanism
alone was present--the preponderance of the physiological and pathological evidence seems to indicate that the angular motion is the
more dangerous and that elimination of head rotation significantly
increases the threshold of concussion. In tests on 11 squirrel
monkeys, all six specimens subjected to rotation exhibited concussion, whereas none of five animals accelerated linearly to similar levels but constrained from rotation by a cervical collar exhibited such syndromes [146]. Concussion was avoided with rotation
permitted when the linear acceleration was reduced from 1230 ($+G_x$)
and 930 ($-G_x$) to 700 ($+G_x$) and 600 ($-G_x$). This relative damage
theory was further supported by data on rhesus monkeys that indicated it was much easier to injure brain tissue by rotationally
induced shear stresses than by translational-motion-induced stresses
of whatever character [148]. On the basis of a tolerance level of
40 krad/s^2 for this animal, the threshold predicted for man obtained from Eq. 6.1 would be 7500 rad/s^2 [79]. Dogs and cats
subjected to translational acceleration without relative head restraint survived levels of 250-500 g (corresponding to intracranial
pressure increase from 0.17-0.66 MPa lasting from 0.5-5 ms) and
280-400 g, respectively, although exhibiting some concussive effects; for cats increased levels of lesions were produced by repeated loading at the same severity level [13,150-151]. Squirrel
monkeys with heads restrained relative to the neck and subjected
to rotational acceleration evidenced no syndromes at 10^5 rad/s^2,
but did not survive levels three times larger. Extensive translational and rotational tests on squirrel monkeys under inertial
loading involving photography, measurement of sensory response and
subsequent pathological examination with particular reference to
the location of focal and the distribution of diffuse lesions
strongly supported the hypothesis that the severity of the injury
is directly proportional to the depth of penetration of lesions
into the brain [54,147].

A different class of experiments have attempted to ascertain
the physiological response of animals subjected to a pressure pulse
on the brain, with the dura intact [13,154-157]. A conduit passing
through a trephinized hole in the skull of rabbits was attached to
a hydraulic system that permitted controlled loading of the brain
through ramming effects of a piston; pressure measurements at
various positions in the system and physiological response data
were determined. Pendulum impacts on the ram yielded rise-time
durations from 0.1-1 ms and peak ram accelerations of 2250 g. These
tests supported the lack of major clinical implications of contrecoup lesions, while indicating noticeable vascular permeability
changes in the brain stem and cervical region, perhaps related to
tissue motion near the cerebrospinal junction. Belgian hares and
a variety of primates have been utilized in a study of whiplash
motion in a vehicular deceleration environment with the employment

of differing restraint systems [158-159]. It was found that the hares proved to be remarkably resistant to severe acceleration pulses, that hyperflexion forces created substantially greater damage to the tissues than hyperextension, and that larger-headed animals were susceptible to greater damage at equal loading levels (in conformity with the scaling hypothesis).

Inanimate model testing for head/neck injury studies has involved the construction of either very simplified versions of the system, such as elastic thin-walled spherical shells for the head or springs for the neck--which are very simple to construct and represent properly in an analytical formulation but do not pretend to closely simulate the prototype--or else complicated devices purporting to replicate the living biological system, such as dummy heads, necks and complete torsos. Most frequently, the response of such dummies has been found not to be sufficiently accurate in at least some respects, as determined by comparison of data from volunteers, and, furthermore, the analytical representation of such devices is almost as complex as that for the living human.

The first mechanical head injury model consisted of a two-dimensional gelatin system surrounded by wax loaded dynamically and examined photoelastically [59]; the results were used to support the rotational acceleration and skull deformation theory of brain damage. This observational technique was later repeated by others to demonstrate the presence of shear strains at the cerebro-spinal junction [160-161]. Clarification of various hypothesized head injury phenomena or substantiation of analytical predictions were sought by experiments where liquid-filled thin spherical or ellipsoidal shells of aluminum, plastic, or glass variously in-strumented with strain- and/or pressure-measuring devices were sub-jected to impact loading [106-107,155,162-166]. Cavitation has indeed been observed in vessels filled with both water and a liquid with a viscosity resembling that of the human brain [164-166] and has also been reported at the opposite pole in water-filled skulls [50]; however, the contrecoup theory of brain damage as the result of cavitation collapse was negated by the observed location of peak pressures in entirely different regions [165], as supported to some extent by analytical considerations [17]. Peak negative pressures were found at the impact site, in contradiction to earlier specu-lations [162-163] which do not consider wave transmission. Surface strains and pressures along the line of action of a radial impact on a freely suspended acrylic shell due to short-duration blows by steel spheres were in excellent correspondence with analytical pre-dictions [106], as was the agreement with respect to the excursion of the head/neck junction, shown in Fig. 4, when this shell was attached to an artificial neck resembling human motion in the sagittal plane [107].

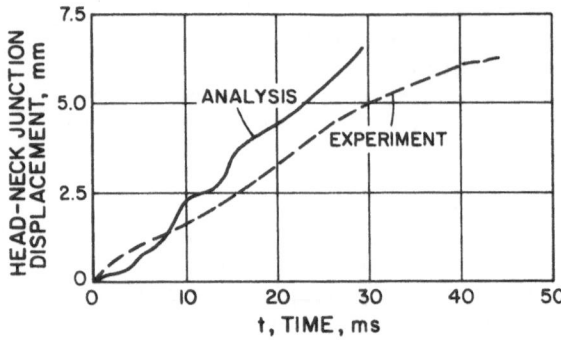

Fig. 4. Head/neck junction motion of Lucite shell on GM artificial
neck loaded horizontally by half-sine pulse of 1272 N
amplitude and 2.5 ms duration.

Efforts to construct replicas of a human skull began with
extensive cataloguing of the anthropometric measurements of the
head [167-170], followed by material selection and construction of
trauma-indicating models [171-173]. A current model consists of a
self-skinning urethane foam skull overlaid by a silicone rubber-
coated skin-simulating cover and exhibiting a silicone gel-filled
cranial cavity with a provision for insertion of a triaxial accelerometer; it was found to be repetitive in impact performance and
to withstand several impacts at human tolerance levels when protected by a helmet. This device represents a substantial improvement over the solid magnesium head specified for impact testing
of vehicular helmets [174]; for the same helmet and impact conditions, the plastic model reduced the measured peak acceleration
from 250 to 145 g, decreased the peak force from 11.6 KN to 5.56 KN
(compared to a cadaver test fracture result of 6.45 KN), and increased the pulse duration by 50%. Another type of anthropometric
head is being constructed that consists of a frangible skull whose
deformation or fracture characteristics might be related to human
head trauma [173]. Heads available commercially for employment in
dummies subjected to biomechanical investigations include the
Sierra 1050, the Alderson and the Hybrid I and Hybrid II model.
A modification of these is represented by a General Motors ATD 502
model, composed of aluminum with a pliable vinyl skin that represents a modification of the Sierra head. The interior is a cavity
accommodating instrumentation and ballast that is accessible through
a back cap [170].

A nylon-filled punch ball served as a head replica for the
extension of boxing data on volunteers [134], struck by a 6 oz
boxing glove on a wooden fist. The mass, natural frequency and
damping characteristics of the human head served to define the
shape and materials employed in the construction of a replica used
to test windshields [84]; the degree of equivalence is based on a

tolerance criterion developed specifically for this evaluation. A recent study of the pressure distribution in the horizontal plane containing the impact axis for a polystyrene-polyvinyl acetate skull simulator filled with water and supported on various types of artificial necks, generated upon impact by a pendulum, shows the need for investigation of this parameter away from the impact axis [175]; however, the tests depended upon repeatability, and no effort was made to assess the presence of the probe on the data obtained.

Endeavors of a similar type have been directed towards the construction of a human-like artificial neck [176-181]. The efficacy of a two-jointed extensible neck subjected to side, oblique and rear impact situations was studied on the basis of a discrete-parameter model including both the spine and musculature [176]; three-dimensional neck replicas should account for coupling between the forces resisting rotations about three orthogonal axes. A further improvement over this model or over a uniform rubber cylinder simulating the neck was represented by a three-jointed structure whose performance was compared both to a mathematical model and the results of volunteer tests [177] and that performed satisfactorily in terms of the range of angular motions of the head relative to the torso, the trajectory of the neck mass center relative to the torso, and the linear and angular accelerations of the head during its motion [178]. Modified neck performance requirements based on the data of [28] have been applied to commercial necks; only the GMR polymeric neck was found to be compatible with these specifications [179], although additional tests were recommended to insure compatibility of such a neck with a total dummy structure and under a wider range of conditions than those for which the model was tested. A further development [180] describes the construction of a four-ball jointed segment and one pin-connected nodding segment neck model that has been used both in sled deceleration tests and in conjunction with model and cadaver head impact studies [107,136]. In addition, a dual-pivot neck containing calibrated lengths of elastic shock cords guided by rotating sectors has been fabricated [181] for the purpose of attaching to a specific head replica, a properly ballasted Alderson VIP-50A model [182]. This device exhibits favorable response relative to known human data whenever motions are involved that are properly transmitted by the attached torso; additional studies are recommended to insure the faithful replication of the external structure to both loading and unloading of the system.

Full-scale vehicular collision testing involving motion and response of anthropometric dummies has been executed by several organizations*; typical results due to frontal impacts of vehicles

---

* Among others, the Institute of Traffic and Transportation, UCLA; General Motors Proving Grounds; Highway Safety Research Institute, University of Michigan.

moving at 11.3-32.2 km/hr with stationary cars result in vehicular and dummy decelerations of 4-7 g and 3-12 g, respectively, with durations of 0.1-0.2 s and a delay of about 100 ms for the dummy [183]. Backward rotation occurred to an extent of 120°, after which rapid deceleration and forward flexion ensued with occasional impact against the windshield and steering wheel. Numerous other situations have been examined, including barrier tests, rear and side collisions. An examination of the influential variables in hyperextension, i.e., seat back rotation, restraint position, and collision speed, has been executed with Sierra dummies in sled tests [184].

Substantial concern has been expressed concerning the validity of the response of dummies in crash environments compared to that of humans. A comparison of the body kinematics and moments about the occipital condyles was obtained from identical sled tests simulating a barrier collision at 17.7 km/hr for a volunteer, cadaver, and anthropomorphic dummy [185]; cinematography revealed similar motions, but the dummy exhibited a maximum acceleration six times larger than that of the volunteer and the torque at the occipital condyles was similarly disproportionate. At the highest impact velocities the dummies exhibited much higher occipital condyle torques than the two cadavers tested. The peak angular acceleration of the head for the volunteer was 250 rad/s^2 at a 16.1 km/hr impact speed, while that for the dummy was 1000 rad/s^2, increased to 2500 when the speed was raised to 37 km/hr. With a head support, identical simulated rear-end collisions indicated the same peak loads of $F_{max} = 33$ a_{sl} , where a_{sl} is the mean sled acceleration, for volunteer, dummy and cadaver.

Comparison of the performance of two different dummies indicated some variability both between samples of the same make and greater variations between different manufacturers [186]. It is concluded that the dummies should be qualified not only on the basis of response duplication, but also with regard to severity level discrimination of the test environment. For this, it is necessary to decide what criteria must be satisfied for the test to be considered repeatable. A controllable crash environment has been developed that should yield reproducible performance regardless of the particular facility employed [187]. This is achieved by pre-tensioned straps constituting the restraint environment. However, a constant comparison must be effected between dummy response and those of volunteers to insure the applicability of the model [188].

7. TOLERANCE LEVELS

Interpretation of any tolerance level must be conditioned by the observation that the mean value quoted is often just slightly larger than the extreme deviation due to the high variability of the strength of biological structures. Data of this type is presented in terms of either regional or whole-body tolerances. Results are ordinarily correlated with severity levels indicative of voluntary exposure, onset of pain, injury threshold, moderate (but reversible) damage, irreversible trauma, and fatality [189]. Data is acquired individually or by a combination of controlled tests with human volunteers, cadaver research, investigations with animals, dummies or other inanimate replicas, clinical and pathological observations, and mathematical models; all techniques have their advantages and shortcomings.

The most common parameter used to indicate head injury potential is linear acceleration; others have included energy, force, pressure, displacement and angular acceleration. The first announced tolerance level for the skull was based on the initiation of single linear fractures produced by the free fall onto metallic anvils of either dry skulls or intact cadaver heads at energies of 4.5 N-m and in the range from 45-102 N-m, respectively, with notice-able variations relative to the position of the impact point [13, 190]. This was translated into an average acceleration of 160 g for a period of 4 ms, a force of 5.8-8.9 KN, and an intracranial pressure increase of 240-280 KPa. The difference in the fracture energies for the two systems is attributed to the protective load-distributing effect of the scalp, although the latter absorbs no more than 13% of the energy of a direct blow [32]. Volunteers sus-tained loads of 1.8 KN for 5 ms and 1.27 KN for 32 ms in the antero-posterior direction without injury; a combination of measurement techniques indicates a peak g value of 60 from speeds of about 20 m/s for the onset of mild concussion [189]. Concussive effects in animals occur generally at substantially higher levels [13,79, 191].

An extensive review of the literature involving forces required to produce fractures of the bare or skin-covered craniums by metallic or foam-covered strikers is given in [32] with a range of peak dynamic loads from 3.1-9.0 KN and durations of 3-5 ms for both local and remote linear fractures. Skull penetration tests with a 12.7 mm diameter impactor quasi-statically and at speeds up to 9 m/s indicated critical loads of 6.4 and 3.9 KN for frontal and parietal embalmed cadaver bone with no observable rate effects. Load tolerances for effective contact areas of 650 mm^2 have been determined as 4.0-4.9 KN, 2.0-2.45 KN and 0.89-1.0 KN for the fron-tal, temporoparietal, and zygomatic areas, respectively [192].

A combination of measured intracranial pressure changes and accelerations generated in cadaver skulls by a blow, data of similar nature and the corresponding physiological response from animals (usually anesthetized), and human voluntary exposure information were employed to construct the Wayne State Tolerance Curve (WSTC)

360

for the human head [193], shown in Fig. 5. This plot is based on
cadaver skull fracture and the onset of concussion in animals and
has been criticized for this basis of discrimination of lethal
dosage in humans, as well as for lack of adequate scaling and
cross-correlation [79,193]. The curve, which is obviously inap-
plicable at either extreme, portrays average acceleration as a
function of pulse duration. It has been supplemented by additional
data, its horizontal asymptote has been raised from 45 to 80 g
[86,195-196], and it has also been modified to account for acceleration of forehead and occiput [84]; nevertheless, it still serves
as the basic criterion for human head tolerance and is widely used
for the even more rudimentary concept of a limiting value of a
mechanical parameter, such as acceleration history or strain, which
separates the region of safety from that of lethality.

These representations, as well as the WSTC, rest upon the
hypothesis that the head and its components can be represented by
one or more lumped masses connected by springs and dashpots. From
mechanical impedance studies, it has been suggested that the rigid-
body motions govern the head for pulse durations of 5 ms or greater,
for which skull frequencies of 200 Hz or less will be excited,
whereas deformation considerations must be included for short rise
times, less than 0.5 ms, when the resonant mode of the skull, about
900 Hz, might be excited [197]. The first such measure was suggested as the area of the acceleration, pressure or force history.
A second attempt to quantify the WSTC and additional data on whole-
body tolerance obtained primarily from military tests [198] involving volunteers and primates subjected to $(-G_x)$ sled tests resulted
in a weighted acceleration integral known as the Gadd Severity
Index (GSI), given by

$$GSI = \int_0^\tau a^n \, dt \quad , \quad n \text{ generally} = 2.5 \tag{7.1}$$

with a as the acceleration in g and τ the pulse duration in
seconds [199]. The original tolerance limit of 1000 was subsequently extended to 1500 as additional data were evaluated. A
further modification of GSI, to more properly account for the
average accelerations inherent in the WSTC and encompassing additional volunteer response under long pulse durations, has been
proposed by [196] and the U.S. Department of Transportation. The
resultant Head Injury Criterion (HIC), adopted as a standard in
certain vehicular impact tests, is given by

$$HIC = [(t_2 - t_1)^{-1} \int_{t_1}^{t_2} a \, dt]^{2.5} (t_2 - t_1) \tag{7.2}$$

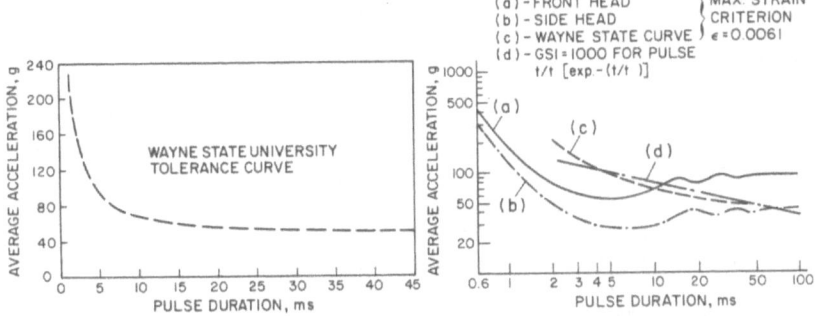

Fig. 5. Wayne State Tolerance   Fig. 6. Comparison of WSTC,
         Curve.   GSI, Maximum Strain
                                               Criterion.

where t_1 is an arbitrary pulse time and t_2 the time which
maximizes HIC, with a tolerance limit established at 1000.

Alternate models proposed thus far are all based on lumped-
mass concepts. The Vienna Institute Index (JIT) [83-84] is based
on a critically damped single-mass system with a natural frequency
of 635 Hz, and leads to a maximum tolerable displacement of 2.35 mm
based on two triangular acceleration pulses, derived from the WSTC,
when used in Eq. 6.4. Impacts are assessed by calculating the
maximum displacement x_m from the given acceleration pulse and
comparison with the cited limit. The Effective Displacement Index
(EDI) [200-201] is similar to JIT with slightly different constants
emphasizing short-duration impact, with a natural frequency of
482 Hz and damping of 0.707 critical; tolerable human displacement
levels were increased to 3.81 mm, with those applicable to dummies
in sled tests ranging to 5.08 mm. The Revised Brain Model [194]
is a further modification of JIT with a natural frequency of 175 Hz,
and a damping constant 0.4 critical. For long-duration inputs, the
recommended tolerance was a brain deformation criterion of 31.75 mm;
for short durations, the tolerance limit was a brain velocity of
3.44 m/s. Based on scaled survival data for the human of a 7.5 ms
acceleration pulse with an amplitude of 56 g, a peak velocity of
6.7 m/s and a peak force of 3.56 KN, values for the damped two-mass
system representing the parietal sector, m_1 , and the rest of the
calvarium, m_2 , have been suggested as follows [85]: (1) for side
impact, m_1 = 0.182 kg, m_2 = 4.09 kg, k = 4.55 MN/m, and c = 420
N-s/m, yielding a resonance and an antiresonance of 812 and 167 Hz,
respectively; (2) for frontal impact, m_1 = 0.273 kg, m_2 = 4.55 kg,
k = 8.76 MN/m, and c = 350 N-s/m, with a resonance of 923 Hz and
an antiresonance of 207 Hz. For both cases, the tolerable mean
strain for the human was found as 0.0061 from cadaver tests.

Comparisons of numerical values determined from the various criteria
for identical input values using dummy windshield impact and volunteer air bag test information leads to close correspondence when the
results are normalized [86,195]. The various criteria have also
been plotted against each other for both average and effective accelerations over the pulse duration range up to 200 ms [85,194,196]
as exemplified by Fig. 6; agreement is not perfect. Finally, the
effect of various pulse shapes exhibiting the same GSI on the response of continuum models of the head has shown almost identical
behavior of the physical system, indicating that such an index,
which is based on a simple spring-mass concept, is a useful device
for representing the severity of a pulse applied to a linear system,
although not necessarily a proper means of identifying the resulting injury potential [31,202].

For comparative purposes, the GSI for punches thrown by a
professional boxer involving a peak acceleration of 260 g with a
duration of 13 ms and an assumed triangular pulse, corresponding
to the conservative value of a fist velocity of 8 m/s, is 3700,
more than twice that considered to be safe [134]. Peak accelerations of 300 g with pulse durations of 300 ms yield values of the
GSI in excess of 10,000, based on the same pulse shape. The lack
of reality of the latter value is probably due to the extremely
sharp spike of the peak acceleration, which is substantially greater
than the average value experienced over the contact interval.

Proposed tolerance levels for the neck in flexion [28] are
given as an equivalent moment about the occipital condyles of
59.7 N-m for the initiation of pain and a value of 88.1 N-m for a
voluntary maximum level; an equivalent moment of 203 N-m and a
2000 N force in the anteroposterior direction is a threshold above
which ligamentous and bone damage is likely. Cadaver tests in extension appear to indicate an upper non-injurious moment limit
about the condyles of 47.5 N-m, with ligamentous damage expected
beyond 57 N-m. The maximum voluntary shear force on the neck was
found to be 845 N-m. Simulated rear-end vehicular impacts of 20 m/s
resulting in a peak force of 1.5 KN did not yield injurious results
for the neck [189]. Dynamic response corridors, i.e., acceptable
moment/head rotation domains, were developed from cadaver and volunteer information, static neck data and dynamic strength data of
others, and are presented in Fig. 7. A full discussion of the
methodology of these curves, their limitations, and their applicability for the performance characteristics of artificial necks
is given in [28]. Other cadaveric tests indicated that the mean
force required to rupture transverse ligaments was 824 N and that
the subsequent force required to produce large anterior displacements of C1 (corresponding to major spinal cord damage) under dynamic loading was 834 N [61].

Several investigators concur that the relative head/neck
motion represents the limiting factor on human tolerance to impact

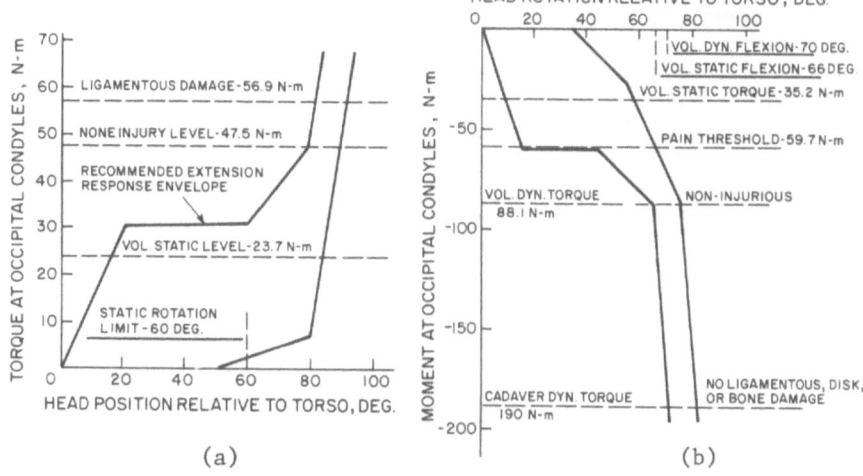

Fig. 7. Head/neck response envelope and tolerance levels for
         (a) extension, (b) flexion.

acceleration. If correct, the tolerance limits of the human head
will be dependent on the level and direction of the applied impulsive load and the degree of restraint present between head, neck,
and torso. Tolerance levels for ($-G_x$) acceleration of belted un-
injured volunteers have been reported at loads up to 14.7 KN, corresponding to 18 peak g, and backwards at 21.13 KN, corresponding
to 30 peak g [203].

   Whole-body tolerances have been primarily obtained from sled
tests of volunteers, cadavers, and animals, and from a study of
accidental falls and their simulation [114-116,204]; [114,116] contain enormous bibliographies and catalogues of physical and physiological characteristics of sled testing. Whole-body tolerance
limits for man are about 50 peak g at 500 g/s for 250 ms duration
with adequate torso restraint under conditions of ($-G_x$) acceleration. For ($+G_x$) acceleration, the most tolerable of major·axis
orientations, levels of 82 g have been survived at 3286 g/s for
40 ms duration; the accepted Air Force limit is 45 g for 100 ms.
Non-reversible injury under conditions of survival are less than
240 g at 11,250 g/s and 350 ms duration for ($-G_x$) orientation when
restrained by a full body harness. In ($+G_x$) tests, unpleasant
physiological reactions were found at 30 peak g and 100 g/s. Lateral tolerances ($\pm G_y$) appear to be substantially lower, of the
order of 20 g at 1200 g/s for 120 ms. Upward vertical acceleration ($+G_z$) appears to have voluntary tolerance limits of 20-30 g
at reasonable rates of onset, whereas downward acceleration ($-G_z$)
along the spinal axis has limited study, although brain hemorrhages
have been reported at over 3 g for more than 1 s [114]. The

tolerance experience for a variety of conditions is represented
in Fig. 8, and that for military sled tests in Fig. 9 [198].

A comprehensive study of free falls shows the greater
survivability of children relative to adults, with peak values of
600 g at an onset rate of 3×10^5 g/s and durations up to 3 ms
(corresponding to a HIC value of 11,000) not resulting in fatality.
The general survival limit for this group of young humans is considered to be 350 peak g with a 2.5-3 ms duration [115].

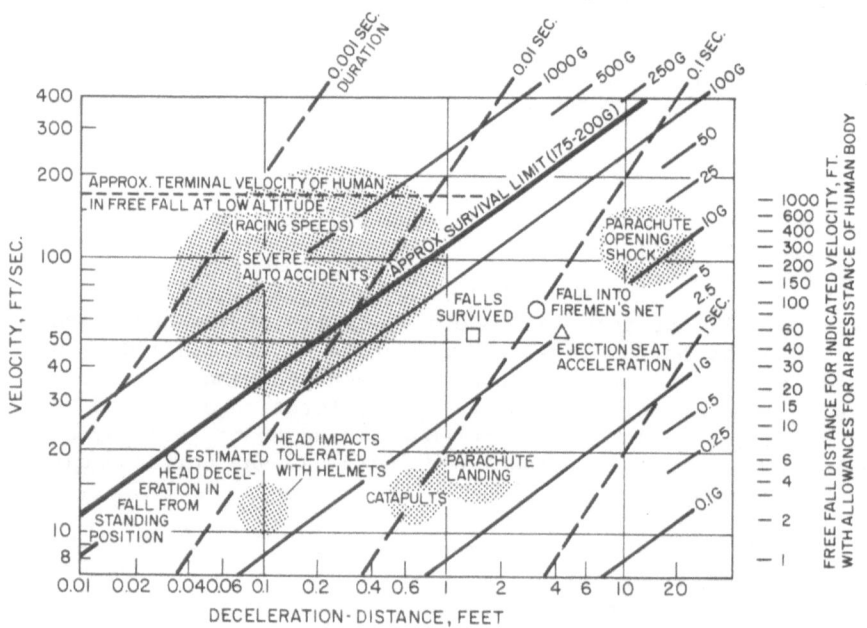

Fig. 8.   Composite of impact experience.

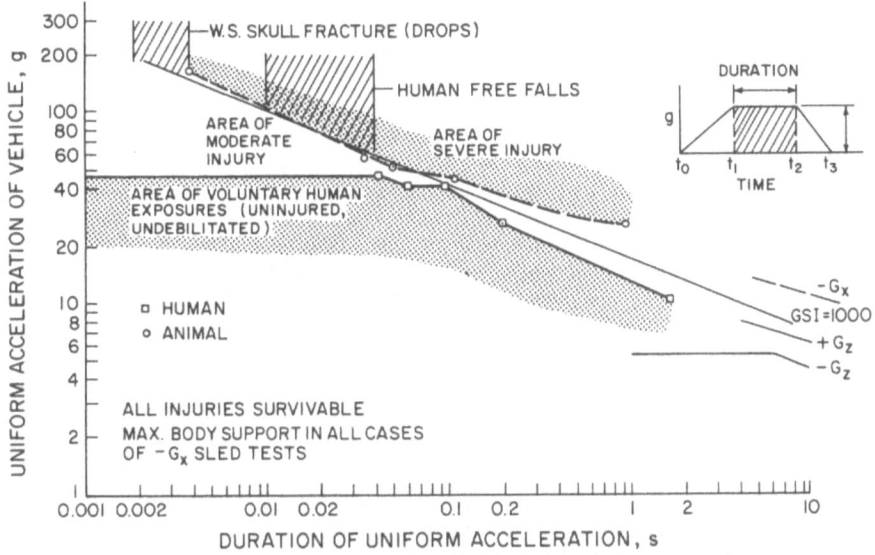

Fig. 9. Tolerance curve for sled tests, cadaver and human falls.

8. PROTECTIVE COVERS

Devices designed to eliminate or mitigate impact or impulsive
loading injury potential can be classified as either external environments or protective covers, i.e., caps or helmets worn by a
victim. The first category, which includes the analysis of the
relative energy absorbing merits of various structures and materials, the proper design of vehicles and their interior surfaces,
the construction and use of both active and passive restraint
systems--belting and air bags--and the general interaction of the
human body with its surroundings under dynamic loading, is too extensive to be covered here and deserves a survey in its own right.
Some information on this topic is contained in [68,93,205-211].
Thus, only the subject of head covers will be briefly addressed
here.

Threats to the head have been identified as due to noise,
electromagnetic waves, extreme climatic conditions, chemicals,
thermal flux, ballistic missiles and collisions [212], with the
latter two of primary interest here. Helmets serve the simultaneous
function of reducing the potential for penetration of the skull,
distributing loads in blunt impact and absorbing a portion of the
energy of a blow. This is accomplished by the presence of an outer
shell and an interior lining and/or suspension system; however, the
benefits of a helmet with respect to head protection are at least
partly balanced by the increased risk of neck injury due to the
presence of a larger mass or inertial moment. In addition to

biomechanical considerations, helmet construction must consider anthropometry, human factors, heat transfer, acoustics and design methodology [212].

Helmets are designed for specific operational uses which include vehicular types (motorcycle and bicycle), sports (football, baseball, ice hockey, riding, mountain climbing, sparring, fencing, etc.), industrial hard hats, and military (infantry, tank, air crew), each having special requirements and some needing to meet specific standards for acceptance. The criteria thus far delineated apply to vehicular and industrial helmets; they were initially determined by an industrywide consensus and promulgated in the form specifications for protective headgear for vehicular users, ANSI Z90.1, and the safety requirements for industrial head protection, Z89.1, issued by the American National Standards Institute [174,213]. The first delineates limitations on the construction, materials employed, labeling, extent of protection, sampling and conditioning for testing. It also provides for impact tests consisting, first, of two successive drops at the same point at four separate positions on the helmet with an energy of 67.8 N-m when striking a hemispherical steel anvil with a radius of 48 mm, and, second, of a similar series involving impact on a flat steel base with an energy of 89.5 N-m. The helmet is to cover a standard 5 kg magnesium alloy headform; any acceleration in excess of 400 g, acceleration of more than 200 g for more than 2 ms, or 150 g for more than 4 ms shall be considered cause for failure. The shell is also to resist penetration by the point of a 60° cylindro-conical striker of 3.0 kg mass, whose tip has a hardness of at least R_C 60, when dropped from a height of 3 m; tensile tests for the retention system were also specified. These requirements were incorporated in the 1973 U.S. Federal Motor Vehicle Safety Standards for Motorcycle Helmets [214]. Additional guidelines concerning the employment of other standard headforms and a limit of acceptance based on a HIC value (1000) have since been considered.

The industrial helmet test procedures, Z89.1, involve an impact test of a 12.7 mm diameter steel ball bearing dropped from a height of 1.524 m on several different points of the shell, with the applied load calculated from the measured diameter of the indentation using the Brinell formula. The helmets are not to transmit more than an average force of 3781 N or a maximum of 4448 N. Shell penetration must also be avoided upon impact by a 0.4545 kg steel plumb bob with a tip angle of 35° when dropped from a height of 3.048 m.

Corresponding types of standards do not exist for other helmets, although some military specifications and guidelines are in force regarding helmet impact tests similar or identical to ANSI Z90.1. The National Operating Committee for Standards in Athletic Equipment, an ad hoc group of industrial representatives and other interested participants, has thus far failed to come to an agreement on appropriate tests and acceptance limits of sports helmets, even though they have been proposed and, to some extent, documented for at least baseball and football helmets [215-217]. Peak energies in football impacts are assessed at 542 N-m involving speeds of 10 m/s. Comparative evaluations of football helmets mounted on a metallic headform have been performed by occipital impacts at a speed of 3.05 m/s against both a metallic anvil and synthetic turf, and by vertex impacts at the same speed against synthetic turf. The result is interpreted in terms of the rise time and peak force when compared to each other and to impacts involving the bare headform [218]. All helmets provided some protection, yielding a reduction from 40% in the peak force to more than a factor of 5 for various conditions. The maximum forces and durations for the helmet tests ranged from about 5.78 KN and 9 ms to 1.68 KN and 12.5 ms for occipital, and from 14.2 KN at 19.3 ms to 9.12 KN at 29.5 ms for vertex collisions; the corresponding data for the bare headform were 10.4 KN at 4 ms and 17.75 KN at 8.4 ms, respectively. Several football helmets exhibited a bottoming-out phenomenon during vertex impact. However, comparative ratings of such helmets under laboratory conditions with maximum applied energies of 100 N-m before initiation of failure have been attacked on the basis that this does not duplicate field experience when the device must withstand a forty-fold energy level, particularly when the apparatus employed does not simulate either the human head or the type of physical insult actually encountered [128-129]. The author can attest to the fact that sports helmets mounted on anthropometrically realistic heads and subjected to the actual collision condition to be examined react totally different than those attached to metallic heads dropped from a given height onto some target in an attempt to simulate the actual event. The effectiveness of helmet suspensions to resist impact of an ice hockey puck formed the subject of one experimental and theoretical (two-mass lumped-parameter system) study where it was found that a massive, flexibly suspended helmet provides maximum protection from fracture-inducing blows, but is impractical for other reasons [217]. The transmission of force to the goaltender's face mask in the same sport was also experimentally investigated [220].

The design and effectiveness of military helmets has been more thoroughly investigated, in the U.S. primarily at the Natick Laboratories, Aberdeen Proving Ground and Edgewood Arsenal. An excellent summary of a Conference to assess the military implications of protective devices designed to prevent or ameliorate head and neck injuries, principally for air crewmen, gives a thorough accounting of the state of the art and directions for future research as of the year 1966 [221]. Three alternatives for the practical construction of helmets are suggested: (1) gross compromises with each of the individual desirable aims of adequate ballistic protection, comfort, compatibility with life-support systems

and eye shielding, to achieve a single device representing some
capability in each of these areas; (2) design of helmets according
to the need of each wearer; and (3) adoption of man/machine compatibility in aircraft (or vehicular or other crash environment)
design. For aircraft crash injuries, studies of the form and composition of helmets included a review of design progress, testing
methodology, liner characteristics and impact environment, basic
structural considerations (single vs. multiple shell, repeated impact and rebound), the retention system and visor design problems.
Body retention systems were examined, and ballistic protection
problems were addressed, including the relative protective effect
of specific shell liner materials. It was concluded that head
impact protection against rigid surfaces could be achieved with
helmets of reasonable thickness (32 mm) for speeds up to 7 m/s,
and that design g levels for helmets should be in the range from
90-160 g. A substantial number of recommendations for improvements
in helmet design were indicated.

The limitations in helmet construction are due to the
restricted stopping (or crushing) distance permitted for deceleration of an object. Thus, the deceleration time for the 32 mm
thickness is less than 6 ms, corresponding to only about 80 g according to WSTC [222]. For a 25.4 mm thick liner permitted to
crush to 30% of its original thickness, the upper limits of deceleration permitted for cushioning helmet materials of 400 g
and 500 g specified by U.S. and British military standards, respectively, correspond to energy absorptions of 316 N-m and 395 N-m,
respectively, and transmitted impulses 57.8 and 53.4 N-s for the
two cases. However, these are regarded as injurious from the
viewpoint of the WSTC which provides a safe energy absorption level
of only 47.5 N-m at a deceleration of 60 g.

The history of research and development of the infantry helmet
is presented in [223] which incorporates a substantial bibliography.
A description of the present and past protective helmets of NATO
and other countries, largely based on responses to questionnaires,
is presented in [224]. This covers infantry, flight, combat vehicle
crewman, parachutist, and other headgear and indicates ballistic
test methods and new developments. For the infantry, Hadfield, Mn
or special steel shells with a mass ranging from 1.14-1.45 kg are
employed; liners consist of polycarbonate, polyethylene, polyamide
or other plastic. American helmets are generally considered too
heavy. The problem of fitting three sizes of helmets to a variety
of personnel is addressed in [225], while the development of a
three-sized, one-piece helmet is considered in [226] with due regard for ballistic protection and human factors.

Very few specific analytical investigations of biomechanical
head/helmet responses to direct or impulsive loading are available
in the literature. In addition to the lumped-parameter system of

[219], finite-element models of concentric spherical shell systems
enveloping a central fluid sphere have been evaluated for specified
loads distributed over a small cap area [227-228]. The major difficulty in these evaluations is the correct delineation of the material characteristics and the proper representation of the actual
intermittent contact between shell, liner, and head. Data obtained
from oblique impact on shell-covered cadaver heads have been related to the predictions for normal impact for this type of analysis
[229].

9. CLOSURE

A dramatic improvement in our knowledge of the biomechanics of
head/neck injury has occurred since this author proposed the first
deformable model of head impact 12 years ago [16]. The mechanical
properties of the tissues of the system, particularly of the cranial
region, have been determined or at least characterized within
limits, numerous analytical and numerical models of head impact,
with or without neck constraint, have been proposed and evaluated,
continuing investigations involving volunteer, cadaver, animal and
other model research have been refined, tolerance limits have been
better quantified and applied to the evaluation of helmets, and
other protective environments have been altered to provide greater
safety to potential victims. Of course, further efforts are needed
in all these categories, but directions have been delineated, and
more attention can be paid to detail rather than to the understanding of overall phenomena.

There are still some aspects of injury hazard and damage to
the structure above the torso that are relatively untouched and
that should be analyzed biomechanically. The first of these is
the area of penetrating cranial wounds where, to the best of the
author's knowledge, no well-known attempt to properly quantify and
predict the process has been undertaken. The approach here might
well parallel the theoretical study of the hydraulic ram phenomenon
occurring in the perforation of fuel tanks, a subject that has attracted considerable attention recently. A second category is a
proper structural representation of impact to the facial region of
the head; while the incidence of fatality under these circumstances
is substantially lower than for direct impact to the skull--although
still demonstrably present--this event is very often disabling as
well as cosmetically destructive. Personal recent research on neck
response has revealed the appalling lack of information on the basic
behavior of the tissues of the neck, particularly muscles, ligaments
and vertebral bodies; much more is known about these for the thoracic and lumbar regions. Neck and spinal analysis under combined
motions needs substantial scrutiny. Finally, improvements are required in the correlation of analytical and laboratory results on
one hand and physiological and pathological findings by the medical

370

profession on the other. Perhaps the next decade will see the same
highly satisfactory rate of progress as had occurred during the past
ten years in the field of head impact.

1. Y.C. Fung, et al., eds., Biomechanics: Its Foundations and Objectives, Prentice-Hall, Englewood Cliffs, N.J., 1972.
2. E.S. Gurdjian, et al., eds., Impact Injury and Crash Protection, C.C. Thomas, Springfield, Ill., 1970.
3. N. Perrone, ed., Dynamic Response of Biomechanical Systems, Shock and Vibrations Committee, AMD, ASME, New York, 1970.
4. W.F. King and H.J. Mertz, eds., Human Impact Response: Measurement and Simulation, Plenum, New York-London, 1973.
5. Y.C. Fung, ed., Biomechanics, ASME, New York, 1966.
6. A.E. Walker, et al., eds., The Late Effects of Head Injury, C.C. Thomas, Springfield, Ill., 1969.
7. W.F. Caveness and A.E. Walker, eds., Head Injury Conference Proceedings, J.B. Lippincott, Philadelphia-Toronto, 1966.
8. E.S. Gurdjian and J.E. Webster, Head Injuries, Little, Brown & Co., Boston, 1958.
9. R.L. McLaurin, ed., Head Injuries, Grune and Stratton, New York, 1976.
10. Head Injuries, Proc. Int. Symp. held in Edinburgh and Madrid, 2nd to 10th, April 1970, C. Livingstone, Edinburgh-London, 1971.
11. W. Lewin, The Management of Head Injuries, Baillière, Tindall & Cassell, London, 1966.
12. G.F. Rowbotham, Acute Injuries of the Head, 4th ed., E. & J. Livingstone, Edinburgh-London, 1964.
13. E.S. Gurdjian, Impact Head Injury, C.C. Thomas, Springfield, Ill., 1975.
14. R.M. Kenedi, ed., Perspectives in Biomedical Engineering, McMillan, London, 1973.
15. H.W. Randel, ed., Aerospace Medicine, Williams & Wilkins, Baltimore, 1971.
16. W. Goldsmith. In: [7], 350.
17. W. Goldsmith. In: [1], 585.
18. A.I. King and C.C. Chou, J. Biomech., 9, 1976, 301.
19. Y.K. Liu. In: Proc. Symp. Biodynamic Models and Their Applications, 1970, Aerosp. Med. Res. Lab., Wright-Patterson AFB, Ohio, AMRL-TR-71-29, 1971, 701.
20. Y.K. Liu, J. Eng. Mech. Div., ASCE, 104, 1978, 131, EM 1, Paper 13540.
21. J.P. Schaeffer, ed., Morris' Human Anatomy, 10th ed., Blakiston, Philadelphia, 1942.
22. G.R. Cokelet. In: [1], 63.
23. R. Cailliet, Neck and Arm Pain, F.A. Davis, Philadelphia, 1975.
24. J.H. McElhaney, et al., Biomechanics of Trauma, Duke University Press, Durham, N.C., 1976, Chapter VI, 691.

25. H.J. Mertz, Neck Injury, GM Res. Publ. 1318, 1973.
26. L.B. Walker, et al., Anat. Rec., 169, 1971, 448.
27. L.B. Walker, et al., SAE Paper 730985, Proc. 17th Stapp Car Conf., 1973, 525.
28. H.J. Mertz and L.M. Patrick, SAE Paper 710855, Proc. 15th Stapp Car Crash Conf., 1971, 207.
29. J.H. McElhaney, et al., J. Biomech., 3, 1970, 495.
30. J.H. McElhaney, et al. In: [14], 215.
31. S.H. Advani and R.P. Owings, SAE Paper 740083, Trans. SAE, 83, 1974, 411.
32. J.W. Melvin and F.G. Evans, SAE Paper 710871, Proc. 15th Stapp Car Crash Conf., 1971, 666.
33. J.L. Wood, J. Biomech., 4, 1971, 1.
34. R.P. Hubbard, J. Biomech., 4, 1971, 251.
35. D.R. Carter and W.C. Hayes, J. Biomech., 9, 1976, 27; 10, 1977, 325.
36. K. Piekarski, J. Appl. Phys., 41, 1970, 215.
37. M.H. Pope and J.O. Outwater, J. Biomech., 5, 1972, 457.
38. T.M. Wright and W.C. Hayes, J. Biomech., 10, 1977, 419.
39. E.S. Gurdjian, et al., J. Biomech., 3, 1970, 239.
40. M. Yamada, Strength of Biological Materials, ed. by F.G. Evans, Williams & Wilkins, Baltimore, 1970.
41. J.E. Galford and J.H. McElhaney, J. Biomech., 3, 1970, 211.
42. H. Metz, et al., J. Biomech., 3, 1970, 453.
43. R.L. McLaurin. In: [8], 233.
44. C.H. Daly, et al. In: Proc. Symp. Biodynamic Models and Their Applications, 1970, Aerosp. Med. Res. Lab., Wright-Patterson AFB, Ohio, AMRL-TR-71-29, 1971, 501.
45. A.C. Knoell, J. Biomech., 10, 1977, 159.
46. P.L. Blanton and N.L. Biggs, J. Biomech., 3, 1970, 181.
47. S.A. Glantz, J. Biomech., 10, 1977, 5.
48. W. Lange. In: Proc. Symp. Biodynamic Models and Their Applications, 1970, Aerosp. Med. Res. Lab., Wright-Patterson AFB, Ohio, AMRL-TR-71-29, 1971, 141.
49. J. Reber, A Lumped Parameter Model of Whiplash, Thesis (M.S.), University of California, Berkeley, 1978.
50. L.M. Thomas. In: [2], 27.
51. E.S. Gurdjian. In: [10], 17.
52. J.D. States, et al., SAE Paper 710873, Proc. 15th Stapp Car Crash Conf., 1971, 710.
53. R. Hooper, Patterns of Acute Head Injury, E. Arnold, London, 1969.
54. A.K. Ommaya and T.A. Gennarelli. In: [9], 49.
55. E.S. Gurdjian, et al., Gen. Practice, 37, 2, 1968, 78.
56. D.H. Robbins and V.L. Roberts, SAE Paper 710872, Proc. 15th Stapp Car Crash Conf., 1971, 686.
57. J.K. Kihlberg. In: [2], 5.
58. A.K. Ommaya and P. Corrao. In: Accident Pathology, ed. by K.H. Brinkhaus, U.S. Government Printing Office, Washington, D.C., 1971, 160.

59. A.H.S. Holbourn, Lancet, 2, 1943, 438.
60. S. Strich. In: [6], 501.
61. C.L. Ewing. In: Aircraft Crashworthiness, University Press of Virginia, Charlottesville, 1975.
62. A.K. Ommaya, et al., SAE Paper 660804, Proc. 10th Stapp Car Crash Conf., 1966, 197.
63. H.D. Portnoy, et al., Proc. 15th Cong. Amer. Assoc. for Automotive Med., 1972, 58.
64. P. Prasad, et al., J. Appl. Mech., 41, 1974, 321.
65. A.I. King, et al., Orthop. Clin. North Amer., 6, 1, 1975, 19.
66. A.K. Ommaya, J. Trauma, 10, 1970, 981.
67. J.H. Field, Epidemiology of Head Injuries in England and Wales, Willsons Printers, Leicester, 1976.
68. E. Gögler, Road Accidents, Ser. Chirurgica Geigy No. 5, 1962.
69. R.C. Schneider, Head and Neck Injuries in Football, Williams & Wilkins, Baltimore, 1973.
70. F.J. Unterharnscheidt. In: Handbook of Clinical Neurology, 23, ed. by P.J. Vinkin, et al., North-Holland, Amsterdam, 1975, 527.
71. J.L. Bleustein, ed., Mechanics and Sport, AMD 4, ASME, 1973.
72. A.K. Ommaya and A.E. Hirsch, Neurosurg., 37, 1972, 95.
73. I. Sunshine, et al., Head Trauma: Analysis of 120 Casualties in Vietnam from July 1967 to January 1968, Dept. of Army, Edgewood Arsenal, EATR 4359, March 1970.
74. R.G. Bernier and H.C. Smith, U.S. Army Casualties Aboard Aircraft in the Republic of Vietnam (1962 through 1967), BRL Memo. Rep. 2030, March 1970.
75. J.T. Purvis and A.B. Clark, USAF, Craniocerebral Injuries due to Missiles and Fragments, Personal Communication.
76. C.L. Ewing and F. Unterharnscheidt, Neuropathology and Cause of Death in U.S. Naval Aircraft Accidents, AGARD Conf. Proc. No. 190, Dec. 1976, B16-1.
77. W.F. Caveness, et al., Combat Head Injuries with and without Helmet "Protection," Trans. Amer. Neurol. Assoc., 97, 1972, 250.
78. P. Harris. In: [10], 42.
79. A.K. Ommaya, et al., SAE Paper 670906, Proc. 11th Stapp Car Crash Conf., 1967, 47.
80. A.I. King. In: Aircraft Crashworthiness, University Press of Virginia, Charlottesville, 1975, 83.
81. A.I. King and C.C. Chiu, J. Biomech., 9, 1976, 301.
82. G.D. Frisch, et al., SAE Paper 760774, Natl. Automobile Eng. and Manuf. Meet., 1976, SP-412.
83. A. Slattenscheck and W. Tauffkirchen, SAE Paper 700426, Intern. Automobile Safety Conf. Compendium, 1970, 280.
84. A. Slattenscheck, et al., SAE Paper 710879, Proc. 15th Stapp Car Crash Conf., 1971, 742.
85. R.L. Stalnaker, et al., ASME Paper 71-WA/BHF-10, 1971.
86. J. McElhaney, Mekh. Polimerov, No. 3, 1976, 465.
87. S.B. Roberts, et al., ASME Paper 69-BHF-11, 1969.

88. J.A. McKenzie and J.F. Williams, J. Biomech., 4, 1971, 477.
89. J.F. Williams, J. Biomech., 8, 1975, 257.
90. G.D. Frisch, et al., Av. Space and Environ. Med., 48, 1977, 223.
91. N.M. Alem, SAE Paper 741192, Proc. 18th Stapp Car Crash Conf., 1974, 579.
92. R.L. Huston, et al., Av. Space and Environ. Med., 49, 1978, 205.
93. G.A. Thurston and R.J. Fay, Denver Res. Inst., Mech. Sci. and Environ. Eng. Dept., June 1974, ONR Contract N00014-67-A-0395-003.
94. P. Prasad and A.I. King, J. Appl. Mech., ASME 41, 1974, 546-550.
95. D. Orne and Y.K. Liu, J. Biomech., 4, 1971, 49.
96. T. Belytschko, et al., Av. Space and Environ. Med., 49, 1978, 158.
97. R.J. Arvikar and A. Seireg, Av. Space and Environ. Med., 49, 1978, 166.
98. P. Prasad, et al., SAE Paper 751172, Proc. 19th Stapp Car Crash Conf., 1975, 869.
99. R.R. McHenry and K.N. Naab, Cornell Aeron. Lab. Rep. YB-21260V-IR, 1966.
100. D.J. Segal. In: [3], 24.
101. J.A. Bartz, SAE Paper 720961, Proc. 16th Stapp Car Crash Conf., 1972, 105.
102. S.B. Roberts and R.B. Thompson, J. Biomech., 7, 1975, 523.
103. I. Kaleps, et al. In: Proc. Symp. Biodynamic Models and Their Applications, 1970, Aerosp. Med. Res. Lab., Wright-Patterson AFB, Ohio, AMRL-TR-71-29, 1971, 211.
104. R.L. Huston, et al., SAE Paper 740275, 1974.
105. R.D. Young, et al., Paper 27, Proc. 3rd Intern. Cong. Automotive Safety, II, 1974.
106. V.H. Kenner and W. Goldsmith, J. Biomech., 6, 1973, 1.
107. B. Landkof, et al., J. Biomech., 9, 1976, 141.
108. T.A. Shugar, A Finite Element Head Injury Model, I and II, Civ. Eng. Lab., Port Hueneme, Ca., USN, TR R 854-1 and R 854-II, July 1977.
109. C.C. Ward, et al., Av. Space and Environ. Med., 49, 1978, 136.
110. T.B. Khalil and R.P. Hubbard, J. Biomech., 10, 1977, 119.
111. Y.K. Liu and J.D. Murray. In: [5], 167.
112. T.F. Li, et al., Proc. Symp. Biodynamic Models and Their Applications, 1970, Aerosp. Med. Res. Lab., Wright-Patterson AFB, Ohio, AMRL-TR-71-29, 1971, 553.
113. J.F. Soechting and P.R. Paslay, J. Biomech., 6, 1973, 195.
114. R.G. Snyder, SAE Paper 700398, Intern. Automobile Safety Conf. Compendium, P-30, 1970, 712.
115. D.R. Foust, et al., SAE Paper 770915, 1977.
116. R.G. Snyder. In: Bioastronautics Data Book, 2nd ed., ed. by J.F. Parker, Jr., and V.R. West, NASA SP-3006, 1973, 221.

117. C.L. Ewing, et al., SAE Paper 680792, Proc. 12th Stapp Car Crash Conf., 1968, 26; SAE Paper 690817, Proc. 13th Stapp Car Crash Conf., 1969, 28.

118. C.L. Ewing and D.J. Thomas, AGARD Conf. Proc. No. 88, 1971, 11-1.

119. C.L. Ewing and D.J. Thomas, Nav. Aerosp. Med. Res. Lab. Detachment, New Orleans, Monograph 21, August 1972.

120. C.L. Ewing and D.J. Thomas, SAE Paper 730976, Proc. 17th Stapp Car Crash Conf., 1973, 309.

121. C.L. Ewing, et al., SAE Paper 751157, Proc. 20th Stapp Car Crash Conf., 1975, 487.

122. W.H. Muzzy, III, and L. Lustick, SAE Paper 760801, Proc. 20th Stapp Car Crash Conf., 1976, 45.

123. G.D. Frisch and C. Cooper, Av. Space and Environ. Med., 49, 1978, 196.

124. L.W. Schneider and B.M. Bowman, Av. Space and Environ. Med., 49, 1978, 211.

125. D.E. Smith and W.R. Anderson, Av. Space and Environ. Med., 49, 1978, 224.

126. H.J. Mertz and L.M. Patrick, SAE Paper 670919, Proc. 11th Stapp Car Crash Conf., 1969, 175.

127. V.L. Roberts and D.H. Robbins. In: [4], 381.

128. S.E. Reid, et al., Selling Sporting Goods, 25, 9, Sept. 1972.

129. S.E. Reid, et al., The Physician and Sportsmedicine, 2, 1974. 32.

130. J.R. Hughes and D.E. Hendrix, Electroenceph. Clin. Neurophysiol., 24, 1968, 183.

131. S.E. Reid, et al., Trauma, 15, 1975, 150.

132. D.W. Moon, et al., Med. Sci. in Sports, 3, 1971, 44.

133. F. Unterharnscheidt, Texas Rep. Biol. Med., 28, Winter 1970, 421.

134. J. Johnson, et al., Med. Biol. Eng., 13, 1975, 396.

135. V.L. Roberts, et al., ASME Paper 66HUF-1, 1966.

136. W. Goldsmith, et al., J. Biomech. Eng., 100, 1978, 25.

137. S.O. Lindgren, Acta Phys. Scand. Suppl., 360, 1966.

138. E.S. Gurdjian, et al., Surg. Gyn. Obst., 113, 1961, 185.

139. L.M. Patrick, Plast. Reconst. Surg., 37, 1966, 314.

140. J.M. Douglass, et al., SAE Paper 680786, Proc. 12th Stapp Car Crash Conf., 1968, 317.

141. F.G. Evans, et al., J. Appl. Physiol., 17, 1962, 405.

142. L.M. Patrick, et al., Proc. 8th Cong. Societé int. de chirurgie orthopédique et de traumatologie, 1960, 781.

143. C.L. Ewing, et al., U.S. Nav. Aerosp. Med. Lab., March 1973, NAMRL-1178.

144. H.J. Clemens and K. Burow, SAE Paper 720960, Proc. 16th Stapp Car Crash Conf., 1972, 76.

145. R.H. Pudenz and C.H. Shelden, J. Neurosurg., 3, 1946, 487.

146. T.A. Gennarelli, et al., Proc. 15th Stapp Car Crash Conf., 1971, 797.

147. A.K. Ommaya and T.A. Gennarelli, Brain, 97, 1974, 633.

148. D.J. Sass, et al., *J. Biomech.*, 4, 1971, 331.
149. F. Unterharnscheidt and L.S. Higgins, *Texas Rep. Biol. Med.*, 27, 1969, 127.
150. F. Unterharnscheidt, SAE Paper 710880, *Proc. 15th Stapp Car Crash Conf.*, 1971, 767.
151. F.J. Unterharnscheidt and E.A. Ripperger. In: [3], 46.
152. V.R. Hodgson. In: [2], 275.
153. J.L. Martinez, ASEE Ann. Meet. Paper No. 167, Michigan State University, June 1967.
154. L. Rinder, *Acta Physiol. Scand.*, 76, 1969, 352.
155. S. Lindgren and L. Rinder, *Acta Physiol. Scand.*, 76, 1969, 340.
156. L. Rinder, *Experimental Brain Concussion by Sudden Intra-cranial Input of Fluid*, Dept. Hygiene, University of Göteborg, 1969.
157. D.A. Stalhammer, *Experimental Brain Damage from Fluid Pressure due to Impact Acceleration*, Dept. of Neurosurg., University of Göteborg, 1974.
158. J. Wickstrom, et al. In: *Proc. 7th Stapp Car Crash Conf.*, ed. by D.M. Severy, C.C. Thomas, Springfield, Ill., 1965, 284.
159. J. Wickstrom, et al. In: *Acceleration Injuries of the Head and Neck, Prevention of Highway Injury*, Highway Safety Res. Inst., University of Michigan, 1967, 182.
160. E.S. Gurdjian and H.R. Lissner, *J. Neurosurg.*, 18, 1961, 58.
161. P.D. Flynn. In: [7], 344.
162. K. Sellier and F.J. Unterharnscheidt, *Excerpta Medica. Int. Cong. Ser.*, 93, 1963, 55.
163. F. Unterharnscheidt and K. Sellier. In: [7], 321.
164. A.G. Gross, *J. Neurosurg.*, 15, 1958, 548.
165. A.G. Gross, *Aviat. Med.*, 29, 1958, 725.
166. C.C. Suh, et al., *J. Biomech.*, 5, 1972, 181.
167. B.G. Master and K.J. Saczalski, ASME Paper 72-WA/BHF-7, 1972.
168. W.D. Claus, et al., U.S. Army Natick Labs., CE & MEL-131, TR75-23 CEMEL, June 1974.
169. R.P. Hubbard and D.G. McLeoad. In: [4], 129.
170. R.P. Hubbard and D.G. McLeoad, SAE Paper 741193, *Proc. 18th Stapp Car Crash Conf.*, 1974, 599.
171. V.R. Hodgson. In: [4], 113.
172. V.R. Hodgson, et al., SAE Paper 720969, *Proc. 16th Stapp Car Crash Conf.*, 1972, 1.
173. D.G. McLeoad and C.W. Gadd. In: [4], 153.
174. Amer. Nat. Stand. Inst., New York, American National Specification for Protective Headgear for Vehicular Users, ANSI Z90.1, 1971.
175. R.D. Marangoni, et al., *J. Eng. Mech. Div.*, ASCE, 104, 1978, 153, EM1, Paper 13526.
176. B.M. Bowman and D.H. Robbins, SAE Paper 720957, *Proc. 16th Stapp Car Crash Conf.*, 1972, 14.

177. J.W. Melvin, et al., SAE Paper 720958, <u>Proc. 16th Stapp Car Crash Conf.</u>, 1972, 45.
178. J.W. Melvin, et al. In: [4], 247.
179. H.J. Mertz, et al. In: [4], 263.
180. C.C. Culver, et al., SAE Paper 720959, <u>Proc. 16th Stapp Car Crash Conf.</u>, 1972, 61.
181. M.P. Haffner and G.B. Cohen. In: [4], 289.
182. S.W. Alderson, SAE Paper 670908, <u>Proc. 11th Stapp Car Crash Conf.</u>, 1967, 62.
183. D.M. Severy, et al., <u>Canad. Serv. Med. J.</u>, <u>11</u>, 1955, 727.
184. R.J. Berton, SAE Paper 680080, 1968.
185. L.M. Patrick. In: [4], 17.
186. H.T. McAdams. In: [4], 35.
187. A.M. Thomas. In: [4], 69.
188. E.B. Becker. In: [4], 321.
189. L.M. Patrick and T.B. Sato. In: [2], 259.
190. E.S. Gurdjian, <u>Head Injury from Antiquity to the Present with Special Reference to Penetrating Head Wounds</u>, The Beaumont Lecture, C.C. Thomas, Springfield, Ill., 1973.
191. A.K. Ommaya and A.E. Hirsch, <u>J. Biomech.</u>, <u>4</u>, 1971, 13.
192. A.M. Nahum, et al., SAE Paper 680785, <u>Proc. 12th Stapp Car Crash Conf.</u>, 1968, 302.
193. E.S. Gurdjian, et al., <u>J. Amer. Med. Assoc.</u>, <u>182</u>, 1962, 509.
194. W.S. Fay, SAE Paper 710870, <u>Proc. 15th Stapp Car Crash Conf.</u>, 1971, 645.
195. J.H. McElhaney, et al. In: [4], 85.
196. J. Versace, SAE Paper 710881, <u>Proc. 15th Stapp Car Crash Conf.</u>, 1971, 771.
197. E.S. Gurdjian, et al., <u>J. Biomech.</u>, <u>3</u>, 1970, 239.
198. A.M. Eiband, <u>Human Tolerance to Rapidly Applied Accelerations: A Summary of the Literature</u>, NASA Memo 5-19-59E, 1959.
199. C.W. Gadd, SAE Paper 660793, <u>Proc. 10th Stapp Car Crash Conf.</u>, 1966, 95.
200. J. Brinn and S.E. Staffeld, SAE Paper 700902, <u>Proc. 14th Stapp Car Crash Conf.</u>, 1970, 188.
201. J. Brinn and S.E. Staffeld, <u>Proc. 15th Stapp Car Crash Conf.</u>, 1971, 817.
202. J.V. Benedict and C.J. Lin, ASME Paper 71-WA/BHF-6, 1971.
203. J.L. Stapp. In: [2], 308.
204. R.G. Snyder, <u>AGARD Conf. Proc. No. 88</u>, 1971, 4-1.
205. L.M. Patrick and G. Grime. In: [2], 444.
206. W.A. Lange and D.J. Van Kirk. In: [2], 475.
207. R.G. Snyder. In: [2], 496.
208. G.R. Smith, et al., SAE Paper 720443, <u>Proc. 2nd Int. Conf. on Passive Restraints</u>, 1972.
209. B. Altman, <u>Acta Phys. Scand.</u>, <u>36</u>, Suppl. 192, 1962.
210. N. Perrone. In: [3], 1.
211. N. Perrone. In: [1], 567.
212. W.D. Claus, <u>J. Biomech. Eng.</u>, <u>99</u>, 1977, 20.

213. Amer. Nat. Stand. Inst., New York, American National Standard Safety Requirements for Industrial Head Protection, ANSI Z89.1, 1969.
214. Nat. Highway Traffic Safety Adm., U.S. Dept. of Transportation, Part 571, Federal Motor Vehicle Safety Standards--Motorcycle Helmets, Fed. Register, 38, No. 160, August 1973, 22390.
215. V.R. Hodgson, Med. and Sci. in Sports, 7, 1975, 225.
216. V.R. Hodgson, The Problem of Head/Neck Injury in Football, Personal Communication.
217. V.R. Hodgson, Standard Method of Impact Test and Performance Requirements for Baseball Helmets, Personal Communication.
218. G.W. Kindt, et al. In: [57], 228.
219. M.A. Townsend, et al., Med. Biol. Eng., 13, 1975, 405.
220. Y. Sze, et al. In: [71], 175.
221. Life Sci. Res. Off., Federation of Amer. Societies for Exp. Biol., Washington, D.C., prepared by Wendell H. Griffith. Summary of Conference: The Study of Military Implications of Protective Devices Designed to Prevent or Ameliorate Head and Neck Injuries, Sept. 12, 1966.
222. A.E. Hirsch. In: [7], 37.
223. C.W. Houff and J.P. Delaney, Historical Documentation of the Infantry Helmet, Research and Development, AMCMS, Human Engineering Lab., Aberdeen Proving Ground, T.M. 4-73, 1973.
224. L.R. McManus, Protective Helmets of NATO and Other Countries, U.S. Army Natick Labs., C & PLSELIOZ, TR73-29CE, 1973.
225. L.R. McManus, et al., Verification Fit Test of Three Size Infantry Helmet, U.S. Army Natick Labs., CEMEL-143, TR75-79, 1975.
226. L.R. McManus, et al., Development of a One Piece Infantry Helmet, U.S. Army Natick Labs, CEMEL-152, Rep. 76-30, 1976.
227. T. Khalil, et al., Int. J. Mech. Sci., 16, 1974, 609.
228. K.J. Saczalski and E.Q. Richardson, Av. Space and Environ. Med., 49, 1978, 115.
229. B. Simpson, et al., Int. J. Mech. Sci., 18, 1976, 337.

379

SHORT CONTRIBUTIONS

PATHOPHYSIOLOGY OF TRAUMATIC BRAIN EDEMA

A. Baethmann
Inst. for Surgical Research, Dept. of Surgery
University of Munich, Nussbaum str. 20
8000 München 2, W. Germany

Brain edema caused by injury to cerebral tissue primarily is
of vasogenic nature. It is characterized by damage of the blood-
brain-barrier leading to uptake of fluid into the parenchyma.
Cerebral tissue becomes not only mechanically damaged by the
traumatic impact, but also by secondary processes, as e.g. hemorrhage
and a rise in intracranial pressure, or brain distortion and
herniation. Formation of edema may have different but interdependent
cause: e.g. circulatory leading to enhanced fluid-filtration,ischemia
together with tissue hypoxia, compression of cerebral tissue by
hematoma, tissue necrosis, and finally formation or release of toxic
compounds. The vasogenic edema fluid spreading through the extracellular space of brain tissue may constitute a toxic environment
for the parenchyma. It may lead to release or activation of active
compounds causing swelling of cells. Swelling may result from an
abnormal extracellular fluid-composition and constitute the basis
for nerve cell dysfunction and even cell death. What is required
is a more detailed understanding of the mechanisms of traumatic
brain edema for the development of specific methods of edema
treatment.

ORTHOSTATIC FUNCTION DISORDERS IN CASE OF POST-CONCUSSIONAL
SYNDROMA FOLLOWING HEAD OR WHIPLASH INJURY

J.B. Baron
Lab. de Statokinésimétrie
Centre Hospitalier Sainte-Anne
1 rue Cabanis, Paris 14, France

Body at rest is never immobile, it swings continuously. The
amplitude and frequency of the displacement give an information on
the different sensori-motor loops. The oculomotor loop plays an
important part in this mechanism. In case of head injury or whiplash
injury, midbrain lesion, producing a small deviation of one eye
never more than 4^0, occurs very often. The introduction of this
error in the oculomotor loop provocates a correction by nucal
muscles. A conflict between the oculomotor systemand the information
starting from the semi-circular canals occurs in this condition.
The body gravity center displacement mechanism is perturbated. Each
loop produces a safety level non-integrated in the minimal scheduled
program. A correction of the error resolves the conflict and
restores the normal schdule.

HUMAN ORTHOSTATIC TONIC POSTURAL ACTIVITY TRANSFER FUNCTION

G. Bizzo
Lab. de Statokinésimétrie
Centre Hospitalier Sainte-Anne
1 rue Cabanis, Paris 14, France

The purpose is to point out the interest of the qualification of the man standing up posture behavior, stimulated by electrical labyrinthine stimulation, for determining a mathematical relationship between the stimulus and the postural reaction provocated. In the first phase, sinusoidal or rectangular stochastic frequency stimuli generator entirely external to the subject is used. In the second phase, the subject body oscillation as stimuli generator through nonlinear or linear reaction loops is used.

MONITORING OF BONE IMPLANTS AND BONE DEFORMATIONS, IN VIVO

F. Burny, R. Burgois and M. Donkerwolcke
Interdisciplinary Centre of Bone Biomechanics
Dept. of Traumatology and Orthopaedic Surgery
Cliniques Universitaires de Brussels
Route de Lennick 808, 1070 Brussels, Belgium

The deformation of an implant, measured in vivo by means of strain gauges, produces useful information on the actual mechanical characteristics of the complex "bone-callus-implant". 1. Measurement of fracture healing. From readings from a strain gauge glued on the fixation beam of an external fixation device, stabilizing a fracture of a limb, for a given load, applied to the extremity of the limb, the recorded deformation will be proportional to the mechanical characteristics of the callus. The method was used in more than 350 patients and was useful in predicting the course of the healing process. 2. Monitoring of nail plate deformation. Using strain gauges glued at the critical point of a nail plate, it was possible to adapt the actual rehabilitation program to the mechanical response of the implant. The critical values of the deformations of the implant obtained experimentally showed good agreement with theoretical calculations. The method was used in 40 patients without any significant complications. Early weight bearing was possible without any risk to the majority of the patients. A composite strain gauge transducer was also manufactured satisfying the requirements for long term implantation. The two components of this transducer are a strain gauge incorporated in a medium of biocompatible resin and a surrounding porous shell. The anchorage of the transducer in the bone is obtained by bone ingrowth into the porous shell. The transducer was tested in two situations simulating the conditions of use in vivo and then implanted in the lateral cortex of the femur of a dog. After one month, deformations of the bone during walking were succesfully recorded.

THE EFFECT OF EXTERNALLY APPLIED DC CURRENT ON THE CALLUS FORMATION

D. Demetriades, K. Piekarski and D.A. Mackenzie
26 A Analipseos Str., Vrilissia, Athens, Greece

Electrical stimulation for callus formation in vivo has been introduced experimentally, with a new noninvasive technique . DC current in the range of densities 123-53 $\mu A/cm^2$ was applied on the skin over the osteotomised radius in 36 rabbits for a period of 2 and 3 weeks. It was observed that the volume of formed callus was directly proportional to the applied current. The orientation of the trabeculae was also affected by the direction of the applied potential.

SIMULATION PROBLEMS IN MECHANICAL TESTS ON TOTAL HIP JOINT REPLACEMENTS

A.M. Gatti
Clinica Ortopedica Istituti Rizzoli
via S.S. Annunziata 13, Bologna, Italy

In hip joint prosthesis, one of the problems is the choice of the mating materials. The coefficient of friction between cup surface and surface of the head should be very small and have wear as minimal as possible. Failures of some types of hip joint prostheses let us carry out a series of simulation tests. For evaluation of mating materials, two different lines of investigations were followed. 1. The interaction between two materials having a relative motion is faced by Tribology. By suitable tests, it is tried to determine and evaluate the typical parameters of this interaction. 2. Simulating devices have been developed to test the prostheses under working conditions. The present work considers these two different cases. The analysis of the different hip joint simulators showed that it is not possible to compare the results, that there are not suitable simulators and that the few suitable simulators can be used to obtain a better surface finish, especially for ceramic materials, before the implantation.

SYSTEMATIC CALIBRATION OF 6-DOF TRANSDUCERS : APPLICATION TO A FORCE PLATE

M.M. Gola
Politecnico di Torino, Ist. Motorizzazione
10100 Torino, Italy

A new force plate, easy and inexpensive to manufacture, is presented. It has 6 DOF and is suspended on six strain-gaged chain-like elements. It has been calibrated via a systematic approach, with a mathematical model of the second order. Results show that the quadratic and cross-talk coefficients are three to four order of magnitudes less than the linear ones.

ANATOMICAL GEOMETRY AND PHYSICAL PROPERTIES BY COMPUTERIZED
TOMOGRAPHY

H.K. Huang
Georgetown University Medical School
3900 Reservoir Road N.W.
Washington D.C. 20007, USA

This paper is to report on a non-destructive method to
generate from cadaveric computerized tomographic (CT) scans a
comprehensive data base of 3D geometry and physical properties
of the human body. The first step is to acquire a suitable specimen
who is, then, placed in a supine position on a computerized
tomographic scanner. Beginning at the cranium and ending at the
ankle joints, scans are taken at one cm intervals. The 3D body
and anatomical component geometry can be obtained from the CT
scans by an interactive computer graphic system. The mass density
of each point from a CT scan can be evaluated by an experimental
procedure. The mass, center of gravity, and inertial tensor of a
cross section or an anatomical component can be computed. These
data are important input parameters in car crash studies using
the simulation method. They also serve as a general human data
base for other biomechanics research.

PHYSIOLOGICAL RESPONSE OF UNSUPPORTED AND SUPPORTED SPINE

S. Kumar
Faculty of Rehabilitation Medicine
University of Alberta
Edmonton, Alberta, Canada

The pattern of physiological response to a standard stress
applied to unsupported and supported spine in sagittal, lateral
and oblique planes was studied. The spinal appliances used were
sacro-iliac belt, lumbo-sacral corset, Harris, Macnab, Knight
and Taylor braces. The electromyographic activity of erector
spinae and external oblique was recorded, and intra-abdominal
pressure was measured by radio-telemetry. The responses for
sagittal plane activity were significantly lower than and statistically different from lateral and oblique plane activities. The
lateral and oblique plane activities were not always significantly
different from each other. The extent of mechanical support forth-
coming from the six spinal appliances as indexed by increased
intra-abdominal pressure did not differ significantly. The
prescription of spinal appliance should be based on stability and
the physiological cost of wearing the device rather than consideration of mechanical support.

BIOMECHANICS OF SWIMMING

L. Lewillie
Unité de Recherche de Biomécanique du Mouvement,
Université Libre de Bruxelles
1050 Bruxelles, Belgium

The hydrodynamic drag of the human body has been measured. The direct application of the hydrodynamic principles is not possible. The principal component is the turbulent flow. The passive hydrodynamic resistance depends on the morphology of the subject. The active resistance is not a function of the passive one. When trailed sidewards ($45°$), the resistance is lower than that in the ventral position until 1.7 m/sec. The resistance at 60 cm below the surface is greater than that at the surface. The water temperature has a great influence on the total body resistance. Telemetry of the EMG has been used to study muscle activity during swimming. Quantification has been made by reference to the maximum isometric contraction. It allows to compare styles, speeds, bevels of qualification, handicap.

THE PRESSURE - VOLUME RELATIONSHIP OF THE CRANIOSPINAL CAVITY

Y. King Liu
Biomechanics Laboratory
Tulane University, School of Medicine
New Orleans, Louisiana, USA

BIOMECHANICS OF LYMPH PROPULSION

N.P. Reddy
Cardiovascular Research Inst.
Univ. of California, San Francisco, Cal., USA

Lymph flow in Lymphatics is governed by certain intrinsic and extrinsic forces. The former is due to muscle contractions. The latter is due to organ movements and skeletal muscle contractions. There are numerous valves along the lymphatics. A mathematical model of the lymphatic system has been developed. The flow and pressure patterns, derived from the model simulation, are consistent with the experimental results. An experimental model using thoracic duct perfusion in anesthetized dogs is developed to study the factors regulating intrinsic contractions. The results confirmed that distention is necessary for motility and indicate a nonlinear relationship between transmural pressure and flow due to motility, and that intrinsic forces can be modulated by several vasoactive substances.

ADVANCED DESIGN TELESCOPIC PROSTHESIS FOR ABOVE KNEE AMPUTEES

C. Rigas
Bioengineering Unit, Univ. of Strathclyde
Glasgow, UK

The Telescopic Prosthesis for AK amputees aims primarily at function, stability and dynamic symmetry. It is a single member assembly hinged at the vicinity of the hip joint and capable of shortening during the swing phase. The shortening is achieved by energy stored in a self-energised system during the stance phase. The author's new design is practical and offers a desirable combination of voluntary and involuntary control for which the prosthesis is also called "Voluntarily Controlled Telescopic". The advantages are : Decrease in the vertical displacement of the hips, more symmetrical kinematics. of gait and decrease of the moment applied at the hip of the prosthetic side. Stability and proprioception have been reported by the wearers to be better than those with their conventional limbs.

THE FRACTURE PATTERN AS AN INDICATOR OF IMPACT LOADING OF THE THORAX

G. Schmidt
Director, Inst. für Rechtsmedizin
Univ. of Heidelberg, W. Germany

The hardness and loading capacity of hundreds of rib pairs (6th and 7th) have been tested in comparison with the results of about 200 acceleration tests concerning belt protected human cadavers. Rib fractures have some individual aspects indicating the direction and strength of the. impact. So we can differentiate between static and dynamic loading. Elasticity and loading capacity of ribs decrease with advancing age.

THE PREVENTATION OF SOME DORSAL COMPLAINTS

C.J. Snijders
Eindhoven and Twente Universities of Technology
Eindhoven, The Netherlands

The proas muscles play a dominating role of maintaining postural equilibrium. A study is presented on the change in the form of the spine as a consequence of pregnancy. Certain exercises have been critisized. The Proas muscles which are usually sufficiently strong have the tendency of spontaneously shortening which influences the posture and the spine. Good postures are related to good chair design. Desk design is also important especially when reading and writing are involved. Anteflexion (school-) headache and dorsal complaints are common with children, students and adults and are related to horizontal desks. A slanted desk will prevent large loading of postural muscles as well as some ligamentous structures.

CLINICAL AND LABORATORY EVALUATION OF PROSTHETIC/ORTHOTIC DEVICES

S.E. Solomonidis
Bioengineering Unit, Univ. of Strathclyde
Glasgow, Scotland

Evaluation of prosthetic or orthotic devices before they are
introduced to clinical use is mandatory. Safe and effective
performance is of primary importance. Factors such as supply,
storage, assembly, fitting, maintenance are also relevant. Based
on our experience, a philosophy and methodology has been evolved.
This includes mechanical and functional testing and clinical trials.
Using the evaluation programme of Above Knee modular artificial
limbs, the philosophies, techniques and implementation were discussed.

EXACT GEOMETRY FINITE ELEMENT MODELS FOR CLOSED HEAD IMPACT INJURY

C. Ward
Civil Engineering Laboratory
Port Hueneme, California, USA

Finite element idealizations of the human skull and brain were
presented. In these models, linear elastic brick elements are used
to represent the soft tissue and skull, and membrane elements
simulate the internal folds of dura, the falx and tentorium. The
pressurized human cadaver experiments used to substantiate these
models were described. The importance of brain volume distensibility
and relative unimportance of skull deformation were shown. Measured
and model predicted intracranial pressures for frontal head impact
were compared, and a relationship between frontal pressure and
frontal lobe injury was presented.

A FIBRE MODEL DESCRIPTION OF THE ALINEAR VISCOELASTIC PROPERTIES
OF THE HUMAN SKIN IN VIVO FOR SMALL DEFORMATIONS

P.F.F. Wijn
Lab. of Medical Physics and Biophysics and
Dept. of Dermatology, Univ. of Nijmegen
Nijmegen, The Netherlands

The alinear viscoelastic properties of the human skin on the
calf are examined in vivo for small deformations using two different
measuring techniques in the plane of the skin: uniaxial strain and
torsion. The response of the skin to a stepwise load consists of
an instantaneous, a delayed elastic and a permanent deformation.
In uniaxial strain experiments tne skin shows a high anisotropy
with respect to Langer's lines. Since the alinearity of the stress-
strain curves appears to be independent of the measuring direction,
the anisotropy can be characterized by the initial coefficients of
elasticity in the principle directions. Within the theory of homogeneous isotropic medium, it appears to be impossible to relate
the results found. The results can be related using a fibre model
based on the structure of the skin. In this model, the summated

properties of the elastin fibres determine the instantaneous
deformation of the skin. Using this model, quantitative, qualitative and structural data about the elastin fibres can be derived.

MOTION ANALYSIS IN TRAFFIC ACCIDENTS

P. Niederer
Inst. for Biomedical Engineering
Swiss Fed. Inst. of Technology
Moussonstrasse 18, 8044 Zürich, Switzerland

Reliable traffic accident reconstruction methods are of
importance for safety, legal as well as scientific reasons.
In recent years several motion analysis computer programs have
been developed which are of help in analysing accidents.
In the case of car-to-car crashes, the SMAC program (Simulation
Model of Automobile Collisions) supports the reconstruction of
planar motions of up to two interacting vehicles. Based on this
method, an approximate motion analysis of a car occupant model can
be performed with the aid of a human body simulation program.
Whenever an accident analysis is performed using computer simulations, a sensitivity analysis with regard to model parameters as
well as initial conditions has to be made, because situations may
arise in which the motion under consideration is so instable in
the sense of Lyapunov that mathematical simulations are no longer
meaningful.

LIST OF PARTICIPANTS

Prof. N. Akgün, Turkey
Dr. N. Akkaş, Turkey
Dr. O. Aksoğan, Turkey
Dr. H. Alp, Turkey
Prof. M. Anliker, Switzerland
Dr. A. Baethmann, W. Germany
Dr. J.B. Baron, France
Dr. N. Berme, U.K.
Mr. L. Bingöl, Turkey
Mr. G. Bizzo, France
Prof. M. Bracale, Italy
Dr. F. Burny, Belgium
Prof. E.F. Byars, USA
Dr. G. Çelebi, Turkey
Dr. S. Çelebi, Turkey
Ms. M. Del Comente, Belgium
Dr. D. Demetriades, Greece
Dr. H. Demiray, Turkey
Prof. E. Deniz, Turkey
Prof. B. Eckstein, W. Germany
Prof. A.E. Engin, USA
Dr. Ü. Erdem, Turkey
Dr. Y. Ersoy, Turkey
Dr. A. Gatti, Italy
Prof. T. Gibson, UK
Dr. M. Gola, Italy
Prof. W. Goldsmith, USA
Dr. N. Güzelsu, Turkey
Dr. M.T. Hatiboğlu, Turkey
Dr. H.K. Huang, USA
Dr. J.M.M. Huijgens, Holland
Dr. B. Jessen, Denmark
Mr. F.B. Jessen, Denmark
Prof. R.M. Kenedi, UK
Dr. E. Kıral, Turkey
Prof. Z. Korkusuz, Turkey
Dr. S. Kumar, Canada
Dr. G. Kurap, Turkey
Prof. L. Lewillie, Belgium
Prof. Y. King Liu, USA
Dr. G.A. Maugin, France
Dr. P.F. Niederer, Switzerland
Prof. C. Pallotti, Italy
Prof. J.P. Paul, U.K.
Prof. K. Piekarski, Canada
Dr. N.P. Reddy, USA
Dr. C. Rigas, Greece and UK
Dr. V.M. Santana Carlos, Portugal

Mrs. E. Schmidt, W. Germany
Prof. G. Schmidt, W. Germany
Dr. E. Selçuk, Turkey
Dr. C.J. Snijders, Holland
Mrs. E. Solomonidis, U.K.
Mr. S.E. Solomonidis, Greece and U.K.
Prof. Ü. Tan, Turkey
Dr. A.B. Thornton-Trump, Canada
Mrs. B.M. Thornton-Trump, Canada
Prof. K.T. Vardar, Turkey
Mr. G. Veres, Norway
Prof. A. Viidik, Denmark
Dr. C. Ward, USA
Mr. P.F.F. Wijn, Holland
Dr. Ç. Yılmaz, Turkey
Dr. Ö. Yüzügüllü, Turkey